CLINICAL HANDBOOK
FOR GERONTOLOGICAL NURSING

For Reference

Not to be taken from this room

CLINICAL HANDBOOK
FOR GERONTOLOGICAL NURSING

Patricia A. Tabloski, Ph.D, APRNBC, FGSA

PEARSON
Prentice
Hall

Upper Saddle River, New Jersey 07458

Library of Congress Cataloging-in-Publication Data
Tabloski, Patricia A.
Clinical handbook for Gerontological nursing / Patricia A. Tabloski.
    p. ; cm.
  Includes bibliographic references and index.
  ISBN 0-13-094224-3
1. Geriatric nursing—Handbooks, manuals, etc.
[DNLM: 1. Geriatric Nursing—Handbooks. 2. Geriatric Nursing—
methods—Handbooks. WY 49 T114c 2007] I. Tabloski, Patricia A.
Gerontological nursing. II. Title.
RC954.T32 2006
618.97'0236—dc22   2005036327

Notice: Care has been taken to confirm the accuracy of information
presented in this book. The authors, editors, and the publisher, however,
cannot accept any responsibility for errors or omissions or for
consequences from application of the information in this book and make
no warranty, express or implied, with respect to its contents.

    The authors and publisher have exerted every effort to ensure that
drug selections and dosages set forth in this text are in accord with
current recommendations and practice at time of publication. However, in
view of ongoing research, changes in government regulations, and the
constant flow of information relating to drug therapy and drug reactions,
the reader is urged to check the package inserts of all drugs for any
change in indications of dosage and for added warnings and precautions.
This is particularly important when the recommended agent is a new
and/or infrequently employed drug.

Pearson Prentice Hall™ is a trademark of Pearson Education, Inc.
Pearson® is a registered trademark of Pearson plc
Prentice Hall® is a registered trademark of Pearson Education, Inc.

Pearson Education Ltd.
Pearson Education Singapore Pte. Ltd.
Pearson Education Canada, Ltd.
Pearson Education—Japan
Pearson Education Australia Pty. Limited
Pearson Education North Asia Ltd.
Pearson Educacíon De Mexico, S.A. de C.V.
Pearson Education Malaysia Pte. Ltd.
Pearson Education Upper Saddle River, NJ

10 9 8 7 6 5 4 3 2 1
ISBN: 0-13-094224-3

Contents

Preface

The *Clinical Handbook for Gerontological Nursing* is a handy, pocket-sized reference that can assist the student in the clinical setting when caring for older patients. It has been developed as a supplement to the first edition of *Gerontological Nursing* and is cross-referenced by chapter. It provides easy-to-follow information that the student can use at the bedside and the goal is to reduce to a minimum the time needed to gain information to make appropriate clinical decisions. As a result, not much detail is provided. This *Clinical Handbook* will help the student to organize his/her thinking when confronting a new clinical situation or to respond quickly to a change in an older person's condition. Please refer to the textbook for more comprehensive information and references.

ORGANIZATION

The *Clinical Handbook* covers the most common health problems nursing students are likely to encounter when providing care to older persons. The conditions appear in order and are organized by system of the body.

KEY FEATURES

The *Clinical Handbook* presents relevant information about each condition the student will most likely encounter in the clinical setting.

- Overview including the definition of the condition, its presentation in the older patient, incidence and basic underlying pathophysiology
- Risk factors and causes when known
- Diagnostic tests most frequently helpful for diagnosing the condition and interpretation of abnormal findings
- Nursing assessment instruments and best practices in the care of older patients
- Nursing management techniques most commonly used and reporting guidelines
- Teaching guidelines appropriate for older persons and their families

Every effort has been made to ensure that the *Clinical Handbook* is current and accurate in order to be most helpful to the nursing student. It is strongly recommended that the nurse check drug insert information to verify drug dosages.

CHAPTER 1

PRINCIPLES OF GERONTOLOGY

IMPLEMENTING THE NURSING PROCESS

An accurate and complete nursing assessment forms the basis for the nursing care plan. Follow the steps listed below to assure an accurate assessment.

ASSESSMENT

Comprehensive geriatric evaluation is essential to fully understand the health needs of an older person. A key part of the geriatric evaluation is the **functional assessment** or systematic evaluation of the older person's level of function and self-care. The comprehensive evaluation is usually interdisciplinary and multidimensional and will address function in the physical, social, and psychological domains. Key members of the interdisciplinary team are the gerontological nurse, the social worker, and the geriatric physician. Other healthcare professionals can be included in the evaluation or consulted depending on the needs and problems exhibited by the older patient. Sometimes physical therapists, occupational therapists, clinical pharmacists, psychologists, psychiatrists, podiatrists, dentists, and other professionals are called in to consult and evaluate an older patient with complex needs.

It is recommended that a comprehensive geriatric evaluation be carried out on a regular basis, including:

1. After hospitalization for an acute illness.
2. When nursing home placement or a change in living status is being considered.
3. After any abrupt change in physical, social, or psychological function.
4. Yearly for the older person with complex health needs during the annual visit for routine health maintenance with the primary healthcare provider.
5. When the older patient or family would like a second opinion regarding an intervention or treatment protocol recommended by the primary care provider.

The Health History

The health history should include emphasis on the following:

- Review of acute and chronic medical problems
- Medications
- Disease prevention and health maintenance review: vaccinations, PPD (tuberculosis), cancer screening
- Functional status (activities of daily living)
- Social supports (family, caregiver stress, safety of living environment)
- Finances
- Driving status and safety record
- Geriatric review of symptoms (patient/family perception of memory, dentition, taste, smell, nutrition, hearing, vision, falls, fractures, bowel and bladder function) (Stanford University Geriatric Education Resource Center, 2000)

Often, a standardized form is used to guide and direct the obtaining of the health history. The gerontological nurse should be aware of potential difficulties in obtaining health histories from older persons, including:

- *Communication difficulties.* Decreased hearing or vision, slow speech, and use of English as a second language have an effect on communication.
- *Underreporting of symptoms.* Fear of being labeled as a complainer, fear of institutionalization, and fear of serious illness can influence symptom reporting.
- *Vague or nonspecific complaints.* These may be associated with cognitive impairment, drug or alcohol use or abuse, or atypical presentation of disease.
- *Multiple complaints.* Associated "masked" depression, presence of multiple chronic illnesses, and social isolation are often an older person's cry for help.
- *Lack of time.* New patients scheduled for geriatric assessment should have the minimum of a 1-hour appointment with the gerontological nurse. Shorter appointments will result in a hurried interview with missed information (Kane, Ouslander, & Abrass, 1999).

Functional Ability

Ability to perform essential elements of self-care and activities of daily living should be assessed as baseline data; periodically to determine effectiveness of treatment; whenever there is a change in medical diagnosis or overall condition in order to determine need for further services or need for change in living environment. Functional status measures include ADLs and IADLs. ADLs include the necessary elements of self-care such as: bathing, dressing, ability to use the toilet, transfer ability, continence, and eating skills. Inability to perform these skills independently may indicate a need for additional assistance. IADLs include: ability to use the telephone, shopping, food preparation, housekeeping, laundry, transportation, taking medicine, and managing money. Ability to perform IADLs is necessary for independent community living.

ACTIVITIES OF DAILY LIVING, OR ADLs

In each category, circle the item that most closely describes the person's highest level of functioning and record the score assigned to that level (either 1 or 0) in the blank at the beginning of the category.

A. Toilet _____

1. Care for self at toilet completely, no incontinence..1
2. Needs to be reminded, or needs help in cleaning self, or has rare (weekly at most) accidents 0
3. Soiling or wetting while asleep more than once a week 0
4. Soiling or wetting while awake more than once a week..0
5. No control of bowels or bladder 0

B. Feeding _____

1. Eats without assistance 1
2. Eats with minor assistance at meal times and/or with special preparation of food, or help in cleaning up after meals 0
3. Feeds self with moderate assistance and is untidy 0
4. Requires extensive assistance for all meals 0
5. Does not feed self at all and resists efforts of others to feed him or her 0

C. Dressing _____

1. Dresses, undresses, and selects clothes from own wardrobe 1

---

2. Dresses and undresses self, with minor
   assistance 0
3. Needs moderate assistance in dressing
   and selection of clothes. 0
4. Needs major assistance in dressing, but
   cooperates with efforts of others to help 0
5. Completely unable to dress self and resists
   efforts of others to help 0

D. Grooming (neatness, hair, nails, hands, face, clothing)   _____

1. Always neatly dressed, well-groomed,
   without assistance.....................................1
2. Grooms self adequately with occasional
   minor assistance, eg, with shaving 0
3. Needs moderate and regular assistance
   or supervision with grooming 0
4. Needs total grooming care, but can remain
   well-groomed after help from others...................0
5. Actively negates all efforts of others to
   maintain grooming.....................................0

E. Physical Ambulation   _____

1. Goes about grounds or city 1
2. Ambulates within residence on or about
   one block distant 0
3. Ambulates with assistance of (check one)
   a ( ) another person, b ( ) railing, c ( ) cane,
   d ( ) walker, e ( ) wheelchair 0
   1.____Gets in and out without help. 2.____Needs
   help getting in and out
4. Sits unsupported in chair or wheelchair, but
   cannot propel self without help........................0
5. Bedridden more than half the time....................0

F. Bathing   _____

1. Bathes self (tub, shower, sponge bath)
   without help...1
2. Bathes self with help getting in and out
   of tub 0
3. Washes face and hands only, but cannot
   bathe rest of body.....................................0

(continued)

4. Does not wash self, but is cooperative with those who bathe him or her. 0
5. Does not try to wash self and resists efforts to keep him or her clean. 0

For scoring interpretation and source, see note following the next instrument.

INSTRUMENTAL ACTIVITIES OF DAILY LIVING SCALE (IADLs)

In each category, circle the item that most closely describes the person's highest level of functioning and record the score assigned to that level (either 1 or 0) in the blank at the beginning of the category.

A. Ability to Use Telephone _____
1. Operates telephone on own initiative; looks up and dials numbers. 1
2. Dials a few well-known numbers. 1
3. Answers telephone, but does not dial. 1
4. Does not use telephone at all. 0

B. Shopping _____
1. Takes care of all shopping needs independently. 1
2. Shops independently for small purchases. 0
3. Needs to be accompanied on any shopping trip. 0
4. Completely unable to shop. 0

C. Food Preparation _____
1. Plans, prepares, and serves adequate meals independently. 1
2. Prepares adequate meals if supplied with ingredients. 0
3. Heats and serves prepared meals or prepares meals, but does not maintain adequate diet. 0
4. Needs to have meals prepared and served. 0

D. Housekeeping _____
1. Maintains house alone or with occasional assistance (eg, heavy-work domestic help). 1

2. Performs light daily tasks such as dishwashing, bedmaking. 1
3. Performs light daily tasks, but cannot maintain acceptable level of cleanliness. 1
4. Needs help with all home maintenance tasks. 1
5. Does not participate in any housekeeping tasks. 0

E. Laundry _____
1. Does personal laundry completely. 1
2. Launders small items; rinses socks, stockings, etc. 1
3. All laundry must be done by others. 0

F. Mode of Transportation _____
1. Travels independently on public transportation or drives own car. 1
2. Arranges own travel via taxi, but does not otherwise use public transportation. 1
3. Travels on public transportation when assisted or accompanied by another. 1
4. Travel limited to taxi or automobile with assistance of another. 0
5. Does not travel at all. 0

G. Responsibility for Own Medications _____
1. Is responsible for taking medication in correct dosages at correct time. 1
2. Takes responsibility if medication is prepared in advance in separate dosages. 0
3. Is not capable of dispensing own medication. 0

H. Ability to Handle Finances _____
1. Manages financial matters independently (budgets, writes checks, pays rent and bills, goes to bank); collects and keeps track of income. 1
2. Manages day-to-day purchases, but needs help with banking, major purchases, etc. 1
3. Incapable of handling money. 0

Scoring Interpretation: For ADLs, the total score ranges from 0 to 6, and for IADLs, from 0 to 8. In some

(*continued*)

Social History

Holistic evaluation is not complete without an assessment of the social support system. Many frail older persons receive support and supervision from family members and significant others to compensate for functional disabilities.

Key elements of the social history include the following:

- Past occupation and retirement status
- Family history (helpful to construct a family genogram)
- Present and formal marital status, including quality of the relationship(s)
- Identification of family members, with designation of level of involvement and place of residence
- Living arrangements
- Family dynamics
- Family and caregiver expectations
- Economic status, adequacy of health insurance
- Social activities and hobbies
- Mode of transportation

- Community involvement and support
- Religious involvement and spirituality

If there is a social worker on the assessment team, the gerontological nurse may work closely to identify and address social problems. Older patients with inadequate health insurance can often be helped by accessing community services, hospital free care, hardship funds established for indigent patients by major drug companies, and referrals to community-based free clinics.

Psychological History

Another key component of the holistic geriatric assessment is evaluation of psychological and cognitive function. A significant proportion of older patients with mental illness remain unrecognized and untreated; when treated, the use of healthcare services decreases (Health Resources and Services Administration, 1996). The reported range of adults over the age of 65 with mental disorders, both in institutions and in the community, is estimated to be between 20 and 30%.

Mental and emotional problems are not a normal part of aging. When mental health problems manifest themselves in the older adult, they should be evaluated, diagnosed, and treated. By forming a trusting therapeutic relationship, the gerontological nurse can demonstrate caring, warmth, respect, and support for the older person who may be hesitant to verbalize feelings of low self-esteem, depression, bizarre thought patterns, or phobias and anxieties.

Key elements of the psychological history include:

- Any history of past mental illness.
- Any hospitalizations or outpatient treatments for psychological problems.

- Current and past stress levels and coping mechanisms.
- Current level of alcohol or recreational drug use.
- Medications taken for anxiety, insomnia, or depression.
- Identification of any problems with memory, judgment, or thought processing.
- Any changes in personality, values, personal habits, or life satisfaction.
- Identification of feelings regarding self-worth and hopes for the future.
- Feelings of appropriate emotions related to present life and health situation (feelings of sadness regarding losses, etc.).
- Presence of someone to love, support, and encourage the older patient.
- Feelings of hopelessness or suicidal ideation.

Instruments commonly used in clinical practice to assess psychological function include the following:

- *Geriatric Depression Scale* (Yesavage & Brink, 1983). The short form includes 15 questions and measures depression in the older adult. Scores over 5 indicate probable depression.

MENTAL STATUS

Many factors can affect mental status including age, level of education, acute and chronic illness, pain and ability to see and hear. The nurse must assess mental status in order to devise a nursing care plan that adequately addresses patient safety, detects changes in mental status due to adverse drug reactions and promotes rehabilitation.

- The Mini Mental State Examination (MMSE) is often used in the clinical setting to screen for cognitive impairments. It assesses orientation to time, place person, short term memory, ability to follow a three

The Geriatric Depression Scale (GDS)
By: Lenore Kurlowicz, PhD, RN, CS

The GDS is not a substitute for a diagnostic interview by mental health professionals. It is a useful screening tool in the clinical setting to facilitate assessment of depression in older adults especially when baseline measurements are compared to subsequent scores.

Patient_____   **Examiner**_____   **Date**_____

Directions to Patient: Please choose the best answer for how you have felt over the past week.
Directions to Examiner: Present questions VERBALLY. Circle answer given by patient. Do not show to patient.

1.	Are you basically satisfied with your life?	yes	no (1)
2.	Have you dropped many of your activities and interests?	yes (1)	no
3.	Do you feel that your life is empty?	yes (1)	no
4.	Do you often get bored?	yes (1)	no
5.	Are you hopeful about the future?	yes	no (1)
6.	Are you bothered by thoughts you can't get out of your head?	yes (1)	no
7.	Are you in good spirits most of the time?	yes	no (1)
8.	Are you afraid that something bad is going to happen to you?	yes (1)	no
9.	Do you feel happy most of the time?	yes	no (1)
10.	Do you often feel helpless?	yes (1)	no
11.	Do you often get restless and fidgety?	yes (1)	no
12.	Do you prefer to stay at home rather than go out and do things?	yes (1)	no
13.	Do you frequently worry about the future?	yes (1)	no
14.	Do you feel you have more problems with memory than most?	yes (1)	no

(continued) 11

15.	Do you think it is wonderful to be alive now? ....yes	no (1)
16.	Do you feel downhearted and blue? ....yes (1)	no
17.	Do you feel pretty worthless the way you are now? ....yes (1)	no
18.	Do you worry a lot about the past?...yes (1)	no
19.	Do you find life very exciting? ....yes	no (1)
20.	Is it hard for you to get started on new projects?...yes (1)	no
21.	Do you feel full of energy?.......................yes	no (1)
22.	Do you feel that your situation is hopeless? ....yes (1)	no
23.	Do you think that most people are better off than you are? ....yes (1)	no
24.	Do you frequently get upset over little things?.......................................yes (1)	no
25.	Do you frequently feel like crying?........yes (1)	no
26.	Do you have trouble concentrating ....yes (1)	no
27.	Do you enjoy getting up in the morning ....yes (1)	no
28	Do you prefer to avoid soial occasion? ....yes (1)	no
29.	Is it easy for you to make decision? ......yes (1)	no
30.	Is your mind as clear as it used to be..yes (1)	no

TOTAL: Please sum all bolded answers (worth one point) for a total score._____

Scores 0–9 Normal 10–19 Mild Depressive
20–30 Severe Depressive

Source: Adapted by a series provided by The Hartford Institute for Geriatric Nursing (hartford.ign@nyu.edu)www.hartfordign.org

stage command, reading, writing, drawing and ability to engage in abstract thinking (Folstein, Folstein & McHugh, 1975). A perfect score is 30 and scores below 24 suggest dementia (Annals Internal Medicine, 1991).

Home Environment

The adequacy of the home environment and the available resources should be assessed for older persons living at home in order to maintain adequate levels of function.

Factors to be considered when assessing the home environment include:

- *Stairs.* Narrow stairs with poor lighting, inadequate railings, and uneven steps are fall risks. Does the older person have the strength and balance to climb stairs? If a wheelchair or walker is used, are there ramps present or space for them to be added?
- *Bathing and toileting.* Can the older person safely transfer on and off the toilet? Is a raised toilet seat needed? Are grab bars present? Is there an adequate bath mat in the tub? Is a shower seat needed? Is lighting adequate?
- *Medications.* Where are medications stored? Are there grandchildren in the home who are at risk because of open storage or nonreplacement of caps? Are old and outdated medications disposed of to prevent accidents? Are medications refilled on time to prevent on-off dosing patterns? Is there a list of medications available for use in emergencies?
- *Predetermined wishes.* Has the older person named a health proxy or established a living will? If so, does the family and primary care provider have a copy? Is the healthcare proxy knowledgeable regarding the patient's preferences? Is the proxy's number posted in an easily visible position (e.g., on the refrigerator)? Is the value quality of life or length of life specified?

- *Nutrition and cooking.* Is there adequate food in the home? Is there a stove or microwave to cook? Are any safety problems reported with the stove or microwave? If a gas stove, is it safe? Is the pilot functioning properly? Are there gas leak detectors? Is food storage adequate? Is spoiled food present? Is the food preparation environment clean? Who does the grocery shopping?
- *Falls.* Are the floors free of cords, debris, and scatter rugs? Is there adequate lighting? Are there nightlights? Are there pets who dart around quickly? If there is a history of falls, would the older person consider wearing an emergency alert system around the neck?
- *Smoke detectors.* Are there functioning smoke detectors? Are batteries changed yearly?
- *Emergency numbers.* Are emergency phone numbers posted or preprogrammed into the phone?
- *Temperature of home.* Is there adequate heat in the winter and cooling in the summer?
- *Temperature of water.* Is the hot water set below 120°F?
- *Safety of the neighborhood.* Can the older person venture outside without fear of becoming a crime victim? Are there adequate door locks and latches? How close is the nearest neighbor? Is there nearby help if it is needed?
- *Financial.* Are there piles of unpaid bills? Are services such as phone and electricity in good working order? Are there large amounts of cash hidden or stored around the house?

Culture and Education

Assess cultural background and educational level and consider how to develop a treatment plan to avoid misunderstanding or ineffective care. Some instruments such as the MMSE have developed and validated scoring norms based upon level of education. Low scores could falsely be attributed to cognitive impairment rather than low reading literacy. Consider and assess educational level, language barriers, reading levels, and cultural background before using standardized instruments.

Understand and elicit the beliefs, attitudes, values, and goals of older people relating to their lives, illness, and health states in order to provide culturally appropriate care. Cultural competence in healthcare consists of at least three components:

1. Knowing the prevalence, incidence, and risk factors (epidemiology) for diseases in different ethnic groups
2. Understanding how the response to medications and other treatments varies with ethnicity
3. Eliciting the culturally held beliefs and attitudes toward illness, treatment, and the healthcare system (Mouton & Espino, 2000)

There is heterogeneity within various ethnic groups, and the provision of culturally sensitive care dictates that each person be approached as a unique individual. Patient age, place of birth, where childhood was spent, and how the older person was socialized to American culture can all affect performance on standardized assessment instruments.

Minimum Data Set

Assessment of an older person for appropriate placement within the nursing home or within the long-term care system is done using the Minimum Data Set (MDS).

The MDS is a comprehensive multidisciplinary assessment that is used throughout the United States. It was devised and passed into law because of the belief that a better, more holistic patient assessment will facilitate improved patient care. The Omnibus Budget Reconciliation Act of 1987 (OBRA 87) contained a provision mandating that all residents of facilities that collect funds from Medicare or Medicaid be assessed using the MDS. The MDS is used for validating the need for long-term care, reimbursement, ongoing assessment of clinical problems, and assessment of and need to alter the current plan of care.

The MDS consists of a core set of screening, clinical, and functional measures. It is used with the Resident Assessment Protocols (RAPS), the Resident Utilization Guidelines (RUGS), and the Resident Assessment Instrument (RAI).

Categories of data gathered for the MDS include the following:

- Patient demographics and background
- Cognitive function
- Communication and hearing
- Mood and behavior patterns
- Psychosocial well-being
- Physical function and activities of daily living
- Bowel and bladder continence
- Diagnosed diseases
- Health conditions (weight, falls, etc.)
- Oral nutritional status
- Oral and dental status
- Skin condition
- Activity pursuits
- Medications
- Need for special services
- Discharge potential

Certain information gathered for the MDS such as functional decline or a poorly managed chronic disease may trigger the need for further assessment using the RAP. The MDS can be viewed as a start in acquiring the broad base of clinical information necessary to provide quality long-term care. See Appendix B for the MDS.

Assessing Capacity

The gerontological nurse will want to assess the older person for capacity to provide consent and ability to make treatment decisions. To be considered capable of providing consent, older patients should have the ability to:

- Comprehend information (understand).
- Contemplate options (reason).
- Evaluate risks and consequences (problem solve).
- Communicate that decision (make their decision known).

While competence is a legal term, capacity is a clinical term. When a patient lacks decisional capacity because of severe illness, sedating drugs, or cognitive impairment, there are mechanisms and laws that dictate who may make a decision for the patient. If the patient has a living will, a healthcare proxy or surrogate decision maker, durable power of attorney, or involved family member, these persons or documents will be used to decide whether to proceed with the treatment or procedure in question. For those with no predetermined wishes, family, or healthcare proxy, the care facility may seek a court-appointed guardian. A guardian is appointed by a judge to act on behalf of a *ward* when the judge has determined that the ward is incapacitated and in need of a decision maker. Guardians may be relatives, friends, or strangers.

Usually wards are people with advanced dementia, untreated mental illness, developmental disabilities, head injuries, strokes, or long-standing drug addictions (Johns & Sabatino, 2002).

Assessment of decisional capacity is an ongoing dynamic process. Patients have the right to make decisions that do not follow the recommendations of healthcare providers and to change their mind at any time. Even if patients have dementia or cognitive impairments, it does not mean that they should not be consulted regarding treatment decisions. Often, while true consent cannot be obtained from an older person, *assent* should be sought. If the older person does not assent to the care to be given, it ethically cannot be offered. To avoid conflict and the risk of potential harm to the patient, assent for all procedures should be obtained from the older patient before beginning any treatment or procedure.

FUNCTIONAL HEALTH PATTERNS AND NURSING DIAGNOSIS

A systematic nursing assessment is necessary to provide holistic care to the older person (ANA, 2004). This nursing assessment must go beyond physical function and the diagnosis of disease (the medical model) by also focusing on the interaction of the older person with the environment. Gordon (1994) developed a set of health-related behaviors that form an assessment framework for nurses. This framework consists of 11 **functional health patterns** that can interact and form the basis for an older person's lifestyle. Although these functional health patterns were not specifically developed for use with older patients, they are ideally suited for use by gerontological nurses. An older person's functional status is a primary concern because it addresses key issues, including how the patient sees his or her present level of health, usual and preferred lifestyle and activities, demands of daily life and existing support systems, and functional ability. Each of the 11 functional areas guides the nurse to seek information about the older patient and forms a crucial foundation to the care-planning process and diagnosis of the patient's nursing needs.

The 11 functional health patterns include the following:

- *Health perception–health management.* The older individual's perceived health and well-being along with self-management strategies.
- *Nutritional-metabolic.* Patterns of food and fluid consumption relative to metabolic need and nutrient supply.
- *Elimination.* Patterns of excretory function and elimination of waste (bowel, bladder, etc.).
- *Activity-exercise.* Patterns of exercise and daily activity. Includes leisure and recreation.
- *Sleep-rest.* Patterns of sleep, rest, and relaxation.
- *Cognitive-perceptual.* Patterns of thinking and ways of perceiving the world and current events.
- *Self-perception–self-concept.* Patterns of viewing and valuing self (body image and psychological state, self-image, etc.).
- *Roles-relationships.* Patterns of engagement with others, ability to form and maintain meaningful relationships, assumed roles.
- *Sexuality-reproductive.* Patterns of sexuality and satisfaction with present level of interaction with sexual partners.
- *Coping–stress tolerance.* Patterns of coping with stressful events and level of effectiveness of coping strategies.

- *Values-beliefs.* Patterns of beliefs, values, and perception of the meaning of life that guide choices or decisions (Gordon, 1994).

Please refer to Appendix A for the NANDA-approved list of nursing diagnoses.

FORMULATING THE NURSING CARE PLAN AND THE NURSING DIAGNOSIS

The interventions are selected on the basis of the needs, desires, and resources of the older adult and accepted nursing practice (ANA, 2004). Appropriate nursing interventions may include the following:

- Assisting the older patient to a higher level of function or self-care
- Identifying health promotion activities
- Identifying disease prevention and screening activities
- Health teaching
- Counseling
- Seeking consultation
- Collecting data on an ongoing basis and refining the initial nursing assessment
- Exploring treatment choices, including pharmacological and non-pharmacological options
- Implementing palliative care and holistic care of the dying or seriously ill patient
- Referring the patient to community resources
- Managing the patient's case
- Evaluating and educating ancillary caregivers and family (ANA, 2004)

Nursing interventions will be selected based upon the following:

1. Linkage to the desired outcome
2. Characteristics of the nursing diagnosis

APPENDIX A

2005–2006 NANDA-APPROVED NURSING DIAGNOSES

Activity Intolerance
Activity Intolerance,
 Risk for
Adaptive Capacity:
 Intracranial, Decreased
Adjustment, Impaired
Airway Clearance,
 Ineffective
Anxiety
Anxiety, Death
Aspiration, Risk for
Attachment, Parent/
 Infant/Child, Risk for
 Impaired
Body Image, Disturbed
Body Temperature:
 Imbalanced, Risk for
Bowel Incontinence
Breastfeeding,
 Effective
Breastfeeding, Ineffective
Breastfeeding,
 Interrupted
Breathing Pattern,
 Ineffective
Cardiac Output,
 Decreased
Caregiver Role Strain
Caregiver Role Strain,
 Risk for
Communication,
 Readiness for Enhanced
Communication: Verbal,
 Impaired
Confusion, Acute

Confusion, Chronic
Constipation
Constipation, Perceived
Constipation, Risk for
Coping: Community,
 Ineffective
Coping: Community,
 Readiness for
 Enhanced
Coping: Defensive
Coping: Family,
 Compromised
Coping: Family, Disabled
Coping: Family,
 Readiness for
 Enhanced
Coping (Individual),
 Readiness for
 Enhanced
Coping, Ineffective
Decisional Conflict
 (Specify)
Denial, Ineffective
Dentition, Impaired
Development: Delayed,
 Risk for
Diarrhea
Disuse Syndrome,
 Risk for
Diversional Activity,
 Deficient
Dysreflexia, Autonomic
Dysreflexia, Autonomic,
 Risk for
Energy Field Disturbance

(continued)

Environmental Interpretation Syndrome, Impaired

Failure to Thrive, Adult

Falls, Risk for

Family Processes, Dysfunctional: Alcoholism

Family Processes, Interrupted

Family Processes, Readiness for Enhanced

Fatigue

Fear

Fluid Balance, Readiness for Enhanced

Fluid Volume, Deficient

Fluid Volume, Deficient, Risk for

Fluid Volume, Excess

Fluid Volume, Imbalanced, Risk for

Gas Exchange, Impaired

Grieving, Anticipatory

Grieving, Dysfunctional

Grieving, Risk for Dysfunctional

Growth, Disproportionate, Risk for

Growth and Development, Delayed

Health Maintenance, Ineffective

Health Seeking Behaviors (Specify)

Home Maintenance, Impaired

Hopelessness

Hyperthermia

Hypothermia

Identity: Personal, Disturbed

Infant Behavior, Disorganized

Infant Behavior: Disorganized, Risk for

Infant Behavior: Organized, Readiness for Enhanced

Infant Feeding Pattern, Ineffective

Infection, Risk for

Injury, Risk for

Knowledge, Deficient (Specify)

Knowledge (Specify), Readiness for Enhanced

Latex Allergy Response

Latex Allergy Response, Risk for

Lifestyle, Sedentary

Loneliness, Risk for

Memory, Impaired

Mobility: Bed, Impaired

Mobility: Physical, Impaired

Mobility: Wheelchair, Impaired

Nausea

Neurovascular Dysfunction: Peripheral, Risk for

Noncompliance (Specify)

Nutrition, Imbalanced: Less than Body Requirements

Nutrition, Imbalanced: More than Body Requirements

Nutrition, Imbalanced: More than Body Requirements, Risk for

Nutrition, Readiness for Enhanced

Oral Mucous Membrane, Impaired

Pain, Acute

Pain, Chronic

Parenting, Impaired

Parenting, Readiness for Enhanced

Parenting, Risk for Impaired

Perioperative Positioning Injury, Risk for

Poisoning, Risk for

Post-Trauma Syndrome

Post-Trauma Syndrome, Risk for

Powerlessness

Powerlessness, Risk for

Protection, Ineffective

Rape-Trauma Syndrome

Rape-Trauma Syndrome: Compound Reaction

Rape-Trauma Syndrome: Silent Reaction

Religiosity, Impaired

Religiosity, Readiness for Enhanced

Religiosity, Risk for Impaired

Relocation Stress Syndrome

Relocation Stress Syndrome, Risk for

Role Conflict, Parental

Role Performance, Ineffective

Self-Care Deficit: Bathing/Hygiene

Self-Care Deficit: Dressing/Grooming

Self-Care Deficit: Feeding

Self-Care Deficit: Toileting

Self-Concept, Readiness for Enhanced

Self-Esteem, Chronic Low

Self-Esteem, Situational Low

Self-Esteem, Risk for Situational Low

Self-Mutilation

Self-Mutilation, Risk for

Sensory Perception, Disturbed (Specify: Visual, Auditory, Kinesthetic, Gustatory, Tactile, Olfactory)

Sexual Dysfunction

Sexuality Patterns, Ineffective

Skin Integrity, Impaired

Skin Integrity, Risk for Impaired

Sleep Deprivation

Sleep Pattern Disturbed

Sleep, Readiness for Enhanced

Social Interaction, Impaired

Social Isolation

Sorrow, Chronic

Spiritual Distress

Spiritual Distress, Risk for

Spiritual Well-Being, Readiness for Enhanced

(continued)

Spontaneous Ventilation, Impaired

Sudden Infant Death Syndrome, Risk for

Suffocation, Risk for

Suicide, Risk for

Surgical Recovery, Delayed

Swallowing, Impaired

Therapeutic Regimen Management: Community, Ineffective

Therapeutic Regimen Management, Effective

Therapeutic Regimen Management: Family Ineffective

Therapeutic Regimen Management, Ineffective

Therapeutic Regimen Management, Readiness for Enhanced

Thermoregulation, Ineffective

Thought Processes, Disturbed

Tissue Integrity, Impaired

Tissue Perfusion, Ineffective (Peripheral)

Tissue Perfusion, Ineffective (Specify: Renal, Cerebral, Cardiopulmonary, Gastrointestinal, Peripheral)

Transfer Ability, Impaired

Trauma, Risk for

Unilateral Neglect

Urinary Elimination, Impaired

Urinary Elimination, Readiness for Enhanced

Urinary Incontinence, Functional

Urinary Incontinence, Reflex

Urinary Incontinence, Stress

Urinary Incontinence, Total

Urinary Incontinence, Urge

Urinary Incontinence, Risk for Urge

Urinary Retention

Ventilation, Impaired Spontaneous

Ventilatory Weaning Response, Dysfunctional

Violence: Other-Directed, Risk for

Violence: Self-Directed, Risk for

Walking, Impaired

Wandering

3. Strength of the research associated with the intervention
4. Probability of successfully implementing the intervention
5. Acceptability of the intervention to the older person and others involved in the plan of care
6. Assurance that the intervention is safe, ethical, culturally competent, and appropriate
7. Documentation of the intervention
8. Knowledge, skills, experience, and creativity of the nurse

EVALUATION

Evaluation is the final component of the nursing process during which the nurse will compare the patient's response to the activities identified in the nursing care plan to the established outcome criteria. The nurse will seek input from the patient, family, and others involved in the care. It is important to consider information from the physical, social, and psychological assessment of the patient; information from diagnostic testing; level of satisfaction with care; and documentation of the costs and benefits associated with the treatment. The initial assessment and nursing diagnosis may be revised with new goals and nursing interventions specified if appropriate. Either the problem has been resolved and the plan should be continued as specified, the problem has been resolved and the nursing interventions can be revised or discontinued, or the problem still exists. If the problem still exists despite implementation of the nursing care plan, that may indicate the interventions were not carried out as specified, the interventions were not effective in alleviating the problem, or there was an error or omission in the initial nursing assessment and diagnosis. At this point, the nurse has the opportunity to modify and revise the nursing care plan.

COMMUNICATING WITH THE OLDER PATIENT

Communication is an ongoing, continuous dynamic process including verbal and nonverbal signals. Nonverbal communication is thought to make up 80% of the communication process and includes body language such as position, eye contact, touch, tone of voice, and facial expression. Nurses should follow these guidelines for verbal communication:

- Do not yell or speak too loudly to patients. Not all older people are hard of hearing. If they are wearing a hearing aid, yelling can be disturbing.
- Try to be at eye level with the patient. Sit down if the patient is sitting or lying down.
- Try to minimize background noise as it can make it difficult for the patient to hear.
- Monitor the patient's reaction. A puzzled look may mean the patient cannot hear but is ashamed to interrupt.
- Touch the patient if appropriate and acceptable. Many older patients report that they are hardly touched by their caregivers and they appreciate the human contact.
- Supplement verbal instructions with written instructions as needed.
- Do not give long-winded speeches or complicated instructions to persons with cognitive impairment, anxiety, or pain.
- Ask how the patient would like to be addressed. Avoid demeaning terms like *sweetie, honey,* or *dearie.*

CHAPTER 2

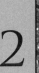

CULTURAL DIVERSITY

Cultural background and language have a considerable impact both on how patients access and respond to healthcare services and on how the caregivers work within the system. There are two main goals:

1. To develop cultural and linguistic competence by nurses and other healthcare providers
2. For healthcare organizations to understand and respond effectively to the cultural and linguistic needs brought by both patients and caregivers to the healthcare experience

BEST NURSING PRACTICES

The Hartford Institute for Geriatric Nursing (1999) has recommended recognition of cultural and religious beliefs, practices and life experiences of ethnic groups, and the influence of these on attitudes toward aging and healthcare. It is important for nurses to understand the following categories of belief from the perspective of their older patients:

- *Respect.* What does this person from another culture believe about the roles and responsibilities of older persons, children, doctors, nurses, and others?
- *Death and dying.* What are the cultural perspectives regarding death, life-sustaining treatments, treatment of the body after death, and funeral rituals?

National Standards for Culturally and Linguistically Appropriate Services in Health Care

Health care organizations should:

1. Ensure that patients/consumers receive from all staff members effective, understandable, and **respectful care** that is provided in a manner compatible with their cultural health beliefs and practices and preferred language.

2. Implement strategies to recruit, retain, and promote at all levels of the organization a diverse staff and leadership that are representative of the demographic characteristics of the service area.

3. Ensure that staff at all levels and across all disciplines receive ongoing education and training in culturally and linguistically appropriate service delivery.

4. Offer and provide language assistance services, including bilingual staff and interpreter services, at no cost to each patient/consumer with limited English proficiency at all points of contact, in a timely manner during all hours of operation.

5. Provide to patients/consumers in their preferred language both verbal offers and written notices informing them of their right to receive language assistance services.

6. Assure the competence of language assistance provided to limited English proficient patients/consumers by interpreters and bilingual staff. Family and friends should not be used to provide interpretation services (except on request by the patient/consumer).

7. Make available easily understood patient-related materials and post signage in the languages of the commonly encountered groups and/or groups represented in the service area.

8. Develop, implement, and promote a written strategic plan that outlines clear goals, policies, operational plans, and management accountability/oversight mechanisms to provide culturally and linguistically appropriate services.

9. Conduct initial and ongoing organizational self-assessments of CLAS-related activities and are encouraged to integrate cultural and linguistic competence-related measures into their internal audits, performance improvement programs, patient satisfaction assessments, and outcomes based evaluations.

10. Ensure that data on the individual patient's/consumer's race, ethnicity, and spoken and written language are collected in health records, integrated into the organization's management information systems, and periodically updated.

11. Maintain a current demographic, cultural, and epidemiological profile of the community as well as a needs assessment to accurately plan for and implement services that respond to the cultural and linguistic characteristics of the service area.

12. Develop participatory, collaborative partnerships with communities and utilize a variety of formal and informal mechanisms to facilitate community and patient/consumer involvement in designing and implementing CLAS-related activities.

13. Ensure that conflict and grievance resolution processes are culturally and linguistically sensitive and capable of identifying, preventing, and resolving cross-cultural conflicts or complaints by patients/consumers.

14. Make available to the public information about their progress and successful innovations in implementing the CLAS standards and to provide public notice in their communities about the availability of this information.

Source: National Standards for Culturally and Linguistically Appropriate Services in Health Care. (2001). *Final report.* Washington, DC: U.S. Department of Health and Human Services.

- *Pain.* What is the cultural perspective toward pain? Is there a view that it is punishment for past behaviors? What are the socially accepted behaviors of a person in pain (crying, wailing, moaning, stoicism, etc.)?

- *Medicines and nutrition.* What is the role of folk and home remedies and caregiving practices?
- *Independence.* How does the culture value independence in old age? Are older people expected or encouraged to stay active in their healthcare and living arrangements?

The nurse is urged to discuss these key issues with the older patient and the family. It would be wrong to make assumptions based on stereotypes, so each person should be approached as a unique individual.

It is important to avoid assuming that all people of the same ethnic, religious, or national background have the same cultural beliefs and values. Similar questions as those listed above may be asked in conversation. When there is knowledge of the patient's and caregiver's ethnocultural heritage and life trajectories, mutual respect between patient, caregiver, and nurse is more likely to develop. The triad can become more unified.

PATIENT-FAMILY TEACHING GUIDELINES

The following are guidelines that the nurse may find useful when instructing older persons and their families about cultural competence in healthcare.

Cultural Competence

1. As a person from a different culture, what can I expect of my healthcare provider?

   You can expect to receive culturally competent care. This means that you will be provided the highest quality of care, regardless of your race, ethnicity, cultural background, English proficiency, or literacy. Some common services provided may include:

- Interpreter services.
- Attempts to recruit persons from your culture (if possible) to work in health facilities in your area.
- Coordination with traditional healers.
- Respect for your values, beliefs, and traditions.
- Printed health information in your language and appropriate to your reading level (Georgetown University, 2004).

2. Why is culturally competent care important?

A culturally competent healthcare system can help improve health outcomes and quality of care, and can contribute to the elimination of racial and ethnic health disparities. It is both to your advantage and to the advantage of your healthcare providers to eliminate any barriers that stand in the way of improving your health and caring for you when you are ill.

3. What can I do to increase my chances of obtaining culturally competent healthcare?

Try to find a healthcare provider to whom you can relate. People who do not have a regular doctor or healthcare provider are less likely to obtain preventive services, or diagnosis, treatment, and management of chronic conditions. Health insurance coverage is also an important determinant of access to healthcare. People without healthcare insurance often wait longer to seek healthcare, delay treatment once diagnosed with an illness, and as a result suffer more serious health problems. Social workers and community clinics often have services for persons without health
(continued)

insurance and can direct you to receive free or low-cost care. Once you have located a healthcare provider, inform him or her about yourself and your culture. If your provider recommends an intervention that is not consistent with your beliefs, discuss this right away. Let your provider know if you cannot understand written material given to you, if verbal instructions contain too much medical jargon that you cannot understand, or if you are given forms to fill out that are inconsistent with your level of reading in English. Providing culturally competent healthcare is an ongoing learning process. Your healthcare provider will be grateful to hear your constructive comments and receive your support.

CHAPTER 3

NUTRITION

NORMAL AGING AND NUTRITION
Changes in Body Composition

Lean muscle mass diminishes with aging. The term **sarcopenia** refers to these age-related phenomena.

Loss of muscle can lead to a functional decline as strength and endurance become affected by specific loss of type II muscle fibers (Evans, 1997).

The loss of muscle leads to lower total body water in the older person.

Unintentional weight loss of 5% of body weight in one month or 10% in one year should not be considered a normal part of aging and requires intervention.

Bone mineral density commonly is lost with age in both men and women.

Oral and Gastrointestinal Changes with Aging
Dentition

By the age of 65 years, 33.1% of Americans suffer from **edentulism** (Hutton, Feine, & Morais, 2002). Poor dental health, missing or loose teeth, and ill-fitting dentures can affect the type and amount of food eaten and interfere with proper nutrition.

Xerostomia

Lack of sufficient saliva production is termed **xerostomia** and can affect taste perception, hinder swallowing, and cause insufficient retention of poorly fitting dentures (Ship, 2002).

Atrophic Gastritis

In the stomach, decreases in size and number of glands and mucous membranes can lead to **achlorhydria**, or lack of hydrochloric acid production, with the aging process. Iron and vitamin B_{12} require an acid medium in the stomach to begin absorption; lack of adequate hydrochloric acid production can limit absorption of both nutrients.

Medications that alter gastric pH such as antacids, proton pump inhibitors, H_2 receptor blockers, and potassium salts may also alter iron and B_{12} absorption due to alkalinizing effects of these medications (White & Ashworth, 2000).

Gastric production of intrinsic factor, which is necessary for vitamin B_{12} absorption in the ileum, may also decrease.

Appetite Dysregulation

Cholecystokinian production increases with age and can cause early satiety as a result. These physiological changes have been called the **anorexia of aging.**

Constipation

Slowed intestinal peristalsis, inadequate intake of fluid and fiber, illness, medications, and a sedentary lifestyle are contributing factors to the prevalence of constipation in the older person.

Thirst Dysregulation

Symptoms of dehydration such as confusion or lethargy can go unrecognized while hydration status continues to worsen without a strong thirst response. Dehydration risk can be worsened by voluntary fluid restriction in the older person trying to cope with incontinence, nocturia, or the need for assistance with toileting.

Sensory Changes

Age-related changes in vision, hearing, taste, and smell can have a negative impact on nutrition.

Vision

Poor vision is associated with a decline in protein and energy intake in functional, community-dwelling older persons (Payette, Gray-Donald, Cyr, & Boutier, 1995). Individuals with poor vision can benefit from mealtime assistance using the clock analogy with their dinner plate: "Your carrots are at two o'clock and the chicken is at six o'clock."

Hearing

Hearing losses that occur with age can make social dining a difficult experience. Social isolation is considered a risk factor for undernutrition in the older person.

Taste and Smell

Taste and smell diminish with age, and the decline has been associated with reduced pleasure with eating (Bromley, 2000; Murphy et al., 2002). Medications are responsible for some taste alterations. Dentures, zinc deficiency, smoking, and neurodegenerative disease, such as Parkinson's disease, are also associated with loss of taste (Bromley, 2000). Some older persons experience **dysgeusia,** or altered taste perception, and complain of metallic and chalky taste transmissions.

Social and Economic Changes Affecting Nutrition

Retirement, social isolation, loneliness, loss of a spouse, bereavement and poverty can introduce additional influences that can alter adequacy of diet. Poverty or near poverty affects 19% of older persons with African American and Hispanic older persons at disproportionate risk compared with White older persons.

Nutrition-Related Changes Associated with Aging

- ↓Lean body mass
- ↓Metabolic rate
- ↓Bone mineral density
- ↑Cholecystokinin and early satiety
- ↓Saliva production
- ↓Thirst perception
- ↓Taste and smell
- ↓Production of gastric acid and fluids

NUTRITIONAL AND DISEASE-RELATED HEALTH CHANGES

Many medications commonly used in older persons can negatively impact appetite, taste, nutrient absorption, and metabolism; diminish saliva production; and cause gastrointestinal side effects. Numerous other diseases and medications have nutritional implications. Table 3–1 outlines some common medications with nutritional implications.

Table 3–1 Medications with Nutritional Implications

Drug	Side Effect	Explanation
ACE inhibitors	Altered taste, dry mouth	Causes metallic taste/reduced taste perception
Alcohol	↓ Absorption and metabolism	Thiamin, folic acid, B_{12}, magnesium, B_6 affected
Antacids	↓ Absorption, constipation	Iron, B_{12} need acid pH
Antianxiety agents	Dry mouth	Affects taste and swallowing
Antidepressants and antipsychotics	↓ Intake and dry mouth	Affects taste, smell, swallowing
Antiparkinson agents	↓ Intake and dry mouth	Nausea, vomiting, taste changes
Colchicine	↓ Absorption	B_{12}, calcium, and iron affected
Corticosteroids	↓ Intake, ↓ nutrition	Nausea, vomiting; affects calcium, vitamin D, B_6, folate
Digoxin	↓ Intake	Anorexia and nausea
Isoniazid	Altered metabolism	Vitamin B_6 affected
KCl (potassium chloride)	↓ Intake, ↓ absorption	Nausea; B_{12} and iron affected
Metformin	↓ Intake, ↓ absorption	Anorexia; B_{12} affected
Methotrexate	↓ Intake, ↓ absorption	Nausea; folate, B_{12} calcium affected
Narcotics and sedatives	↓ Intake, constipation	Nausea, vomiting, sedation
Penicillamine	↓ Intake, ↓ nutrition	Anorexia, B_6 affected

(continued)

Table 3-1 Medications with Nutritional Implications (*continued*)

Drug	Side Effect	Explanation
Phenytoin	↓ Intake, ↓ nutrition	Altered taste and smell; folate, B_6, vitamin D affected
Sulfasalazine	↓ Absorption	Folate and iron affected
Theophylline	↓ Intake, ↓ nutrition	Nausea, vomiting, anorexia; B_6 affected

Source : Adapted from Gazewood, J. D., & Mehr, D. R. (1998); Bromley, S.M. (2000); White, R., & Ashworth, A. (2000).

NUTRITIONAL REQUIREMENTS AND AGING

Unique Nutrient Recommendations

The Modified Food Guide Pyramid recommends protein foods in the fourth tier of the pyramid with three dairy servings per day and at least two servings in the meat-poultry-fish-dry beans-eggs-nuts group.

Vitamin D

Vitamin D is required for its role in maintaining bone mineralization and proper serum calcium levels. Adults over age 70 require 600 IU (or 15 μg) of vitamin D while adults 51 to 70 years of age require 400 IU (or 10 μg) (Institute of Medicine, 1997).

Vitamin E

High vitamin E intake can interact with anticoagulant therapy as well as potentiate the antiplatelet effects of other supplements such as ginkgo biloba, ginger,

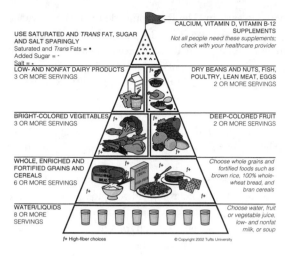

Figure 3–1 ■ TUFTS Modified Food Guide Pyramid for persons over 70 years of age.
Source: Russell, R. M., Rasmussen, H., & Lichenstein, A. H. (1999). *Journal of Nutrition, 129,* 751–753.

ginseng, and garlic (Ang-Lee, Moss, & Yuan, 2001; Fairfield & Fletcher, 2002; Norred & Brinker, 2001). The Tolerable Upper Limit (TUL) of vitamin E is 1,000 mg/day (Institute of Medicine, 2000).

Calcium

Calcium in the diet is required for the maintenance of bone mineral density and plasma calcium levels. The recommended intake for calcium in adults over 50 years of age is increased to 1,200 mg compared to 1,000 mg for adults 19 to 50 years of age (Institute of Medicine, 1997).

Vitamin B₁₂

Vitamin B_{12} (cyanocobalamin) is required in cell division and to maintain the myelin sheaths of the central nervous system. The Recommended Daily Allowance (RDA) for vitamin B_{12} is 2.4 µg. A vitamin B_{12} supplement is recommended because of decreased absorption of the vitamin associated with atrophic gastritis and altered gastric pH (Institute of Medicine, 1998; Russell, Rasmussen, & Lichtenstein, 1999).

Symptoms of vitamin B_{12} deficiency include macrocytic anemia and neurological problems such as peripheral neuropathy, irritability, depression, and poor memory.

Folic acid supplementation can mask a B_{12} deficiency. However, neurological symptoms will continue to progress without adequate B_{12}. A B_{12} assessment should be part of any workup for symptoms or dementia (Eastley, Wilcock, & Bucks, 2000).

Vitamin B_6

Vitamin B_6 (pyridoxine) is required as a coenzyme in metabolism of protein, fat, and other biochemical reactions. The dietary reference intakes (DRI) for B_6 in adults over 50 years of age is 1.5 mg per day for women and 1.7 mg per day for men. Symptoms of deficiency include an inflamed tongue and oral mucosa, called **glossitis and cheilosis**, depression, and confusion. The TUL for B_6 is 100 mg.

Fluid

Specific daily total water recommendations for adults older than 51 years, including water from all foods and beverages, are 3.7 L and 2.7 L for men and women, respectively (Institute of Medicine, 2004). This includes a recommendation that daily total water from beverages alone reach 13 cups for men and 9 cups for women. Symptoms of dehydration include: dark urine, dry mucous membranes, confusion, postural changes in pulse and blood pressure, and sunken eyes.

NUTRITIONAL ASSESSMENT

Both undernutrition and overnutrition in the older person can affect quality of life, morbidity, and mortality. Malnutrition is associated with adverse outcomes such as poor wound healing, skeletal muscle loss, functional decline, altered immune response, altered pharmacokinetics, and increased risk of institutionalization (Sullivan, Bopp, & Roberson, 2002; Covinsky, 2002; Covinsky, Covinsky, Palmer, & Sehgal, 2002). Overnutrition can also affect quality of life in the older person when it is manifested as obesity, degenerative joint disease, diabetes, hypertension, and cardiovascular disease.

Nutritional Assessment Parameters

A comprehensive nutritional assessment reviews anthropometric measurements, laboratory values, and clinical findings from the physical examination and patient history.

Anthropometrics

Anthropometric measurements include height, weight and weight history, muscle mass, and fat mass measurements are included.

Weight

Recorded weights on admission and at regular intervals are essential for all older patients. Individuals should be weighed with a minimum of clothing and after voiding. The nurse should note any presence of edema. A weight history that reveals unintentional weight loss of 5% body weight over a month or 10% over 6 months is clinically significant and should trigger further investigation.

Height

Height can be measured using a standing measure or in a recumbent position. Recumbent measurements can be made with an individual lying flat and straight in bed with light pencil marks made on bed linens at head and heel to then be measured with a cloth tape. Generally bed height measurements are 1.5 in. longer than standing height (American Medical Directors Association, 2001).

Body Mass Index

Body mass index is derived using measured height and weight with the following formula: BMI = weight (kg)/height^2 (m). Decreased BMI below 22 in the older person is predictive of undernutrition and associated with mortality (Sullivan et al., 2002). While a BMI over 25 is considered overweight and carries an increased mortality risk for the general population, the relative risk of death associated with being overweight decreases after age 65 (Calle et al., 1999; Stevens et al., 1998).

Laboratory Values

Several laboratory parameters are used to assess nutritional status.

Plasma Proteins

Albumin, prealbumin, and transferrin are all used to assess visceral protein status. An albumin $\leq$ 3.5 mg/dl is considered indicative of mild malnutrition.

Folate and Vitamin B_{12} Assessment

Evaluation of vitamin B_{12} and folic acid status is particularly pertinent due to the effects of aging, disease, and medications on absorption and metabolism of both vitamins. A high red blood cell mean cell volume

(MCV) should be followed up by assessments of plasma folic acid and vitamin B_{12}.

Cholesterol

It is debated whether low serum cholesterol concentration, defined as < 160 mg/dl, is an independent risk factor for malnutrition or just an indicator of an existing medical condition (Hu, Seeman, Harris, & Reuben, 2003; Volpato, Leveille, Corti, Harris, & Guralnik, 2001). The increased use of pharmacological interventions for elevated serum cholesterol may further complicate the usefulness of low cholesterol levels as a nutritional indicator.

Nursing Assessment

The nursing assessment should focus on skin condition, including turgor, lesions, nonhealing ulcers, color variations, and excessive dryness or cracking.

The oral cavity is inspected for tooth or denture condition, oral lesions, hyperplasia of the gums, fissures around the lips, oral hygiene, and any coatings on the tongue. The abdomen should be palpated for firmness or tenderness. The bowel record should be checked for date of the last bowel movement, as constipation and fecal impaction will inhibit appetite. The nurse should observe the patient eating and drinking, note any swallowing difficulties or positioning problems, and consult with occupational therapy as needed.

It is important to assess pain levels and administer prn (as needed) medications 1 hour before mealtime if unrelieved pain appears to be a factor.

Finally, the medication list should be reviewed for any medications (long-standing or newly prescribed) that could be causing anorexia or depression. Many medications have the side effects of early satiety,

Common offenders are digoxin, diuretics, chemo-therapy agents, some antibiotics, and some anti-depressants.

Nutritional History
Diet Recall
A 24-hour dietary recall can be done during an office visit or as part of an admission interview.
Food Frequency
A food frequency assessment is an excellent tool to use with a 24-hour recall to fill in the gaps of missing in-formation that occur with a one-day snapshot.

Screening Tools
Nutritional screening and assessment tools exist to streamline the incorporation of nutritional status into routine healthcare processes. It is essential that any tool be used in the context for which it was developed and validated.

Mini Nutritional Assessment and Subjective Global Assessment
Both the Mini Nutritional Assessment and Subjective Global Assessment tools have been validated as clinical tools for use in screening nutritional status in the older person (Vellas et al., 1999; Persson, Bris-mar, Katzarski, Nordenstrom, & Cederholm, 2002; Covinsky et al., 2002).

Minimum Data Set
The MDS includes nutritional components that must be assessed for all residents (Centers for Medicare and Medicaid Services, 2002). Important criteria that can

MINI NUTRITIONAL ASSESSMENT
MNA®

Last Name: _____ First Name: _____ M.I. _____ Sex: _____ Date: _____

Age: _____ Weight, kg: _____ Height, cm: _____ Knee Height, cm: _____

Complete the form by writing the numbers in the boxes. Add the numbers in the boxes and compare the total assessment to the Malnutrition Indicator Score.

ANTHROPOMETRIC ASSESSMENT

	Points
1. Body Mass Index (BMI) (weight in kg) / (height in m)²	
a. BMI < 19 = 0 points	
b. BMI 19 to < 21 = 1 point	
c. BMI 21 to < 23 = 2 points	
d. BMI ≥ 23 = 3 points	□
2. Mid-arm circumference (MAC) in cm	
a. MAC < 21 = 0.0 points	
b. MAC 21 – 22 = 0.5 points	
c. MAC > 22 = 1.0 points	□.□
3. Calf circumference (CC) in cm	
a. CC < 31 = 0 points b. CC ≥ 31 = 1 point	□

4. Weight loss during last 3 months
   a. weight loss greater than 3 kg (6.6 lbs)   = 0 points
   b. does not know   = 1 point
   c. weight loss between 1 and 3 kg
      (2.2 and 6.6 lbs)   = 2 points
   d. no weight loss   = 3 points

□

GENERAL ASSESSMENT

5. Lives independently (not in a nursing home
   or hospital)
   a. no = 0 points   b. yes = 1 point

□

(continued)

	Points
6. Takes more than 3 prescription drugs per day a. yes = 0 points b. no = 1 point	☐
7. Has suffered psychological stress or acute disease in the past 3 months a. yes = 0 points b. no = 2 points	☐

8. Mobility
  a. bed or chair bound = 0 points
  b. able to get out of bed/chair but does not go out = 1 point
  c. goes out = 2 points
	☐

9. Neuropsychological problems
  a. severe dementia or depression = 0 points
  b. mild dementia = 1 point
  c. no psychological problems = 2 points
	☐

10. Pressure sores or skin ulcers a. yes = 0 points b. no = 1 point	☐

DIETARY ASSESSMENT

11. How many full meals does the patient eat daily?
  a. 1 meal = 0 points
  b. 2 meals = 1 point
  c. 3 meals = 2 points
	☐

	Points

12. Selected consumption markers for protein intake
  • At least one serving of dairy products (milk, cheese, yogurt) per day?   yes ☐ no ☐
  • Two or more servings of legumes or eggs per week?   yes ☐ no ☐
  • Meat, fish, or poultry every day?   yes ☐ no ☐
  a. if 0 or 1 yes = 0.0 points
  b. if 2 yes = 0.5 points
  c. if 3 yes = 1.0 points
	☐.☐

13. Consumes two or more servings of fruits or vegetables per day? a. no = 0 points b. yes = 1 point	☐

14. Has food intake declined over the past three months due to loss of appetite, digestive problems, chewing or swallowing difficulties?
  a. severe loss of appetite = 0 points
  b. moderate loss of appetite = 1 point
  c. no loss of appetite = 2 points
	☐

15. How much fluid (water, juice, coffee, tea, milk, . . .) is consumed per day? (1 cup = 8 oz.)
  a. less than 3 cups = 0.0 points
  b. 3 to 5 cups = 0.5 points
  c. more than 5 cups = 1.0 points
	☐.☐

16. Mode of feeding
  a. unable to eat without assistance = 0 points
  b. self-fed with some difficulty = 1 point
  c. self-fed without any problem = 2 points
	☐

ASSESSMENT TOTAL (max. 30 points):

MALNUTRITION INDICATOR SCORE		
≥ 24 points	well-nourished	□
17 to 23.5 points	at risk of malnutrition	□
< 17 points	malnourished	□

Ref: Guigoz Y, Vellas B and Garry PJ. 1994. Mini Nutritional Assessment: A practical assessment tool for grading the nutritional state of elderly patients. *Facts and Research in Gerontology.* Supplement #2: 15–59.

SELF-ASSESSMENT

17. Do they view themselves as having nutritional
problems?
    a. major malnutrition   = 0 points
    b. does not know or moderate malnutrition = 1 point
    c. no nutritional problem   = 2 points   □

18. In comparison with other people of the same age,
how do they consider their health status?
    a. not as good   = 0.0 points
    b. does not know   = 0.5 points
    c. as good   = 1.0 points
    d. better   = 2.0 points   □.□

Figure 3–2 ■ Mini Nutritional Assessment®.

Source: Reprinted from Vellas, B., et al. (1999). The Mini Nutritional Assessment and its use in grading nutritional state of elderly patients. *Nutrition, 15,* 116–122. Used with permission from Elsevier.

signal nutritional problems include weight loss and leaves 25% or more of food uneaten. (See Appendix B for the MDS and nutrition related criteria.)

COMMON NUTRITIONAL CONCERNS IN THE OLDER PERSON

Unintentional Weight Loss

Causes of weight loss include:

Insufficient Intake

Lack of adequate food and fluid intake occurs for multiple physical and psychosocial reasons including:

- **Dehydration**
- **Sadness and clinical depression**
- **Polypharmacy** is associated with undernutrition (Chia-Hui, Schilling, & Lyder, 2001). Many medications can cause lack of appetite directly or from additional side effects, such as sedation.
- **Pain**
- **Chronic diseases** such as chronic obstructive pulmonary disease, congestive heart failure, and cancer can contribute to anorexia.
- **Dysphagia** can result from difficulty chewing or swallowing or both.
- **Dependency on others** for feeding or eating-related activities.
- **Cognitive impairment**. Diminished ability to recognize food, failure to respond to hunger cues, difficulty with chewing and swallowing, and behavioral issues such as agitation can lead to declining intake.
- **Sensory changes** including poor vision, impaired taste and smell, and dry mouth can make eating less pleasurable.

- Overzealous use of therapeutic diets may serve no clinical benefit if they are not eaten. Long-term care residents should be on liberalized diets unless deemed medically contraindicated following an individual assessment (Position of the American Dietetic Association, 2002).
- **Poverty** and food insecurity can lead to poor nutritional health because of diminished intake.

Iatrogenic Practices

Iatrogenic practices can put an individual at risk for undernutrition. As many as 21% of hospitalized older persons were found to have an average intake of less than 50% of their energy needs while in the hospital (Sullivan, Sun, & Walls, 1999). Patients may be NPO for testing followed by an unnecessary delay in returning to a normal diet.

Nutrient Losses

Nutrient losses during absorption or metabolism can lead to undernutrition even with adequate dietary intake. Inflammatory bowel disease, high output ostomies, and radiation treatment can alter nutrient status.

Hypermetabolism

Hypermetabolism warrants intake of increased energy and nutrients. When these increased needs are not met, undernutrition results. Wounds, fever, infections, and cardiopulmonary disease can cause hypermetabolism.

Consequences of Unintentional Weight Loss and Undernutrition

Undernutrition is associated with poor clinical outcomes, including mortality, poor wound healing, development of decubitus ulcers, skeletal muscle loss, functional decline, altered immune response, altered pharmacokinetics, and increased risk of institutionalization (Covinsky, 2002; Covinsky et al., 2002; Sullivan et al., 2002).

A BMI less than 21 is included as a trigger for decubitus ulcer assessment in the MDS for long-term care patients (Centers for Medicare and Medicaid Services, 2002). Vitamins A and C and zinc are necessary for wound closure (Rojas & Phillips, 1999; Thomas, 2001).

Low serum albumin can lead to decreased binding of certain drugs and can lead to multiple drugs competing for diminished protein binding sites and increase the likelihood of adverse drug reactions.

Treatment of Unintentional Weight Loss and Undernutrition

Developing a nutritional care plan for an older person with undernutrition first requires a conversation with the individual or a proxy to determine the extent of personal wishes, quality-of-life issues, and advance directives before any aggressive interventions are begun.

Verbal prompting throughout the day has been shown to increase fluid intake by 78% in long-term care patients.

Flagging the meal tray or door of long-term care patients at risk for dehydration can remind caregivers to provide extra prompting, and food service workers to leave unfinished beverages at the bedside, if safe to do so.

Alter the physical environment by using music to reduce agitated behavior and provide finger foods to improve intake (Manthorpe & Watson, 2003).

Orexigenic medications, such as megestrol acetate, are sometimes considered, but no medication has yet to be approved by the FDA as an appetite stimulant for geriatric use (Council for Nutrition Clinical Strategies in Long-Term Care, 2001).

Commercial oral supplements have been prescribed to boost intake with mixed results. Supplements should be liquid and not solid and should be given more than an hour before meals to minimize satiety (American Medical Directors Association, 2001; Huffman, 2002). Providing a 4-oz serving of liquid supplement instead of other fluids with four medication passes each day can provide almost 500 kcal.

A nasogastric tube may be used for short-term feeding. A more permanent tube, such as a gastrostomy or jejunostomy tube, may be used for long-term feeding. Most formulas that are 1 cal/ml are isotonic in nature, minimizing the osmotic draw of fluid into the gastrointestinal tract during feeding. A registered dietitian will generally make an assessment and recommendation for appropriate formula type and volume. Continuous drip-feeding with the head of the bed or chair upright at least at a 30- to 45-degree angle is necessary when there is risk of aspiration. Feeding tubes should be flushed both before and after giving medications to avoid clogging the tube with precipitate. Nursing interventions for common problems with tube-feedings include frequent hand washing to prevent infection, checking for gastric residual volumes to prevent aspiration, administering feeding at room temperature to avoid diarrhea, treating constipation with added fiber, and careful monitoring of hydration status.

PATIENT-FAMILY TEACHING GUIDELINES

The following are guidelines that the nurse may find useful when instructing older persons and their families about dietary supplements (adapted from NIH, 2000).

Dietary Supplements

1. Do I need a dietary supplement?

   Dietary supplements can consist of vitamins, minerals, fiber, herbs, hormones, or a variety of other substances. While it is generally accepted that taking a multivitamin daily is a good idea, great controversy exists surrounding the use of other supplements. As the FDA does not test or regulate these supplements, there is little evidence to back up these claims. In fact, some of these supplements can hurt you. Your best bet is to talk to your doctor, your nurse, or a dietitian about supplements if you are considering taking one.

2. What about vitamins and minerals?

   Vitamins and minerals are nutrients found naturally in food. The best way to get vitamins and minerals is by eating a balanced diet, not by taking supplements. Try to eat a variety of foods including meats, fruits, whole grains, and vegetables daily. Avoid foods that are low in fiber and high in fat and added sugar. If you occasionally skip meals or do not always eat right, taking a multivitamin may be a good choice for you. Remember:

   - A regular multivitamin will do. It does not have to be a "senior" formula.

- Do not megadose or take large quantities of any vitamin or mineral supplement.
- Generally, store or generic brands are fine and equivalent to more expensive preparations.

3. What vitamins does my body need now that I am older?

Depending on your age and level of health you should take the following amounts of vitamins from food and supplements if needed:

- Vitamin B_{12}—2.4 μg. Some foods, like cereal, are fortified with B_{12}, but many older people cannot absorb the B vitamins from food.
- Calcium—1,200 mg. As you age, you need more calcium to keep your bones strong. Vitamin D helps calcium to be absorbed, so look for a calcium preparation with this vitamin.
- Vitamin D—400 IU daily up to age 70 and 600 IU daily after age 70. It is a vitamin stored in the body, so do not take over 2,000 IU each day.
- Iron—up to 8 mg daily. Normally older people do not lose blood (as do menstruating women) but if you are recovering from surgery or you are a blood donor, be sure to eat foods high in iron or take a supplement. Be careful; it can be constipating.
- Vitamin B_6—1.7 mg for men and 1.5 mg for women. Found in some whole grain products and fortified cereals.

4. How about herbal supplements?

You may have heard of ginkgo biloba, ginseng, echinacea, ephedra, St. John's wort, and black cohosh. These are herbal supplements that are harvested from certain foods and plants. Their ingredients will have some effect on your body,

(continued)

and they may interfere with medications you have been prescribed. Some herbal supplements can also cause serious side effects such as high blood pressure, nausea, diarrhea, constipation, fainting, headaches, seizures, heart attack, or even stroke. Play it safe. Check it out with your healthcare provider before you take any herbal supplement.

5. What is best for me if I am considering taking a dietary supplement?

If you are thinking of taking an herbal supplement for any reason, consider this advice:

- Talk to your doctor, nurse, pharmacist, or dietitian. Do not believe the manufacturer's claims. Be cautious and careful.
- Use only the supplement recommended by your healthcare professional. Treat it as you would a prescription medication with careful dosing, with monitoring for effect and side effects.
- If you decide to stop taking a supplement your doctor has recommended, make sure to let him or her know.
- Learn as much as you can about the supplement before taking it. Buy only from a reputable buyer. Avoid products sold over the Internet.
- If you are not sure, ask questions. Be an informed consumer.

CHAPTER 4

PHARMACOLOGY

PHARMACOKINETIC ALTERATIONS IN THE OLDER PERSON

With aging there is a decrease in body water (as much as 15%) and an increase in body fat. This could result in increased concentration of water-soluble drugs (e.g., alcohol) and more prolonged effects of fat-soluble drugs.

Hepatic blood flow may be decreased by as much as 50% in individuals over 65 years. This could result in increased toxicity when they take usual doses of "first-pass effect" drugs since less of these drugs would be detoxified immediately by the liver.

Decreases in serum albumin levels or binding capacity may result in increased serum levels of the "free" or unbound proportion of protein-bound drugs. This may result in toxic levels of highly bound drugs because more unbound drug is available to produce its effects.

Renal function generally decreases with age. Blood urea nitrogen (BUN) levels are poor indicators of renal function in the older person because of the decrease in muscle mass and other variables affecting BUN levels. Serum creatinine levels can be used to estimate creatinine clearance but are less reliable in older persons than in younger persons because older persons have less muscle mass, and creatinine is a product of muscle breakdown. The following formula (Cockcroft & Gault, 1976), which includes variables of age and for gender, is often used to estimate creatinine clearance:

$$\frac{\text{creatinine}}{\text{clearance}} = \frac{(140 - \text{age}) \times \text{lean wt (kg)}}{72 \times \text{serum creatinine}} \times \begin{array}{l} 0.85 \text{ for} \\ \text{women} \end{array}$$

The rule of thumb for drug prescription in the older person is "start low; go slow." This rule will help prevent toxic side effects and adverse drug reactions.

Drugs requiring special consideration in the elderly include:

1. Drugs expected to be widely used in the elderly population
2. Drugs that affect or are affected by a biological homeostatic mechanism that may be deficient in older adults (e.g., cardiovascular system)
3. Drugs that act in the central nervous system
4. Drugs that have a low therapeutic to safety ratio and:
    a. are excreted largely by kidney
    b. are subject to large first-pass effect
    c. are metabolized by oxidative mechanisms
    d. generate significant metabolites
    e. are highly protein bound

Adverse Drug Reactions and Iatrogenesis

Adverse drug reactions (ADRs) are a particular problem in the older person. Suspect an adverse drug reaction if a patient has cognitive changes, falls, or experiences anorexia, nausea, or weight loss. Encourage the discontinuation of one drug when another is added to a drug regimen.

Adverse Drug Effects of Concern in the Older Person

Cognitive Effects

Cognitive impairment (e.g., delirium, dementia, depression) can be caused by a variety of medications. Delirium may be caused by drugs (including psychotropic medications) with anticholinergic effects. Changes in mood such as anxiety and depression can result from many types of drug therapy, such as antihypertensives (e.g., beta-blockers), antiparkinsonian agents, steroids, NSAIDs, narcotic analgesics, antineoplastic agents, central nervous system (CNS) depressants, and psychotropics (e.g., alcohol, benzodiazepines, and other antianxiety agents).

Anticholinergic Syndrome

Central anticholinergic effects include agitation, confusion, disorientation, poor attention, hallucinations, or psychosis. Peripheral effects include constipation, urinary retention, inhibition of sweating, decreased salivary and bronchial secretions, tachycardia, and mydriasis. Individuals with benign prostatic hypertrophy or other strictures of the urinary urethra may experience increased difficulty in initiating urine flow. Dryness of the mouth can slow the absorption of sublingual medications and may affect the ability to swallow oral preparations. Drugs with anticholinergic effects may also affect vision. Anticholinergic effects on cardiac function may alter cardiovascular drug effects or lead to the possibly unnecessary prescription of cardiovascular drug therapy.

Atropine, a common medication given preoperatively to dry up secretions and prevent aspiration while the patient is under anesthesia, is often associated with anticholinergic side effects. These side effects include bradycardia, dry mouth, decreased sweating, tachycardia, dilated pupils, blurred near vision, decreased intestinal peristalsis, dysphasia, dysphagia, urinary retention, hyperthermia and flushing, ataxia, hallucinations, delirium, and coma. Check each drug for its anticholinergic profile. A useful heuristic to remember anticholinergic effects is "Dry as a bone; Red as a beet; Hot as a hare; Blind as a bat; Mad as a hatter."

Gastric and Esophageal Irritation

Oral drugs that are swallowed but do not reach the stomach can result in esophageal obstruction or irritation of the esophageal lining. Older patients should take medications in an upright position and remain upright for 30 minutes; should not crush tablets without consulting with the pharmacist; swallow medications with at least 8 oz of water; and avoid medications that relax the lower esophageal sphincter muscle if they have gastroesophageal reflux disorder.

Gastric irritation can be caused by a variety of medications. This can lead to not only discomfort ("heartburn") but also gastric bleeding, which could be life threatening. Some drugs that have this effect are produced with an enteric coating that prevents the drug from dissolving until it reaches the alkaline environment in the duodenum. The coating of enteric-coated drugs (e.g., enteric-coated aspirin, erythromycin, oral bisacodyl tablets) may break down prematurely in the stomach if given with other drugs or foods that make the stomach alkaline; therefore, calcium, dairy products, and antacid should not be given with enteric-coated preparations or within 2 hours.

Commonly used medications like aspirin and NSAIDs can cause irritation, and block prostaglandin synthesis, which decreases resistance of the stomach lining to acid and other stomach contents. Additional effects of prostaglandin inhibition include slowing of blood clotting, therefore increasing the danger of gastric bleeding from these drugs. Gastric bleeding in an older person may occur with little or no prior symptoms.

ALTERNATIVE AND COMPLEMENTARY MEDICINE

Herbal medicines have widespread use and availability today. Herbs do interact with medications. If patients are to have anesthesia, it is important that they notify the anesthetist of what herbal remedies they have been using. Table 4–1 highlights the uses and drug therapy concerns of some commonly used herbs.

Over-the-Counter Medications

Patients' use of alcohol should be carefully assessed since alcohol is a CNS depressant, may cause gastric irritation, and interferes with the metabolism of certain medications such as acetaminophen. Decongestants may raise blood pressure, antacids can inhibit the absorption of other medications, and acetaminophen inhibits the absorption of warfarin.

Appropriate Versus Inappropriate Prescribing Practices

Appropriate prescribing may be defined as follows:

- The selection of a medication and instruction for its use that agree with accepted medical standards
- Use of appropriate dose and scheduling guidelines

Table 4–1 Common Herbal Preparations and Interactions With Drugs

Herbal Preparation	Use	Interactions/Precautions
Echinacea	Stimulation of immunity.	Counteracts effects of immunosuppressive drugs (e.g., cyclosporine).
Ephedra (ma huang) (no longer available in U.S.)	Promotion of weight loss, increasing energy, treatment of respiratory condition.	Sympathomimetic effects can cause elevated blood pressure, stroke, and death.
Garlic	Reducing risk of atherosclerosis by decreasing blood pressure, thrombin formation, and lipid and cholesterol levels.	Inhibits platelet aggregation and potentiates effects of platelet inhibitor drugs (e.g., indomethacin, dipyridamole).
Ginseng	Protection against effects of stress, helps to restore homeostasis.	Can cause bleeding problems and hypoglycemia.
Ginkgo	Enhancement of cognitive performance, treatment of peripheral vascular disease, age-related macular degeneration, vertigo, tinnitus, erectile dysfunction, altitude sickness.	Inhibits platelet-activating factor and can cause bleeding.
Kava	Anxiolytic and sedative.	Causes excessive sedation when used with other CNS depressants.

Herbal Preparation	Use	Interactions/Precautions
St. John's wort	Treatment of mild to moderate depression.	May cause excess levels of serotonin if taken with selective serotonin reuptake inhibitors (SSRIs). Can increase the metabolism of many drugs, resulting in reduced effectiveness.
Valerian	Sedative, hypnotic.	Withdrawal from valerian mimics acute benzodiazepine withdrawal syndrome. Potentiates sedative effects of barbiturates and anesthetics and anesthetic adjuvants.

Source: Adapted from Ang-Lee, Moss, & Yuan, 2001. Used with permission of the American Medical Association.

- Agreement of the manufacturer's standards and FDA labeling guidelines, standard medication references, and interpretation of the scientific literature by drug therapy experts (Schmader et al., 1994)

Table 4–2 lists drugs that are considered inappropriate to use in the older person based on the 1997 Beers criteria.

APPROPRIATE USE OF PSYCHOTROPICS IN THE OLDER PERSON

The following are provisions of OBRA 87 regulations as refined by OBRA 91 (Department of Health and Human Services, 2001):

- *Chemical restraint.* The use of a drug to control an individual's behavior and is legally permissible

Table 4–2 Drugs Inappropriate For Use in Older Patients Regardless of Dose, Duration, or Disease Condition

Drug Category	Drug
Analgesics:	meperidine, propoxyphene, pentazocine
Analgesics-NSAIDs:	indomethacin, phenylbutazone*
Antiarrhythmic:	disopyramide
Antidepressants:	amitriptyline and combinations, doxepin
Antihistamines:	chlorpheniramine, cyproheptadine, dexchlorpheniramine, diphenhydramine, hydroxyzine, promethazine, tripelennamine
Antihypertensives:	methyldopa or combinations, reserpine and combinations
Antiemetics:	trimethobenzamide
Dementia drugs:	ergoloid mesylates, cyclospasmol
Gastrointestinal antispasmodics:	belladonna alkaloids, dicyclomine, hyoscyamine, propantheline
Muscle relaxants/ antispasmodics:	carisoprodol, chlorzoxazone, metaxalone, methocarbamol
Oral hypoglycemics:	chlorpropamide
Platelet inhibitors:	dipyridamole, ticlopidine
Sedatives and hypnotics:	diazepam, chlordiazepoxide and combinations, flurazepam, meprobamate, all barbiturates (except pentobarbital)

*Deleted from 2003 consensus criteria.
Source: Beers et al., 1991. Used with permission of the American Medical Association.

only if to ensure the physical safety of residents or other individuals.

- *Unnecessary drug.* Any drug when used in excessive dose (including duplicate therapy), or for excessive duration; or without adequate monitoring; or without adequate indication for its use; or in the presence of adverse consequences, which indicate the dose should be reduced or discontinued; or without specific target symptoms.

Use of Antipsychotic Drugs

The facility must ensure that residents who have not used antipsychotic drugs are not given these drugs unless antipsychotic drug therapy is necessary to treat a specific condition, as diagnosed and documented in the clinical record. Residents who use antipsychotic drugs must receive gradual dose reductions, drug holidays, or behavioral programming, unless clinically contraindicated, in an effort to discontinue these drugs.

As needed (prn) doses of neuroleptics are not to be used more than twice in a 7-day period without further assessment and are to be used only for the purpose of titrating dosage for optimal response or for management of unexpected behaviors that are otherwise unmanageable.

Conditions that are considered to be inappropriate as the sole basis for the use of antipsychotic drugs are wandering, poor self-care, restlessness, impaired memory, anxiety, depression (without psychotic features), insomnia, unsociability, indifference to surroundings, fidgeting, nervousness, uncooperativeness, or agitated behaviors that do not represent danger to the resident or others.

Long-acting benzodiazepines are strictly regulated and should not be used unless:

- There has been an attempt to use a shorter acting drug.
- The possible reasons for a resident's distress have been carefully assessed and treated if at all possible.

Table 4–3   Maximum Daily Doses of Long-Acting Benzodiazepines

Generic Name	Brand Name	Maximum DAILY Oral Dosage
Chlordiazepoxide	Librium	20 mg
Clorazepate	Tranxene	15 mg
Clonazepam	Klonopin	1.5 mg
Diazepam	Valium	5 mg
Flurazepam	Dalmane	15 mg
Prazepam	Centrax	15 mg
Quazepam	Doral	7.5 mg

- The use of a long-acting agent results in maintenance or improvement in the resident's functional status.
- Daily use is less than 4 continuous months, and an attempt at gradual dose reduction has been tried without success.
- Daily use is less than or equal to the total daily doses in Table 4–3. If higher doses (as evidenced by the resident's response or the resident's clinical record) are necessary for the maintenance of or improvement in the resident's functional status, they may be cautiously used with the reasons documented in the medical record by the prescribing physician.

Short-Acting Benzodiazepines and Other Anxiolytics

Drugs such as alprazolam, lorazepam, and oxazepam also have maximum daily dosage limits. These drugs should be used only when (1) evidence exists that other possible reasons for the resident's distress have been considered and ruled out; (2) use results in a maintenance or improvement in the resident's functional status; (3) daily use (at any dose) is less than 4 continuous months unless an attempt at gradual dose reduction is unsuccessful; (4) use is for one of the following indications: generalized anxiety disorder, organic mental syndromes (including dementia) with associated states that are quantitatively and objectively documented and that constitute sources of distress or dysfunction of the resident or represent danger to the resident or others, panic disorder, or symptomatic anxiety that occurs in residents with another diagnosed psychiatric disorder (e.g., depression, adjustment disorder); and (5) use is equal to or less than following the listed total daily doses, unless higher doses as evidenced by the resident response or the resident's functional status.

Evaluating Appropriate Prescribing of Medications

The following questions can guide the clinician in reviewing appropriateness of drug use and could help to assess compliance with OBRA 87 regulations:

1. Is the condition sufficiently problematic to require treatment?
2. Are there nursing or other nonpharmacological treatments that could alleviate the condition, prevent or delay use of a medication, or complement drug therapy?
3. If a drug is indicated for treatment of a specific condition, is the need for the medication documented in the medical record (e.g., an established or working diagnosis for which the drug is approved)?
4. Has informed consent for prescription been obtained from the patient or legally determined surrogate decision maker?

5. Is the prescription likely to be effective in achieving the prescriber's preset goals for therapy (i.e., objective measures of signs or symptoms)?
6. How long should the drug be used before decreasing dosage or discontinuing it? Will this be at a specific time or based on a change in the patient's condition?
7. Is there duplication of the specific drug with other drugs the patient is taking or overlap of therapeutic or adverse effects of other drugs being taken?
8. Are the dose and timing correct? Is the drug being administered correctly?
9. Are there potential drug-drug, drug-disease, or drug-nutritional interactions?
10. Is the patient being adequately monitored for common serious side effects (e.g., periodic blood levels, functional and mental status tests, movement disorder scales)?
11. If side effects are present, is there a positive balance of the risks and benefits? Are the negative effects of treatment outweighed by the positive aspects (e.g., improving, maintaining, or slowing decline of resident function or alleviating suffering)?

PROMOTING ADHERENCE AND COMPLIANCE

Compliance with a prescribed regimen presumably leads to better patient outcomes. Noncompliance with medication regimens results in considerable costs to patients, employers, health insurers, and the healthcare system.

The nurse should assess the following factors:

- Ability to read and comprehend main label (prescription)

- Ability to read and comprehend the auxiliary labels (e.g., warnings)
- Manual dexterity (open vials, remove correct number of tablets, recap medication) (Hartford Institute for Geriatric Nursing, 1999)

Measures to help older persons manage their medications correctly include:

- Simplifying the regimen by decreasing, to the extent possible, the number of drugs and the number of pills to be taken in a day.
- Establishing a routine for taking medications, such as preparing medications for the day in different containers.
- Scheduling medications at mealtime or in conjunction with other specific daily activities (e.g., before brushing teeth at night or before leaving for a daily activity such as exercise or card playing) unless contraindicated.
- Developing a method with the patient for remembering if he or she actually took the medication (e.g., moving the medication to another place).
- Conducting a total assessment of all medications by asking the patient to bring in all medications he or she has at home, including OTC preparations. These can be checked for outdated preparations, unused or unfinished prescriptions, overlap, or duplication of medications.
- Considering the use of telephone reminders (Fulmer et al., 1999) or computer-based or e-mail reminders.

Suggestions to improve medication compliance include:

- Providing careful instruction with written information at about the fifth-grade level

- Providing an audiotape for patients with visual impairment
- Including a description of adverse effects and actions to be taken should they occur
- Providing missed dose instructions
- Including a family member or friend if possible and appropriate
- Encouraging the patient to obtain all prescriptions and OTC drugs from the same pharmacy

ASSESSING OLDER PATIENTS' APPROPRIATE USE OF MEDICATIONS

The nurse should follow these guidelines:

1. Review the patient's medical conditions and allergies. Update the chart when new allergies are reported and document the allergic response. Check patients for MedicAlert jewelry or cards indicating that they are taking certain medications or have certain allergies.
2. Review each drug. If patients are living at home, have them assemble all medications for review whether prescribed or OTC, including vitamins and herbal remedies. This is sometimes called a "brown bag" review because patients often bring their medications in a brown bag.
3. Is the drug considered to be inappropriate for use in older persons?
4. Is the patient taking it as prescribed: dose, route, frequency and timing in relation to food or other medications, method (e.g., with fluid or food), and duration?
5. Is the medication producing the intended therapeutic effect?
6. Is the medication outdated?

7. Does the patient understand what condition the drug is treating and the signs and symptoms that should be reported to a physician immediately?
8. Does the patient have any cognitive or physical condition affecting the ability to safely administer the medication?
9. Does the patient have financial resources for the costs of the medication? Is there a generic version of this drug (or another that is equally effective for the patient's condition) available that would be less expensive?
10. Does the patient have any cultural or ethnic beliefs or practices that might impact compliance?
11. Does the patient have a family member or friend who can help with medication management on a regular basis if needed (e.g., if the patient becomes ill)?
12. Review each drug for:
    Interactions with other drugs.
    Interactions with herbal medicines.
    Interactions with vitamin or foods.
    Allergies.
    Duplicate therapy (from more than one prescriber or from patient's use of OTC medications containing the same or similar ingredients as prescribed medications).

Costs of Medication

Medications can be costly for the older person. Suggestions to patients to reduce costs of medications include the following:

- Ask the physician if the drug is really necessary or if there is a less expensive substitute.
- Ask the physician about free samples.

- Do not order large amounts of newly prescribed medications until you know that it is effective and that you can tolerate it.
- Ask if there is a generic version of the medication.
- Contact different pharmacies; shop around.
- Ask the pharmacist about store-brand substitutes for more expensive brand-name OTC medications.
- Ask for senior citizen discounts.
- Contact AARP or medicare representatives for information about the Medicare D drug benefit.
- Go to the BenefitsCheckUpRx website at the National Council on the Aging to determine eligibility for help from community, state, or federal programs, or from drug companies.
- Try mail-order prescriptions.
- Try Internet pharmacies. Make sure it is a legitimate pharmacy by checking with the National Association of Boards of Pharmacy (NABP) website.

Unsafe Medication Practices

Older patients should be cautioned to avoid certain risky medication behaviors such as:

- *Sharing others' medications.*
- *Using imported medications.*
- *Using outdated medications.*

The medications not only may be ineffective but also can actually cause injury to the heart, liver, or kidneys.

PATIENT-FAMILY TEACHING GUIDELINES

The following are guidelines that the nurse may find useful when instructing older persons and their families about medications and drug safety.

1. I am taking a lot of medications prescribed by my doctor. How do I know if they are all safe?

Medications can be lifesaving and promote health and quality of life. However, you enter into a partnership with your doctor when you agree to take a medication he or she prescribes for you. Here are some suggestions for taking medication safely:

- Inform your doctor of all allergies, medical problems, drug reactions, over-the-counter medications, herbal remedies, and recreational drugs (including tobacco and alcohol) that you use.
- Ask about how to take the drug. Possible questions might include: Does "two tablets a day" mean two in the morning? One in the morning and one at night? Should it be taken with water? Should I sit up after taking the medication? Can I take it at the same time as my other medications? What should I do if I am ill and cannot take the medication?
- Ask about alternatives to the medication. Are there dietary or lifestyle changes that might decrease the need for or dose of the medication?
- What are the common side effects? What should be reported immediately?
- If you are on multiple medications, go over the schedule with your nurse. Write it down so you can keep the schedule in your wallet or pocketbook.
- Take the exact amount as prescribed.
- Do not share medications with others.
- Ask if you can drink alcohol. If so, ask how much is safe.
- Check for expiration dates on your medicine and throw away expired bottles. They may be unsafe to take.

(continued)

- Take all medications as prescribed, even if you are feeling better. Check with your doctor or nurse before stopping a medication in the middle of the treatment.
- Adhere to lab tests, blood pressure checks, and ongoing monitoring so that your doctor can keep track of the effectiveness and safety of your medications.

2. As my nurse, how can you help me to take medications safely?

As your nurse, I would like to review your medications with you at every clinic visit. This should be done on a regular basis and after every acute care hospitalization because many medicines are changed when you go to the hospital. I will also make sure that you have not started taking any new over-the-counter medications or herbal remedies that could interact with your prescription medicine. I will ask you questions regarding dizziness, rashes, constipation, dry mouth, or other changes to make sure you are tolerating your medications without side effects. I will also let you know if there are any warnings or changes regarding the safety or interactions of your medications. If you would like, I will write out medication instructions for you after you have seen the doctor so that you can refer to the instructions at home if you have questions.

3. What is the pharmacist's responsibility?

Tell your pharmacist if you have trouble reading small labels or opening the childproof prescription bottles. If you request non-childproof bottles, store them in a safe place if grandchildren or neighborhood children are visiting your home. Try not to store medications in a bathroom medicine cabinet if you take long steamy showers. The humidity can cause the medication to break down and become ineffective.

Be sure to ask questions about the name of the medication, and go over instructions regarding dosage and how to take it. Check the label before you leave the pharmacy. Make sure you have the correct prescription. If the medication looks different, check with the pharmacist to verify there is no error. Medication safety is a team effort, and you and your family are the key players on the team. Remember, medicines that are strong enough to cure you can also hurt you if they are not used correctly. Do not be afraid to ask questions and advocate for your own safety.

CHAPTER 5

PSYCHOLOGICAL FUNCTION

Older people evidence fewer diagnosable psychiatric disorders than younger persons, excluding cognitive impairment. Only cognitive impairments such as Alzheimer's disease show a definite age-associated increase (American Psychological Association, 2003).

Racial and ethnic minorities and older gay men and lesbians bear a greater burden from unmet mental health needs and thus suffer greater losses that negatively impact their overall health and productivity at all ages. The major barriers include the cost of care, societal stigma, and the fragmentation of services. Additional barriers include healthcare providers' lack of awareness of cultural issues, bias, or inability to speak the older person's language, and the older person's fear and mistrust of treatment (U.S. Surgeon General, 2003). Minority elders may be considered especially vulnerable and at risk for mental health problems because of **ageism** (negative stereotypes toward elderly adults) and cultural bias.

Depression in older adults is often undetected and untreated. The symptoms of depression are often associated with chronic illness and pain. Vague physical decline and somatic complaints may be the only clues of underlying depression.

Certain medications like sleeping pills, tranquilizers, and some pain medications can cause symptoms similar to dementia (confusion, lack of interest, memory impairment) but are not true dementia. These symptoms are called false or pseudodementia.

NORMAL CHANGES WITH AGING

Some general cognitive changes considered to be normal age-related changes include the following:

- Information-processing speed declines with age, resulting in a slower learning rate and greater need for repetition of information.
- The ability to divide attention between two tasks shows age-related decline.
- The ability to switch attention rapidly from one auditory input to another shows age-related decline (visual input switching ability does not change significantly with age).
- Ability to maintain sustained attention appears to decline with age.
- Ability to filter out irrelevant information appears to decline with age.
- Short-term or primary memory remains relatively stable.
- Long-term or secondary memory exhibits more substantial age-related changes, with the decline greater for recall than for recognition. (Cueing improves performance of long-term memory.)
- Most aspects of language are well preserved, such as use of language sounds and meaningful combinations of words. Vocabulary improves with age. However, word finding, naming ability, and ability to generate a word list rapidly decline with age.
- Visuospatial task ability declines with age such as drawing and construction ability.
- Abstraction and mental flexibility show some age decline.

- Accumulation of practical experience, or wisdom, continues until the very end of life.

(American Psychological Association, 1998)

Life satisfaction does not usually decrease as one ages.

Older adults cope with normal aging changes in a variety of ways. Methods for coping with age-associated cognitive changes include:

- Making lists, posting appointments on calendars, and writing "notes to self."
- Memory training and memory enhancement techniques (for instance, when meeting a new person for the first time, trying to link his or her name to a common object or easily remembered item).
- Keeping the mind challenged and mentally active (reading daily, completing a crossword puzzle, playing bridge, etc.).
- Using assistive devices such as pill boxes and reliance on habit such as preprogrammed telephones, parking in the same place in the mall parking lot, and so on, to reduce chances of forgetting vital information.
- Seeking support and encouragement from others.
- Staying positive and hopeful for the future, including laughing at oneself when appropriate. ("You won't believe what I did today. I showed up for my doctor's appointment with one brown and one black shoe! Oh well, at least I'm not a slave to fashion!")

PERSONALITY DISORDERS

Psychiatric symptoms that should be investigated and not written off as normal changes of aging include:

- *Memory and intellectual difficulties. Pseudodementia or cognitive changes due to underlying anx-*

iety, depression, or other potentially treatable psychiatric disorders can masquerade as Alzheimer's disease.

- *Change in sleep patterns.*
- *Changes in sexual interest and capacity.*
- *Fear of death.*
- *Delusions.*
- *Hallucinations.*
- *Disordered thinking.*
- *Problems with emotional expression, such as failure to show emotion, laugh, cry, or make eye contact, or withdrawal from opportunities for human interaction* (Journal of the American Medical Association, 2000; Merck Manual of Geriatrics, 2001).

PSYCHOTIC DISORDERS

Schizophrenia rarely occurs for the first time in old age. Some symptoms of schizophrenia such as hallucinations and delusions appear to decline with age, but other symptoms such as apathy and withdrawal may place the older person at high risk for social isolation and neglect.

The most common form of psychosis in later years is paranoia (American Psychological Association, 2003). Risk factors include hearing loss, social isolation, underlying personality disorder, cognitive impairment, and delirium.

Adjustment Disorder

The most common stressor that leads to adjustment disorder in later life is physical illness. Other stressors that may precipitate adjustment disorders among older adults include forced relocation, financial problems, family problems, and lengthy hospitalizations (American Psychological Association, 2003).

Bereavement

Symptoms of pathological grief among older adults include preoccupation with death, extensive guilt, an overwhelming sense of loss and worthlessness, marked psychomotor retardation, and functional impairment.

Factors that can affect the duration and course of grieving include:

Centrality of the loss.
Health of the survivor.
Survivor's religious or spiritual belief system.
History of substance abuse.
Nature of the death. Sudden deaths that are a result of trauma, natural disaster, or violent acts may be more difficult to bear and prolong the grieving process.

STRESS AND COPING

Symptoms that indicate the older person may be suffering negative effects of stress include the following:

- Sleep problems and insomnia
- Chronic high anxiety levels
- Use or abuse of alcohol, prescription or recreational drugs, or tobacco
- Jumpiness and inability to remain still for long periods of time
- New-onset hypertension, tachycardia, tremors, or irregular heartbeat
- Depression, chronic fatigue, or lack of pleasure in life
- Chronic pain or physical complaints

Suggested nursing actions include:

- Assisting older persons to identify stressors and rate their levels of stress.
- Educating the older person and family about stress theory and the stress cycle.

- Helping the older person identify successful coping mechanisms used in the past during periods of high stress.
- Assisting the older person to examine current coping mechanisms and behaviors and to alter or eliminate negative or maladaptive mechanisms.
- Reinforcing and strengthening positive coping mechanisms.
- Investigating community resources, support groups, stress-reduction clinics, and other stress relievers that may be useful to the older person.

Alternative therapies to relieve stress may be used in conjunction with traditional treatment approaches and counseling. Alternative therapies include biofeedback, massage therapy, progressive muscle relaxation techniques, audiotapes, exercise, and use of calming music.

DEPRESSION

Symptoms of depression may be emotional and physical. Emotional symptoms include sadness, diminished ability to experience joy in life, inability to concentrate, recurrent thoughts of death, and excessive guilt over things that happened in the past. Physical symptoms can include body aches, headaches, pain, fatigue, change in sleep habits, and weight gain or loss. The major clues to depression in the older person include multiple somatic complaints and reports of persistent chronic pain.

The criteria for diagnosis of a major depression as manifested by the *Diagnostic and Statistical Manual of Mental Disorders IV TR* (American Psychiatric Association, 2000) include the following:

- Depressed mood or loss of interest or pleasure
- Duration of symptoms for at least 2 consecutive weeks that represent a change from previous functioning

- At least five of the following (**SIG E CAPS**):
  1. Depressed mood
  2. (**S for Sleep**) Insomnia or hypersomnia (excessive sleepiness)
  3. (**I for Interest**) Diminished interest or pleasure
  4. (**G for Guilt**) Feelings of guilt or worthlessness
  5. (**E for Energy**) Energy loss or fatigue
  6. (**C for Concentration**) Lack of ability to concentrate
  7. (**A for Appetite**) Appetite or weight change (gain or loss)
  8. (**P for Psychomotor**) Psychomotor retardation or agitation
  9. (**S for Suicide**) Suicidal thoughts or attempts, or recurrent thoughts of or desire for death with or without a plan

Women experience depression about twice as often as men (Blehar & Oren, 1997). Men are less likely to admit to depression, and doctors are less likely to suspect it.

Medications such as analgesics, antihypertensives, antipsychotics, anxiolytics, sedative-hypnotics, corticosteroids, and antiulcer medications can cause symptoms of depression in the older person.

Nursing Assessment of Depression

The Geriatric Depression Scale (GDS) is a screening instrument used in many clinical settings to assess depression in older people. The GDS is a 30-item (long version) or 15-item (short version) instrument with questions that can be answered yes or no. Please refer to pages 11–14 in Chapter 1 for the GDS.

Suicide

Older persons age 65 and over have the highest suicide rates of all age groups (Bille-Brahe & Andersen, 2001). A major risk factor for suicide is depression.

Risk factors for suicide that may be determined from the past health history include previous suicide attempt, alcohol or substance abuse, presence of a psychiatric illness, history of a psychiatric illness, presence of auditory hallucinations (hearing voices commanding action), and living alone (Jenike, 1999). Once the suicide intent is verbalized, the means to carry out the plan should be assessed. Older patients who have the means to carry out a suicide attempt should be immediately referred for evaluation. Those perceived to be at risk for suicide will probably be hospitalized for a short period to protect their lives and provide for intensive observation and treatment.

Patients hospitalized with suicidal ideation will be placed on "suicide precautions" that include one-to-one monitoring by an observer, locked window, and removal of items that have potential for self-harm such as belts, sharp knives, medications, and so on. Therapy and treatment of the underlying depression will most often improve the older patient's situation.

Alcohol Abuse

Problems related to excessive or regular alcohol consumption include:

- *Malnutrition.* Failure to prepare and eat an adequate diet.
- *Cirrhosis of the liver.* One of eight leading causes of death for the older person.
- *Osteomalacia.* Thinning of the bones.

- *Decreases in gastric absorption.* Failure to absorb key minerals and vitamins from ingested food.
- *Decline in cognitive function.* Impairment of memory and information processing.
- *Interactions with medications.* Interaction with benzodiazepines greatly increases risk of falls and hip fractures.

(American Psychological Association, 2003; Scott & Popovich, 2001)

The *DSM-IV-TR* criteria for possible **alcohol dependence** include three or more of the following:

- Tolerance (requiring more alcohol to get effect)
- Withdrawal or drinking to ease withdrawal
- Drinking in larger quantities or for longer periods of time than expected
- Persistent desire to drink or unsuccessful efforts to control drinking
- Spending a lot of time obtaining or using alcohol, or recovering from effects
- Giving up important social or recreational activities to pursue drinking
- Drinking despite persistent or recurrent physical or psychological problems caused by alcohol

The *DSM-IV-TR* criteria for possible **alcohol abuse** include one or more of the following:

- Drinking resulting in the failure to fulfill major obligations
- Drinking in situations where it is physically hazardous
- Alcohol-related legal problems
- Continued drinking despite social problems caused or worsened by alcohol

The CAGE (acronym for Cut down, Annoyed by criticism, Guilty about drinking, Eye-opener drink) questionnaire has been validated in the older adult

(Reuben et al., 2002). One positive answer to the CAGE questionnaire suggests the older person is a problem drinker. Additional questions that may provide valuable information to supplement the CAGE include:

- How many days do you drink per week?
- How many drinks do you have per day?
- What is the maximum number of drinks you have per day?
- What type of alcohol do you drink (beer, wine, liquor)?
- What is "a drink"?

More than two drinks per day for women or three for men is considered potentially harmful, depending on the older person's tolerance, physical health, medication use, and living situation (Reuben et al., 2002). It is recommended that older persons consume no more than one drink per day after the age of 65. Red wine consumed in small to moderate amounts has been shown to decrease risk of cardiovascular disease.

Older persons who are hospitalized or institutionalized in long-term care facilities may become delirious during acute alcohol withdrawal. Acute agitation and hallucination may occur (delirium tremens). Non-pharmacological measures to protect patient safety include keeping the room as quiet as possible, avoiding excessive light and stimulation, encouraging family visitation for comfort and reassurance, providing orientation to time and place, communicating directly and succinctly, and providing frequent observation and monitoring of vital signs. Usually the physician will prescribe lorazepam (Ativan) 0.5 to 2.0 mg every 4 to 6 hours to prevent alcohol withdrawal seizures. Adequate hydration and nutrition will ease the withdrawal process (Reuben et al., 2002).

Basic Principles Relating to Psychological Assessment in Older Adults

Psychological testing should be done under the following circumstances:

- When considering admission to a geropsychiatric inpatient unit
- When considering need for and benefit of outpatient geropsychiatric services
- To assist in the diagnosis of dementia versus depression
- To provide information for the legal determination of competency
- When evaluating sudden or severe changes in mood, personality, or psychological function
- To evaluate and monitor response to therapy or psychotropic medication

Observe the older patient carefully. If the patient becomes tired and has difficulty concentrating, take a break and resume testing at another time.

If English is the second language for the older patient, request assistance from a translator rather than asking a family member to translate. The translator has been trained in the precise use of medical terminology.

Older patients should also be asked about obsessions (recurrent, unwanted ideas that cannot be resisted, although they may seem unreasonable) and compulsions (repeated, unwanted behaviors such as hand washing or rechecking a locked door). Compulsions can be elicited by asking, "Must you do certain things (e.g., wash your hands) repeatedly, more than you need to?"

If underlying health problems are influencing psychological function, a referral to an internist for complete assessment of health problems includes a head-to-toe physical examination and a variety of laboratory tests, including a complete blood count (CBC), a chemistry panel (SMA-18), test of thyroid function (TSH), and assessment of serum levels of medications taken on a regular basis (digoxin, warfarin, etc.) is needed.

CULTURAL CONSIDERATIONS

The unique life experiences, values, and beliefs of these minority elders may be very different from those of the larger cohort of older adults.

- The onset of chronic illness is usually earlier than in Caucasian older adults.
- There are frequent delays in seeking health treatment.
- Health problems may be underreported because of lack of trust in healthcare workers.
- Mental health services are underutilized.
- There are higher rates of treatment dropout and medical noncompliance.
- Although longevity for African American men is shorter than that for White men, African American men and women surviving to the age of 75 live longer than Caucasians.
- There is a higher incidence of obesity and type 2 diabetes mellitus.
- A large number of minority elders possess no health insurance.

NURSING INTERVENTIONS
Non-Pharmacological Treatments

Both individual and group psychotherapy, family and couples therapy, self-help groups, educational sessions, reminiscence therapy and behavior modification have all been shown to be effective in treating the older adult's psychological problems. Additional helpful interventions include travel with senior citizens' groups, taking classes at the local college, elder hostels, volunteer work, regular exercise, hobbies and crafts, and increased family involvement. Light therapy has been shown to be effective for older patients diagnosed with **seasonal affective disorder**, a cyclic depression that occurs when hours of daylight are short, usually in the fall and early spring. Older persons with substance abuse problems (drug or alcohol) may attend Alcoholics Anonymous meetings.

Pharmacological Treatments

As many of the antidepressants take 6 to 12 weeks to achieve therapeutic effects and ease depression, the older person and the family should be patient and realistic in their expectations regarding antidepressant therapy. The duration of therapy should be at least 6 to 12 months following remission for older patients experiencing their first depressive episode. Most older patients with a history of major depression require lifelong antidepressant therapy (Reuben et al., 2002). The initial dose should be about one half the usual adult dose, and careful monitoring is needed during the first few days of treatment so that any adverse side effects can be quickly noted. Falls, sedation, urinary retention, constipation, drowsiness, visual changes, appetite changes, tachycardia, and photosensitivity have all been reported as side effects of antidepressants and may pose a significant health and safety risk for older adults. Older patients taking warfarin should be closely monitored during the first few weeks of the initiation of antidepressant therapy. Older patients should be strongly urged to avoid alcohol while taking antidepressant medications.

Because many of the tricyclic antidepressants (TCAs) are associated with anticholinergic side effects such as constipation, urinary retention, dry mouth, hypotension, and tachycardia, some geriatricians prefer to use the selective serotonin reuptake inhibitors (SSRIs) as first-line drugs for many older patients, especially those with the following conditions:

- Heart conduction defects or ischemic heart disease
- Benign prostatic hypertrophy
- Difficult-to-control glaucoma

In general the SSRIs are well tolerated in the older person. Side effects include nausea, diarrhea, headache, erectile dysfunction, insomnia, or somnolence.

Additional drugs sometimes used to treat depression in the older person include bupropion (Wellbutrin). This drug may lower seizure threshold and is contraindicated in older patients with seizure disorders. It is usually started at 37.5 mg bid and titrated to 75 to 100 mg bid. Methylphenidate (Ritalin), a stimulant, has been used in some older people who exhibit marked psychomotor retardation and apathy. It is recommended only for short-term use with careful monitoring of cardiovascular side effects. It is usually dosed at 5 to 10 mg once or twice a day (Jenike, 1999).

Lithium carbonate has been used to treat recurrent bipolar illness. Side effects include bradycardia, hypothyroidism, tinnitus, tremor, ataxia, nystagmus, mental status changes, and seizures (Jenike, 1999). This drug must be used with caution, and blood levels and patient function must be carefully monitored during the initial dosing period.

Monoamine oxidase inhibitors (MAOIs) are sometimes used in older people with dementia and depression and in those who have not responded to other drug therapies. Because these drugs inhibit the metabolism of norepinephrine, hypertensive crisis can occur if they are administered with other drugs or food that raise blood pressure such as anticholinergics, stimulants, and foods containing tyramine (red wine, cheese, etc.).

Electroconvulsive therapy (ECT) is indicated in older patients who do not respond to other antidepressant medications, are diagnosed with delusional depression, or have life-threatening behaviors (suicidal ideation, catatonic, etc.).

PATIENT-FAMILY TEACHING GUIDELINES

Many older people think it is normal to have a variety of physical and mental problems. However, mental health problems, including depression and anxiety, are not part of the normal aging process. If you, a family member, or friend experience a sudden change in mood, the way you think, or your memory, see your healthcare professional as soon as possible.

1. What causes mental health problems?

   Some mild memory or mood problems can occur in healthy older adults, but serious problems can be a sign of underlying mental health disease.

2. What tests are needed to tell if I have a serious mental health problem?

   Your healthcare provider will probably conduct a complete physical examination, ask about your daily function, survey your medications (prescription and over the counter), and obtain some laboratory tests to make sure you are not anemic, to make sure you have adequate levels of B_{12} and folate, or to determine if you are having trouble with your thyroid. Your healthcare provider will also ask a lot of questions about your mood and memory. Sometimes a CT scan of the brain or other tests such as MRI are necessary to detect the source of mental health problems. If further information is needed, you may be referred to a neuropsychologist for more in-depth testing that can give more detailed information about your memory and mood. The results of this test can help your healthcare provider decide if additional testing is needed to diagnose your mental health.

3. How do I know if I have depression?

If you experience feelings of sadness, fatigue, lack of enjoyment of life, sleep problems, feelings of being helpless and hopeless, loss of interest in sex, or difficulty concentrating and making decisions, you may be depressed. Some older people say that they just do not feel like their old self. Others gain or lose weight because they change the way they eat. Others may avoid going out to social events and prefer to stay home alone. Everyone is different, so it is important to think broadly and look for a variety of symptoms.

4. Is suicide a problem with older people?

Yes, some groups of older people (especially older White men) have high suicide rates. If you have persistent thoughts of death or harming yourself or others, seek help immediately. There are mental health professionals who are available to protect your life and help you return to mental health. Do not risk ending your life prematurely.

5. Is treatment available and effective for older people with mental health problems?

(continued)

Yes, there are a variety of pharmacological and non-pharmacological methods to treat mental health problems. The newer antidepressants have fewer side effects and are just as effective in treating depression in older people as they are in treating middle-aged and younger people, so do not be afraid to try them if your doctor thinks it will help you. Mental health professionals such as social workers, psychologists, psychiatrists, and psychiatric–mental health nurses can also provide counseling to help you identify the source of and appropriate intervention for your mental health problems. Non-pharmacological ways to ease depression include exercise, increased social activity, alcohol avoidance, light therapy, and a variety of other methods unique to each older person.

CHAPTER 6

SLEEP AND THE OLDER ADULT

Sleep complaints are common among older people, and the incidence of sleep problems increases with age. Older adults experience age-related changes in the nature of their sleep, including greater difficulty falling asleep, more frequent awakenings, decreased amounts of nighttime sleep, and more frequent daytime napping. Sleep disturbances can exacerbate behavioral problems in older persons with Alzheimer's disease and other cognitive impairments.

Defining characteristics according to the North American Nursing Diagnosis Association (NANDA, 2001) criteria include the following:

- Complaints of difficulty falling asleep (sleep latency greater than 30 minutes)
- Awakening too early in the morning
- Three or more nighttime awakenings
- Changes in behavior and function, including lethargy, listlessness, and irritability
- Decreased ability to function
- Dissatisfaction with sleep and not feeling well rested

Presence of related factors including:

- Physical discomfort/pain
- Psychological discomfort
- **Sleep hygiene** problems
- Environmental factors

Sleep problems can be classified as transient (short term), intermittent (on and off), and chronic (constant). Transient sleep problems may be caused by short-term health problems, stress, worry related to a situational event like a move to a new residence, or changes in sleep schedules such as those due to travel and jet lag. Intermittent sleep problems may be related to exacerbations of chronic illness or recurrent anxiety. **Insomnia** is chronic if it occurs on most nights and lasts a month or more (National Institutes of Health, 2000).

NORMAL SLEEP AND AGING

The amount of time spent in deeper levels of sleep diminishes with aging. There is an associated increase in awakenings during sleep and an increase in the total time spent in bed trying to sleep as sleep becomes less efficient.

Abnormal sleep behaviors are a category of events that can occur at any time throughout the life cycle but become more common with advancing age. According to Merritt (2000), this category includes the following:

- Myoclonus or sudden contractions of muscles and tingling feelings in the legs, also called "restless leg syndrome"
- Sleepwalking or sleep terrors
- Sleep-related epileptic seizures

This group of abnormal sleep behaviors requires evaluation from neurologists or sleep specialists and is usually treated with medications such as antianxiety agents, benzodiazepines, and dopamine agonists (Merritt, 2000).

Most older adults require 6 to 10 hours of sleep nightly. Less than 4 or more than 9 hours of sleep is associated with higher mortality rates than those sleeping 8 hours (Chesson, 2000).

Older persons may nap more often during the day, thus further disrupting normal circadian patterns. While one or two "cat naps" (naps under 50 minutes) a day were found not to disrupt the nighttime sleep of older people, more frequent daytime napping can be disruptive (Floyd, 1999).

Various health problems and the medications used to treat them are associated with sleep disruption in older persons. Pulmonary disease, heart disease, arthritis, dementia associated with Alzheimer's disease, and depression may cause sleep disruption. Diseases of the cardiac and respiratory system are often associated with orthopnea and shortness of breath. Persons with congestive heart failure are often asked "the pillow question" as an indicator of the stability and progression of their disease. Physical discomfort or pain can be a major deterrent for sleep. Acutely ill hospitalized patients may experience pain from surgical incisions, pain from the trauma or injury that was the cause of the hospitalization, or discomfort from intravenous tubing, indwelling urinary catheters, or other instrumentation.

SLEEP DISRUPTION

Sleep disruption is common in older persons with psychosocial problems. Life stresses when combined with predisposing emotional factors such as depression and anxiety may be related to the onset of sleep problems (Jao & Alessi, 2004).

Dementia

Older persons with dementia endure even more sleep disruptions than other older persons. Sleep disruptions common in dementia such as those with Alzheimer's disease include breakdown of the normal sleep-wake cycle with short periods of fragmented sleep occurring throughout a 24-hour period (Jao & Alessi, 2004). Sleep disturbances in older persons with dementia cause caregiver stress, increase the potential for nursing home placement, and cause serious problems for those providing care in the nursing home or home environment. These behaviors may contribute to caregivers' complaints about their own disrupted sleep, daytime sleepiness, and fatigue (Riccio, Knight, & Cody, 1999). In an attempt to promote more normal sleep patterns in those with dementia, psychotropic medications may be administered. These medications are usually indicated for short-term use only. Typical side effects of hypnotic drugs include falls, swallowing difficulties, constipation, dizziness, and daytime sleepiness (Tabloski, Cooke, & Thoman, 1998).

Snoring

Many older people consider snoring a minor annoyance, but it can signal a potentially serious condition known as **sleep apnea,** or temporary interruption of breathing during sleep. For those affected by sleep apnea, there can be many temporary interruptions in breathing, each lasting about 10 seconds throughout the sleep period. These interruptions in breathing can occur as often as 20 to 30 times per hour (Pace, Lynn, & Glass 2001). Symptoms of sleep apnea include the following:

- Heavy snoring, usually on inspiration
- Choking sounds or struggling to breathe during sleep
- Delays in breathing during sleep (usually with a reduction in blood-oxygen saturation), followed by a snort when breathing begins
- Excessive daytime sleepiness
- Morning headaches
- Difficulty with concentration and staying awake during driving or other tasks

Sleep Apnea

Sleep apnea can be caused by problems with the central nervous system and the brain or may be caused by partial obstruction of the airway when the muscles in the throat, soft palate, and tongue relax during sleep (Pace et al., 2001). Risk factors for sleep apnea include obesity (body mass index > 30), hypertension, and anatomical abnormality to the upper respiratory tract. If sleep apnea is suspected, the older person should be referred to a sleep center for an overnight sleep study using polysomnography, a specialized method of sleep testing that measures brain and body activity during sleep.

Treatment for sleep apnea may begin with simple interventions designed to keep the airway open such as weight reduction for the obese, encouraging sleep on the side rather than the back by wearing a tennis ball in a pocket sewn on the back of a nightshirt, avoiding sleeping pills and alcohol before sleeping, and avoiding smoking (Pace et al., 2001). For those with anatomical abnormalities of the upper airway, surgery may be required to restore normal structure and function. The surgery, known as uvulopalatopharyngoplasty, is usually performed to the pharyngeal walls or the base of the tongue to enlarge the pharyngeal air space (Merritt, 2000). However, the most common medical treatment for sleep apnea is continuous positive airway pressure (CPAP). CPAP is a noninvasive treatment administered through a nasal mask. The pressure keeps the airway open, preventing its collapse and allowing the patient to breathe more normally. Usually, between 5 and 20 cm of CPAP is needed to prevent apnea and maintain adequate oxygen saturation (Merritt, 2000).

Older persons with untreated sleep apnea should not use alcohol or sedative-hypnotic medications because of their potential to increase the severity of apneic episodes.

Urinary Problems

Older persons may be awakened from sleep because of the need to urinate. Common age-related alterations in urinary tract function include urinary frequency, nocturia, and incontinence (Miller, 2000). Older men may suffer from benign prostatic hypertrophy, which inhibits complete emptying of the bladder and may be associated with the sensation of always feeling the urge to void. Check a postvoid residual by inserting a urinary catheter immediately after the patient voids to ascertain the amount of urine that is retained in the bladder. Older men who retain more than 50 cc of urine should be referred to a urologist for urological evaluation or cystoscopy and cystometric studies.

Sleep Problems in Hospitals and Nursing Homes

When older persons are institutionalized in the hospital or nursing home, sleep problems are common and the environment may be part of the problem. Waking a patient from deep sleep to provide routine care can result in sleep deprivation, which can delay healing and recovery.

Alcohol and Caffeine

Although many older persons use alcohol to promote sleep, alcohol is a potent disrupter of REM sleep due to its sedative effect on the central nervous system (Brown, 1999). Additionally, caffeine and nicotine can affect the older adult's ability to initiate and maintain sleep. Nicotine extends the time it takes to fall asleep and reduces total sleep time and REM sleep (Brown, 1999). Both caffeine and nicotine increase the number of nighttime awakenings and the length of time it takes to fall back to sleep. Because alcohol, caffeine, and nicotine are typically used in conjunction with one another, the sedating and arousal effects frequently interact, creating multiple sleep disturbances.

Sleeping Medications

Prescription drugs have also been shown to affect sleep. It is generally agreed that long-term administration of hypnotics is an inadequate treatment strategy for chronic insomnia in the older adult (Cheng, Umland, & Muirhead, 2000). Hypnotic medications are generally recommended for short-term use: about 2 weeks or less. Long-term use will blunt the effect of these medications. For those with long half-lives, steady states or relatively high constant blood levels will occur, which can cause excessive daytime sleepiness. These effects can exacerbate an older person's risk of fall and injury.

Drugs used to treat mood disorders such as depression can also affect sleep. Some drugs are sedatives and should be given in the evening, whereas others are stimulants and are best taken in the morning. Sedating antidepressants best taken in the evening include the following:

- Amitriptyline (Elavil)
- Doxepin (Sinequan)
- Nortriptyline (Pamelor)

Stimulating antidepressants best taken in the morning include the following:

- Desipramine (Norpramin)
- Sertraline hydrochloride (Zoloft)
- Paroxetine hydrochloride (Paxil)

Benzodiazepines, even those with short half-lives like lorazepam (Ativan), should be used with caution in older persons. They can exacerbate sleep apnea, suppress deep sleep, increase the likelihood of falling, and cause increased confusion (Tabloski & Church, 1999).

If the medication has been used at least 5 nights a week for greater than 2 weeks, a taper and withdrawal schedule should be followed. By using a gradual withdrawal schedule (one half the dose for 1 week prior to discontinuation), the chances of inducing rebound insomnia and other withdrawal symptoms are lessened (Tabloski et al., 1998).

NURSING ASSESSMENT

The components of a sleep assessment should include a health history, a physical examination, daily sleep diaries, and polysomnography testing if sleep apnea is suspected. Key assessment areas are as follows:

Health History

- Diagnosed acute or chronic illness
- Current medications (including OTC)
- Chronic pain or pruritus
- Psychological problems
- Change in living conditions or sleep routines
- Current stressors or worries
- Nicotine, alcohol, or caffeine use
- Last complete medical examination

NURSING INTERVENTIONS

Sleep hygiene should be encouraged in any older person with a sleep problem. Inadequate sleep hygiene refers to daily activities that interfere with the maintenance of good quality sleep and daytime alertness. Sleep hygiene measures such as limiting time spent in bed to 8 hours a night, avoiding daytime napping, and using the bed only for sleep and sex have been found to be an effective intervention (Beck-Little & Weinrich, 1998).

Additional Non-Pharmacological Measures

Sleep restriction therapy is based on the theory that many older persons with sleep problems spend too much time in bed trying to get 8 hours of satisfactory sleep. After the nurse and the older person have identified an appropriate goal, a schedule is established for time to bed and time to arise. Gradually, older persons will increase their sleep efficiency as their bodies learn to become more sleep efficient. Additional rules to be followed in sleep restriction therapy include:

- Use the bed only to sleep. No reading, TV watching, or eating in bed is allowed. Sexual activity is the only exception to this rule.
- If you are unable to sleep, get up and go to another room. The goal is to learn to associate the bed with restful sleep.
- Get up at the same time every day, regardless of the amount or quality of sleep obtained the night before.
- Do not nap during the day.

Older persons who vigorously adhere to the provisions of sleep restriction therapy may find improved quality and quantity of sleep.

Cognitive therapy focuses on changing the older person's expectations about sleep. **Bedtime rituals** such as progressive relaxation exercises, nature tapes, praying, reading a few pages of a novel, or other relaxing activities may assist the older person who is anxious at bedtime to sleep. Once a satisfactory nighttime ritual is established, it should be maintained to ease the transition from wakefulness to sleep.

Unfortunately, the non-pharmacological interventions mentioned above are not appropriate for the older person with dementia. The following recommendations are made to nurses working in long-term care facilities (Schnelle, Alessi, Al-Samarrai, Fricker, & Ouslander, 1999):

- Establish consistent nighttime routines, which signal to both staff and residents that sleep is to be facilitated.
- Reduce noise and light disruption throughout the night.
- Turn down televisions and radios and ringers on phones.
- Avoid using intercoms and beepers during sleep hours.
- Turn night-lights on at the hour of sleep and turn off overhead lights.
- Keep residents busy and occupied during the daytime with exercise and recreational programs so that long naps are avoided.
- Do not put residents to bed immediately after supper. Try to provide restful evening activities like music or group readings so that gastrointestinal problems such as gastroesophageal reflux disease are avoided.
- If residents are awake and noisy during the night, assist them from bed to a lounge or recreation area where they will not disturb other residents. When they become sleepy, they can return to their beds.

Pharmacological Treatments for Altered Sleep Patterns

Studies have shown that most benzodiazepines are effective for promoting sleep on a short-term basis. However, the nurse should be aware of the lack of evidence that these drugs are effective for long-term use. Benzodiazepine therapy is recommended for short-term use not to exceed 2 weeks. If used long term, it is to be given in intermittent courses. Shorter acting benzodiazepines (half-life 6 hours) like lorazepam are suggested to be the better choice for elderly adults. These drugs have the best effect profile and raise the fewest safety concerns (Cheng et al., 2000).

Sedating antidepressants may also be used if the older person exhibits signs and symptoms of depression. Amitriptyline, doxepin, and nortriptyline may be used cautiously. Generally, lower doses of tricyclic antidepressants are needed for sleep disorders than are needed to treat depression, thereby lessening the risk of adverse side effects (Cheng et al., 2000).

Antihistamines such as diphenhydramine (Benadryl) should not be used because of the anticholinergic side effects and the potential to decrease respiratory drive. Barbiturates, sedatives, hypnotics, opiates, and antipsychotics should not be used for the routine treatment of sleep disorders. The use of barbiturates has fallen out of favor because of the potential for abuse, overdose, and severe withdrawal symptoms (Cheng et al., 2000). Additionally, movement disorders such as tardive dyskinesia are common with antipsychotics.

Many older persons also use herbal or natural remedies. Melatonin is a hormone produced in the pineal gland and plays a role in the regulation of sleep. Doses of 0.5 to 3 mg have been suggested for sleep (Huebscher, 1999). It should be taken approximately 2 hours before bedtime. Melatonin has been found to significantly improve sleep in older persons with insomnia and can even help older persons who are "benzodiazepine addicted" withdraw from these drugs. Because melatonin has a short half-life (about 40 minutes), a controlled-release formulation is recommended to maintain sleep throughout the entire sleep cycle (Garfinkle, Zisapel, Wainstein, & Laudon, 1999). Additional natural remedies include herbal chamomile tea (if no allergies to ragweed or daisies), hops, lemon balm, and valerian (Huebscher, 1999). Valerian root has been used in Europe for the past several years, and a dose of 400 to 450 mg of the extract will shorten sleep latency similar to a short-acting benzodiazepine (Brown, 1999).

PATIENT-FAMILY TEACHING GUIDELINES

1. What is insomnia or disordered sleep?

   These disorders are characterized by the perception or complaint of inadequate or poor quality sleep because of:
   - Difficulty falling asleep (longer than 20 minutes is considered a problem).
   - Waking up often during the night and being unable to fall quickly back to sleep.
   - Waking up too early in the morning and staying awake.
   - Waking up in the morning without feeling refreshed.

2. What causes sleep problems?

   Certain conditions make some older persons more likely to have sleep problems than others.

Examples of these conditions include the following:

- Age over 60
- Female gender
- History of or current diagnosis of depression
- Certain medications (diuretics or long-term use of sleep medications)
- Daytime loneliness or boredom with long naps
- Chronic illness with components of pain or difficulty breathing
- Diagnosis of Alzheimer's disease or other neurological problems
- Situational events like moving to a new home or loss of a loved one

3. What seems to make sleep problems worse?

The following behaviors seem to perpetuate sleep problems and make them more likely to become chronic:

- Worry about sleep and expecting to have problems every night
- Drinking too much caffeine
- Drinking alcohol before bedtime
- Smoking cigarettes before bedtime
- Sleeping longer than 50 minutes during the day
- Being told by a sleep partner that you are snoring and gasping during sleep
- Not seeking medical attention for pain, urinary problems, nighttime gastroesophageal reflux disease, or tingling sensation in the legs

4. Where should the older person go for evaluation and treatment?

An older person who does not have a current healthcare provider should seek evaluation from a primary care physician, geriatrician, or

(continued)

gerontological nurse practitioner. Underlying acute and chronic health problems should always be investigated and ruled out or treated optimally. These providers can then make referrals for polysomnography and sleep laboratory testing if appropriate. It is helpful to keep a sleep diary for a week or so before the medical appointment because this valuable information will encourage better decision making by the healthcare provider.

5. How are sleep problems treated?

Some sleep problems are transient and intermittent and will resolve spontaneously. For instance, jet lag may last only a few days. Pain from a fractured bone may resolve within a week or 10 days. The strangeness of moving to a new home may resolve within a few weeks. For long-term sleep problems, the treatment will depend on the cause. A thorough assessment of sleep problems will guide the competent clinician toward appropriate treatment.

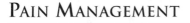

CHAPTER 7

PAIN MANAGEMENT

Pain is a common negative sensation experienced by all human beings during the process of living. Although acute pain can be protective, chronic pain can become an intolerable burden (Thomas, Flaherty & Morley, 2001).

There is increased emphasis on the assessment and treatment of pain, and patients and their families are becoming more aware of the need to treat both acute and chronic pain. Barriers to effective **pain management** include lack of knowledge of the care providers, persistent misperceptions regarding addiction to pain medication, and state and federal regulation of the prescribing of opioid analgesics (American Pain Society Quality of Care Committee, 1995). Further, many older people and their families believe that pain is a normal part of aging and fear that complaining is a sign of weakness.

THE ART AND SCIENCE OF PAIN RELIEF

The goal of ideal pain management is to relieve both acute and chronic pain with appropriate pharmacological and non-pharmacological techniques while minimizing side effects. Older patients are generally more sensitive to opioid analgesics, and most often these patients are started on smaller doses to avoid toxicity. The dose is then titrated upward until effective pain relief is achieved without adverse effects. The titration process may take several days or even longer, especially when drugs with longer half-lives are used.

Greater reductions in pain are seen when pharmacological and non-pharmacological techniques are combined (AGS, 2002). The nurse should assess the older patient's beliefs and willingness to use relaxation techniques, heating pads or cold compresses, biofeedback, music, therapeutic touch, or other methods to enhance or replace analgesic drugs.

Dying patients have special pain and symptom control needs that mandate respectful and responsive care. Concern for the patient's comfort and dignity should guide all aspects of care during the final stages of life. The Joint Commission on Accreditation of Healthcare Organizations (JCAHO, 2003) has proposed the following standards for healthcare organizations providing end-of-life care:

- Providing appropriate treatment for any primary and secondary symptom, according to the wishes of the patient or the surrogate decision maker
- Managing pain aggressively and effectively
- Sensitively addressing issues such as autopsy and organ donation
- Respecting the patient's values, religion, and philosophy
- Involving the patient and, where appropriate, the family in every aspect of care
- Responding to the psychological, social, emotional, spiritual, and cultural concerns of the patient and the family

PHARMACOLOGICAL MANAGEMENT

In most cases, it makes sense to progress from non-opioid analgesics such as acetaminophen to anti-inflammatory drugs, neurotransmitter-modulating and membrane-stabilizing drugs, and opioids to balance the risk and benefits of treating more severe pain (AGS, 2002). Table 7–1 provides information on pharmacotherapeutic agents that may be used to treat chronic pain in elderly patients.

Adjuvant Drugs for Older Patients with Pain

Adjuvant drugs (antidepressants and anticonvulsants) are not typically considered pain medicines, but they may relieve discomfort and potentiate the effect of pain medications to reduce the side effect burden. Examples of adjuvant drugs that nurses may see used in the clinical setting include:

1. *Antidepressants and Anticonvulsants (tricyclics, selective serotonin reuptake inhibitors, carbamazepine, gabapentin)*—helpful for diabetic neuropathy, trigeminal neuralgia, and postherpetic neuralgia.

2. *Topical Analgesics (capsaicin, menthol methylsalicylate, EMLA cream, lidocaine gel)* —helpful for chronic arthritis pain, herpes zoster, and diabetic neuropathy; may be used in anticipation of painful procedures such as venipuncture for blood draws, IV insertion, and so on.

3. *Muscle Relaxants (baclofen, diazepam, carisoprodol)*—helpful when there is significant muscle spasm component to pain; to be used in addition to, not in place of analgesic medications.

4. *Antianxiety Medications (diazepam, doxepin, oxazepam)*—helpful when patient is anxious or agitated.

5. *Medications to Dry Secretions (scopolamine, glycopyrrolate)*—helpful when patient has thick secretions that require frequent suctioning.

Table 7-1 Pharmacotherapeutic Agents and Dosing Suggestions For Management of Persistent Pain in the Older Person

Drug	Starting Doses	Titration	Comments
Non-Opioids			
Acetaminophen	325 mg q4h	After 4–6 doses	Maximum dose 4 g/24 hr. Reduce dose with hepatic disease or history of alcohol abuse.
Ibuprofen	400–600 mg q6h	After 2–3days	Take with food to reduce risk of GI distress.
Corticosteroids	5 mg qd	After 2–3 doses	Use lowest possible dose to avoid chronic steroid side effects.
Tricyclic antidepressants	10 mg hs	After 3–5 days	Significant risk of anticholinergic side effects.
Anticonvulsants			
Carbamazepine	100 mg qd	After 3–5 days	Monitor LFTs, CBC, BUN/creatinine, electrolytes.
Gabapentin	100 mg hs	After 1–2 days	Monitor sedation, ataxia, edema.

Opioids

Morphine sulfate	10–20 mg q4h	After 1 day	Start low and titrate to comfort. Anticipate and treat side effects.
Oxycodone Hydrocodone	5–10 mg q4h	After 1–2 days	Start low and titrate to comfort. Anticipate and treat side effects.
Hydromorphone	1.5 mg q4h	After 1–2 days	Start low and titrate to comfort. Anticipate and treat side effects.
Transdermal fentanyl	25 µg q72h	After 3 days	Apply to clean, dry skin. Peak effects of first dose take 24 hr, so cover with oral meds the first day of application.

6. *Antipruritics (diphenhydramine, hydroxyzine)*—helpful when patient has pruritus secondary to liver disease or other conditions that are itchy and result in scratching.
7. *Diuretics (furosemide, hydrochlorothiazide)*—helpful to ease discomfort from ascites from liver cancer or cirrhosis.
8. *Magic Mouthwash (diphenhydramine elixir/Maalox/viscous lidocaine)*—helpful when patient has mucositis secondary to chemotherapy. Add nystatin if there is evidence of thrush (Thomas et al., 2001; Woods-Smith, Arnstein, Rosa, & Wells-Federman, 2002).

Special Pharmacological Issues Regarding Pain Management in the Older Person

It is becoming more acceptable for physicians and others to manage persistent noncancer pain with the use of opioid analgesics (AGS, 2002). Although true addiction (drug craving to achieve euphoria) to opioid medication in elderly patients is rare, physical dependency is an inevitable consequence over time, especially when patients experience relief from chronic, debilitating pain. Studies indicate that **tolerance** (the need for more drug to get the same therapeutic effect) is slow to develop in the face of stable disease (AGS, 2002).

When mixed drugs containing opioids and acetaminophen or aspirin are used to control pain (acetaminophen with codeine, Oxycodone with aspirin, aspirin with codeine), the nurse should be aware that doses are limited by the toxic effect that can occur as a result of high salicylate or acetaminophen levels. Acetaminophen is hepatotoxic above 4 g/day, and aspirin can cause gastric bleeding and abnormal platelet function at doses above 4 g/day. Special caution is advised in older patients with decreased renal and hepatic function and those currently using alcohol or possessing a history of alcohol abuse.

Propoxyphene is not recommended for treatment of persistent pain in the older person (AGS, 2002). Because of the added burden of serious side effects caused by the accumulation of toxic metabolites. These metabolites can cause delirium, ataxia, and dizziness. Other drugs are suggested for the treatment of persistent pain in the older person.

Pharmacological Principles for Successful Pain Management

Pain medication given by mouth is the preferred way to control pain in the older person. Even patients who cannot swallow can be given concentrated liquid morphine drops by the sublingual or buccal route. It is the safest, least expensive, and easiest route.

Pain medication works best when it is administered around the clock. The nurse should be familiar with the duration of action of analgesics and give the medication routinely to prevent the return of pain. Patients avoid the needless suffering and mental anguish that can occur when medication is given on a prn (as needed) basis. The use of long-acting once-daily medications can control chronic pain very effectively, and immediate-release, short-acting preparations (Roxanol) can be used for breakthrough pain or pain associated with activity or procedures.

If the patient experiences breakthrough pain on a consistent basis, the nurse should notify the physician so that the dose of the long-acting, sustained-release preparation can be increased to more effectively control the pain. The dose may be increased by up to 25%.

NON-PHARMACOLOGICAL METHODS TO MANAGE PAIN IN THE OLDER PERSON

Non-pharmacological methods to control pain can be effective as stand-alone treatments and adjuncts to pharmacological interventions with the potential to lessen dosages of medications and thus reduce the odds of adverse drug reactions. Non-pharmacological methods of pain control include pain education programs, socialization or recreation programs (movies, art therapy, therapeutic use of music), behavior modification (imagery, hypnosis, relaxation), physical therapy (massage, ultrasound, exercise, hot and cold packs), and neurostimulation (acupuncture, transcutaneous nerve stimulation) (Thomas et al., 2001).

CONSEQUENCES OF UNRELIEVED PAIN

Depression, anxiety, decreased socialization, sleep disturbance, impaired ambulation, and increased healthcare costs have all been found to be associated with the presence of pain in older people (AGS, 2002).

Be alert for patients who report that their pain level is tolerable and that it only hurts when they move. Effective pain relief should be provided to encourage movement and participation in rehabilitation activities.

An expert JCAHO (2003) panel developed the Seven Commandments of Pain Management including:

I. Recognize the right of patients to appropriate pain assessment and management. Pain is the fifth vital sign
II. Assess the existence, nature, and intensity of pain
III. Record the results of the assessment in a way that facilitates regular reassessment and follow-up

IV. Determine and assure staff competency in pain assessment and management and orient all new staff to techniques

V. Establish the policies and procedures that support the appropriate prescription or ordering of effective pain medication

VI. Educate patients and their families about effective pain management

VII. Address patient needs for symptom management in the discharge planning process

Acute Pain in Elderly Adults

Acute pain is pain occurring from a time-limited illness, a recent event such as surgery, medical procedures, or trauma (Agency for Health Care Policy and Research, 1995).

Ideally, the nurse should conduct a baseline patient assessment prior to a known painful event such as surgery, an invasive medical procedure, or a planned rehabilitation event such as postoperative physical therapy. This baseline assessment will allow the nurse to (1) investigate pain terminology typically used by the patient and the patient's attitudes toward pain medication and pain relief techniques, (2) identify sociocultural variables that may influence pain behaviors and expression, (3) obtain a health history that can identify accompanying chronic conditions that could contribute to the anticipated pain experience, (4) investigate past methods of pain relief, (5) identify pain medications used effectively in the past and any medication allergies and intolerance, and (6) select an appropriate pain scale and measurement technique for later use (Titler & Mentes, 1999).

If the patient is unable to communicate effectively because of language differences, cognitive impairment, or expressive aphasia after a stroke, the nurse may wish to obtain information from a family member or significant other about the baseline function and pain level of the patient. Observe the patient carefully during the baseline period and document the information in the patient care plan. Important indicators are baseline vital signs; ability to walk, stand, or move about in bed; baseline agitation level; appetite and eating pattern; sleep patterns; elimination habits; and cognitive function and mood. Postoperative or postprocedure assessments can then focus on noting and treating changes from baseline and the identification of new behaviors that may be pain-related such as grimacing, moaning, guarded movements, and bracing.

Emergency relief of pain may best be provided by administration of analgesics by the intravenous or intramuscular route. Slowed intramuscular absorption of analgesics in older patients may result in delayed or prolonged effect, altered analgesic serum levels, and potential toxicity with repeated injections.

The use of patient-controlled analgesia for intravenous analgesics may be less effective in elderly patients, especially those with cognitive impairment. The nurse should carefully monitor the patient during the immediate posttrauma or postoperative period. If acute confusion develops, it is important to assess for other contributing factors such as unrelieved pain before discontinuing analgesic medication. Bowel function and urinary output should be carefully monitored and a constipation protocol put in place to prevent fecal impaction and ileus related to narcotic analgesics (Agency for Health Care Policy and Research, 1995).

Chronic Pain in the Older Person

A comprehensive pain treatment plan is needed to treat the biopsychosocial needs of the older patient. A vicious

chronic pain cycle can occur with negative consequences, including inactivity, withdrawal from daily
life, fatigue, sleep disturbance, irritability and physical
deconditioning, and other signs of stress and depression
(Wells-Federman, 1999).

Pain Assessment Techniques

Pain is measured subjectively according to the patient's
self-report or by careful observation in the nonverbal or
severely cognitively impaired patient.

Sample pain questions include:

Pain history. (When did it start?)
Distinguishing between acute and chronic pain.
(Can you describe the pain? Is it new?)
Location. (Where is it?)
Frequency. (Do you have it every day?)
Intensity. (On a 1 to 10 scale with 10 as the worst
pain ever, please rate your pain.)
Alleviating and aggravating factors. (What
makes it better? Worse?)
Associated symptoms. (Do you have nausea,
vomiting, chills, loss of appetite, etc.?)
**Response to previous and current analgesic
therapy.** (Are you taking pain meds now? Before?
Did it work?)
Meaning of pain. (What does the pain mean to
you? Does your culture or religion influence the
way you respond to pain?)

(Wells-Federman, 1999; American Pain Society,
1999; McCaffery, & Pasero, 1999)

Additional information may be gathered by asking
the patient to complete graphic rating scales such as the
pain intensity scales illustrated in Figure 7–1.

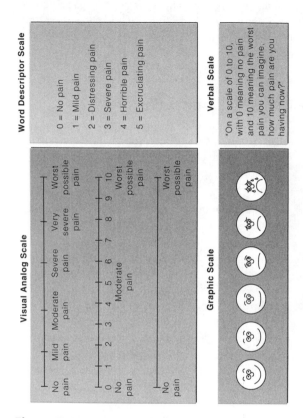

Figure 7–1 ■ Example of pain intensity scales.
Source: Adapted from AGS Panel on Chronic Pain in Older Persons, (1998). The management of chronic pain in older persons. *Journal of the American Geriatrics Society, 46,* 635–651. Used with permission.

Box 7–1 ABCDEs of Pain Assessment

*A*sk about pain regularly. Assess pain systematically.
*B*elieve the patient and family in their reports of pain
and what relieves it.
*C*hoose pain control options appropriate for the patient,
family, and setting.
*D*eliver interventions in a timely, logical, and
coordinated fashion.
*E*mpower patients and families. Enable them to control
their course to the greatest extent possible.

Source: Agency for Health Care Policy and Research, 1995.
Clinical practice guidelines, Acute pain management clinical
guide. Retrieved June 14, 2002, from *www.AHRQ.gov*.

When assessing pain in the older person, the guidelines in Box 7–1 are useful.

Analysis of the Pain Management Plan

When pain persists despite the administration of analgesics, the pain treatment plan can be analyzed to refine
the treatment and successfully manage the pain for
most individuals. The nurse may follow these steps:

1. Review the initial pain assessment. Was anything
   missed? Was any area incomplete? Where is further information needed?
2. Analyze the alignment of the intensity of pain with
   the analgesia provided. Are mild analgesics being
   prescribed for severe pain? Is the patient taking the
   medication properly? If prn medications are available, have they been appropriately administered?
3. Determine the patient's medication requirement.
   Has partial response been achieved at a certain
   dose? Have side effects occurred?

4. Provide feedback and documentation as needed to refine the plan. Are there indications that stronger medications are needed? Are dosing changes indicated? Should more effective relief of breakthrough pain be available? Are there indications that dosing intervals should be shortened?

5. Use nondrug techniques to complement the analgesic regimen. Have heat and cold packs been tried? Have patients had access to social or recreational activities?

6. Use all available resources in the clinical setting. Have pain experts, if available, been consulted? Are there other members of the interdisciplinary team who can offer insight? Are there unaddressed spiritual or religious issues?

(Adapted from Woods-Smith et al., 2002)

PATIENT-FAMILY TEACHING GUIDELINES

1. What is chronic pain?

   Persistent or chronic pain is discomfort that continues for an extended time. Some conditions that cause pain can come and go over a period of years. In addition to pain, you can also suffer from depression, insomnia, problems walking, and difficulty healing from disease. There are treatments for pain that can make you feel better.

2. How can I tell my doctor and nurse about my pain?

   Persistent pain can be reported to your healthcare providers. Be as specific as you can to accurately convey your situation. Keep a diary or pain log for a few days before your visit. Here are things to jot down:

- Where it hurts
- How often it hurts
- What the pain feels like (burning, stabbing, shooting, dull ache, etc.)
- What makes it worse
- What makes it better
- What medications you have tried that work and don't work
- How the pain affects your life

3. Will over-the-counter remedies help?

   Acetaminophen (Tylenol) is a good choice for mild to moderate pain caused by osteoarthritis. Check with your healthcare provider about the dose if you take it for more than a few days. Non-steroidal anti-inflammatory drugs (NSAIDs) such as aspirin and ibuprofen work well also, but are associated with the risk of side effects like stomach upset and ulcer formation. Take NSAIDs with food for a short period of time. If you have or have had ulcers, avoid NSAIDs altogether. The new COX-2 inhibitors are more selective in treating pain without side effects, but their safety is being debated and the cost is high. Vioxx has been withdrawn from the market because of its association with stroke and heart attack, and Celebrex is being studied to establish its safety for long-term use.

4. Will I get addicted to my pain medicine?

   Most older people take painkillers, even narcotics, safely without becoming addicted. It is important not to drive or engage in tasks requiring your full attention (such as babysitting) when you start a new pain medication.

(continued)

5. Once my pain is treated, will I be back to my old self again?

In addition to treating your pain, you may also need treatment for accompanying conditions such as depression. People with chronic pain often complain of feeling blue, and these feelings sometimes hang on even when the pain is gone. Antidepressants can help older people to deal with certain kinds of pain (from nerve diseases or nerve injury) and treat the depression that can result from living with pain. Using a second medication may allow your healthcare provider to prescribe a lower dose of pain medication, thus lessening the risk of side effects.

CHAPTER 8

VIOLENCE AND ELDER MISTREATMENT

Elder mistreatment is the outcome of abuse, **neglect, exploitation,** or **abandonment** of older adults and represents some of the most tragic behavior in the area of family violence. Nurses are in key positions to screen, assess, and intervene for older adults subjected to elder mistreatment (Lachs & Pillemer, 1995).

Legal Issues

Every state in America has mechanisms for reporting elder mistreatment, and **adult protective services** (APS) programs exist in each state. Amendments to the Older Americans Act in 1987 included federal definitions of elder abuse. State to state variations do exist (Capezuti, Brush, & Lawson, 1997). Nursing homes' standards for care are based on policy stipulated in the Nursing Home Reform Act of 1987 (Omnibus Budget Reconciliation Act, 1987). In some states, failure by clinicians to report suspected incidents of mistreatment is a misdemeanor, punishable by fine or penalty (Capezuti et al., 1997).

Categories of Elder Mistreatment

One challenge of understanding elder mistreatment is that the literature proposes a variety of definitions and categories. There are three basic categories of elder mistreatment:

1. Domestic mistreatment generally occurs within the older adult's home dwelling at the hand of significant others (i.e., child, spouse, in-law).
2. Institutional mistreatment occurs when an older adult has a contractual arrangement and suffers abuse (i.e., long-term care facilities, assisted-living facilities, rehabilitation facilities, hospitals).
3. **Self-neglect** occurs when older adults who are mentally competent enough to understand the consequences of their own decisions engage in behaviors that threaten their own safety.

Institutional Mistreatment

Pillemer and Moore (1989) have found that nursing home patient aggressiveness is a predictor of physical and psychological abuse by staff members. Researchers have also speculated that shortages of staff, inadequate training of staff, and staff burnout may be precipitating factors in mistreatment of nursing home residents.

Characteristics of Older Adults at Risk

Older adults who are victimized are more likely to be old-old (75 and above), to be female (Dunlop, Rothman, Condon, Hebert, & Martinez, 2000), and to live with their abusers (Lachs, Williams, O'Brien, Hurst, & Horwitz, 1997; Pillemer & Finkelhor, 1988). Moreover, older adults who suffer from chronic, disabling illnesses that impair function and create care needs that exceed their caregiver's capacity to meet these needs are at higher risk of being mistreated (Fulmer & O'Malley, 1987).

Characteristics of People Who Mistreat Older Adults

Abusers are more likely to be male and suffer from impairments such as substance abuse, mental illness, or dementia (Brownell, 1999). In a majority of cases, family members have been shown to be the abusers (National Center on Elder Abuse at the American Public Human Services Association, 1998). Caregivers of older adults should be assessed for caregiver stress, substance abuse, and a history of psychopathology (Swagerty, 1999).

Cultural Perceptions of Elder Mistreatment

Nurses and other clinicians should be aware of the possibility of differences in perceptions about what constitutes mistreatment based on culture, and should take this into account during assessment and care planning. Cultural and linguistic competences are important for successful intervention in cases of elder mistreatment (Institute of Medicine, 2002).

ASSESSMENT

Screening for domestic violence has been recommended by the American Medical Association (Aravanis et al., 1993) for over a decade. A sample elder assessment instrument is included in the Best Practices feature on pages 124–128.

Ideally, the patient and the suspected abuser should be interviewed separately, which may reveal inconsistencies. Maintaining a nonjudgmental environment will enable the nurse to obtain more accurate data. A caregiver's refusal to allow for separate interviews should increase suspicion of elder mistreatment.

Elder Assessment Instrument (EAI)

The Hartford Institute for Geriatric Nursing (1999) recommends the Elder Assessment Instrument (EAI) for use in the clinical setting. Screening can facilitate accurate assessment, risk categorization, referral for services, and ultimately protection of the older person who is being mistreated or abused.

Various screening instruments have been developed that aid nurses and other clinicians in undertaking a thorough mistreatment assessment. The EAI (Fulmer & Cahill, 1984; Fulmer, Street, & Carr, 1984) assesses signs and symptoms of elder mistreatment. The nurse should first assess general appearance. An older adult appearing disheveled with poor hygiene warrants further investigation. Common signs of abuse include bruising, malnutrition, burns, excoriations, and fractures. Common clinical manifestations of neglect include dehydration, malnutrition, decubitus ulcers, and contractures. Other signs and symptoms of elder mistreatment include delays between the injury or illness and the seeking of medical treatment, frequent visits to the emergency department, and diagnostic testing results inconsistent with the history given (Lachs & Pillemer, 1995).

I. General Assessment	Very Good	Good	Poor	Very Poor	Unable to Assess
1. Clothing					
2. Hygiene					
3. Nutrition					
4. Skin integrity					
5. Additional Comments:					

II. Possible Abuse Indicators	No Evidence	Possible Evidence	Probable Evidence	Definite Evidence	Unable to Assess
6. Bruising					
7. Lacerations					
8. Fractures					
9. Various stages of healing of any bruises or fractures					
10. Evidence of sexual abuse					
11. Statement by elder re: abuse					
12. Additional Comments:					

(continued)

III. Possible Neglect Indicators	No Evidence	Possible Evidence	Probable Evidence	Definite Evidence	Unable to Assess
13. Contractors					
14. Decubiti					
15. Dehydration					
16. Diarrhea					
17. Depression					
18. Impaction					
19. Malnutrition					
20. Urine burns					
21. Poor hygiene					
22. Failure to respond to warning of obvious disease					
23. Inappropriate medications (under/over)					
24. Repetitive hospital admissions due to probable failure of health care surveillance					
25. Statement by elder re: neglect					
26. Additional Comments:					

IV. Possible Exploitation Indicators	No Evidence	Possible Evidence	Probable Evidence	Definite Evidence	Unable to Assess
27. Misuse of money					
28. Evidence of financial exploitation					
29. Reports of demands for goods in exchange for services					
30. Inability to account for money/property					
31. Statement by elder re: exploitation					
32. Additional Comments:					

V. Possible Abandonment Indicators	No Evidence	Possible Evidence	Probable Evidence	Definite Evidence	Unable to Assess
33. Evidence that a caretaker has withdrawn care precipitously without alternate arrangements					
34. Evidence that elder is left alone in an unsafe environment for extended periods of time without adequate support					
35. Statement by elder re: abandonment					
36. Additional Comments:					

(continued)

127

VI. Summary	No Evidence	Possible Evidence	Probable Evidence	Definite Evidence	Unable to Assess
37. Evidence of abuse					
38. Evidence of neglect					
39. Evidence of exploitation					
40. Evidence of abandonment					

VII. Comments: _____

_____

_____

_____

_____

NB: Ther is no "score." A patient should be referred to social services if the following exists:

1) if there is any evidence (±) without sufficient clinical explanation,
2) whenever there is a subjective complaint by the elder of EM
3) whenever the clinician deems there is evidence of abuse, neglect, exploitation, abandonment

Source: Reprinted by permission of SLACK Inc., and *Journal of Gerontological Nursing*.

Physical Examination

The presence of both fresh and healing injuries may suggest ongoing episodes of trauma and represent the need for further investigation to determine whether abuse or neglect may be a contributing factor. Examples include fractures, bruising, and burns (Lachs & Pillemer, 1995). If you suspect elder mistreatment or abuse, a complete visual examination of the older person without clothing is necessary because abusers may strike where clothing hides the resulting bruises. You can protect privacy by viewing the older person's body one area at a time from head to toe.

Laboratory findings that support the presence of dehydration and malnutrition without medical causes also increase suspicion for elder mistreatment. Additional diagnostic studies may include a complete blood count to evaluate for anemia; chemistry studies for dehydration, vitamin B_{12}, folate, total protein, and albumin to evaluate nutritional status; and toxicological screening to assess for evidence of illicit drug use. If sexual abuse is suspected, the nurse may be needed to assist with a pelvic examination that will likely include a Papanicolaou test (Pap smear) and cultures for sexually transmitted diseases. Radiological testing may also be anticipated if there is suspicion of fractures or internal injuries (Wagner, Greenberg, & Capezuti, 2002).

Interventions

Elder mistreatment requires an interdisciplinary team approach. Some forms of elder mistreatment, such as caregiver neglect, may benefit from interdisciplinary interventions. Educational interventions that may assist a stressed informal caregiver include disease management, aging changes, maximizing healthcare services, respite services, behavioral management, or caregiver support groups. In cases where abuse is suspected, an older adult may benefit from a hospital admission to allow the healthcare team to carefully assess and formulate a plan of care.

For the older adult living in longer term care facilities, the *California Advocates for Nursing Home Reform* (2002) recommend the following steps in preventing elder abuse in long-term care settings:

- Residents and significant others should join or form a resident's council.
- Residents and their significant others must stay informed by being active participants in care plan meetings and monitoring care.
- Significant others should stay connected to long-term care residents and visit at varied times.

Documentation

The nurse must clearly provide objective documentation. Documentation that focuses on the older adult's reactions when the suspected abuser is present must be provided in an unbiased manner. Physical indicators of elder mistreatment that are clearly documented will assist interdisciplinary members in discussing and planning goals of patient care. Photo-documentation is especially warranted in cases where there is evidence of physical or sexual abuse.

Implications for Gerontological Nursing Practice

The Joint Commission on Accreditation of Healthcare Organizations recommends the American Medical Association's *Diagnostic and Treatment Guidelines on Elder Abuse and Neglect* (American Medical Association, 1992). These guidelines are presented in Figure 8–1.

Screening and assessment for elder mistreatment should follow a routine pattern.
Assessment of each case should include the following:

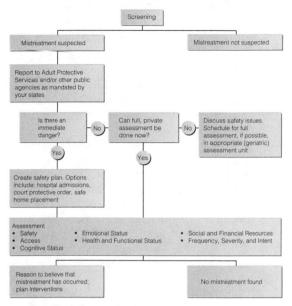

Figure 8–1 ■ Intervention and case management:
Part 1.
Source: Reprinted with permission of the American Medical
Association. (1992). *Diagnostic and treatment guidelines on
elder abuse and neglect,* 13.

PATIENT-FAMILY TEACHING GUIDELINES

Educating About Elder Mistreatment

1. I am worried about my older aunt who may be being abused by her son. What is elder mistreatment?

   Any action or inaction that harms or endangers the welfare of an older adult may be considered elder mistreatment. There are approximately

   (continued)

1.2 million cases of elder mistreatment in the United States each year.

Types of abuse:

- Physical abuse is an intentional infliction of physical injury or pain such as slapping or hitting.
- Psychological or emotional abuse is infliction of anguish such as repeatedly scolding an older individual who cannot perform personal hygiene tasks.
- Sexual abuse is any form of nonconsensual sexual intimacy.
- Financial exploitation is when an older individual is taken advantage of for monetary or personal benefit.
- Neglect may be on the part of a caregiver who intentionally or unintentionally does not provide adequate care or services for an older adult (i.e., not seeking healthcare when needed or withholding prescribed medications). Neglect may also be on the part of the older adult (self-neglect) who exhibits personal disregard or inability to perform self-care.
- Institutional mistreatment occurs when an older adult has a contractual arrangement and suffers abuse or neglect.
- Abandonment is desertion or willful forsaking of an older person. An example of this is when an older individual is "dropped off and left" at the emergency department.

2. If she is being abused, how can I help? I am only a niece.

   If you suspect elder mistreatment, contact your local adult protective services office or the department of human services in your state, county, or local jurisdiction. A case worker will visit your aunt and assess the situation. If help and support for her caregivers is needed, additional services will be brought into the home and the situation will be monitored to protect your aunt's safety.

3. What if abuse or neglect of my aunt is found? Will she be put in a nursing home?

The goal of the case worker's first assessment is to identify if your aunt is in immediate danger. Older people in immediate danger from abuse are removed from the home and temporarily protected in hospitals or safe havens with the authority of a court order. If the abuser needs mental health treatment or detoxification from drugs or alcohol, this will be facilitated. The goal is to improve the situation if possible and return the older person to the home environment when safe. If your aunt is not in immediate danger, resources will be brought into the home to ease the caregiver strain and improve your aunt's safety.

CHAPTER 9

CARE OF THE DYING

The nurse who helps the patient die comfortably and with dignity provides the following benefits of good nursing care:

- Attention to pain and symptom control
- Relief of psychosocial distress
- Coordinated care across settings with high-quality communication between healthcare providers
- Preparation of the patient and family for death
- Clarification and communication of goals of treatment and values
- Support and education during the decision-making process, including the benefits and burdens of treatment

(National Consensus Project [NCP] for Quality Palliative Care, 2004)

Possible barriers to the provision of excellent end-of-life care include failure of healthcare providers to acknowledge the limits of medical technology, lack of training about effective means of controlling pain and symptoms, the unwillingness of providers to be honest about a poor prognosis, discomfort telling bad news, and lack of understanding about the valuable contributions to be made by referral and collaboration with comprehensive end-of-life programs such as hospice or **palliative care** services (Kyba, 1999). All healthcare providers, including nurses, are challenged to address and overcome these barriers to improve the quality of care provided to the dying and their families.

PALLIATIVE CARE

The goals of palliative care are to prevent and relieve suffering and to support the best possible quality of life for patients and their families, regardless of the stage of the disease or the need for other therapies. Although palliative care can be delivered to patients of any age, including children, it is especially appropriate when provided to older people who have:

- Acute, serious, life-threatening illness (such as stroke, trauma, major myocardial infarction, and cancer where cure or reversability may or may not be a realistic goal but the burden of treatment is high).
- Progressive chronic illness (such as end-stage dementia, congestive heart failure, renal or liver failure, and frailty).

Palliative care may take place in hospitals, in outpatient clinics, in long-term care facilities, or in the home. The patient and family are supported during the dying and **bereavement** process. The care provided emphasizes quality of life and living as full a life as possible until the moment of death.

HOSPICE CARE

Hospice care can be defined as the support and care for persons in the last phase of an incurable disease so that they may live as fully and comfortably as possible (National Hospice and Palliative Care Organization, 2000). The Medicare hospice benefit was designed to support dying patients with less than 6 months to live. Many hospices are expanding service options so that patients and families can receive palliative care long before the last 6 months of life to meet the needs of patients dying from chronic illnesses (Dembner, 2004).

A multidisciplinary team of physicians, nurses, therapists, home health aids, pharmacists, pastoral counselors, social workers, and trained lay volunteers assist the family in providing care at home. The hospice nurse assumes the role of specialist in the management of pain and the control of symptoms. Hospice care may be provided at home if someone is available to safely provide care. The hospice nurse assesses the patient's and family's coping mechanisms, the available resources to care for the patient, the patient's wishes, and the support systems in place.

Stages of the Dying Process

Elisabeth Kübler-Ross, a psychiatrist at the University of Chicago, was also a pioneer. Her research identified the stages of dying that are still used as guidelines today including denial, anger, bargaining, depression, and acceptance. It must be remembered that a dying person may not exhibit all of these stages, or may move through a stage, only to return to it at a later time.

COMPLEMENTARY AND ALTERNATIVE CARE

Besides hospice care, the patient or family member may seek other alternative care. Traditional medicine may share the spotlight with acupuncture, massage therapy, Reiki therapy, chiropractors, or herbal medicine. Within the context of quality end-of-life care, the unique needs of each older patient and family (including significant others who may or may not be related to the patient) are respected, and the patient and family constitute the unit of care.

The common fears and concerns of the dying include the following:

- Death itself
- Thoughts of a long or painful death
- Facing death alone
- Dying in a nursing home, hospital, or rest home
- Loss of body control, such as bowel or bladder incontinence
- Not being able to make decisions concerning care
- Loss of consciousness
- Financial costs and becoming a burden on others
- Dying before having a chance to put personal affairs in order

THE NURSE'S ROLE

Core principles for the care of patients at the end of life include the following:

- Respecting the dignity of patients, families, and caregivers
- Displaying sensitivity and respect for patient and family wishes
- Using the most appropriate interventions to accomplish patients' goals
- Alleviating pain and symptoms
- Assessing, managing, and referring psychological, social, and spiritual problems
- Offering continuity and collaboration with others
- Providing access to therapies (including complementary therapies) that may improve the quality of the patient's life
- Providing access to palliative care and hospice services

- Respecting the right of patients and families to refuse treatment
- Promoting and supporting evidence-based clinical practice research

(Adapted from Cassell & Foley, 1999)

Pain Relief at the End of Life

Pain is a distressing sensation that is described as acute or chronic. Pain has the potential to hasten death and is associated with needless suffering at the end of life. People in pain do not eat or drink well, do not move around, cannot engage in meaningful conversations with others, and often become isolated from the world in order to save energy and cope with the pain sensation.

Pain is acknowledged to be a subjective experience. Self-report is the gold standard for measuring pain. When an older person cannot speak or is so cognitively impaired that he or she cannot report the level of pain, in addition to questioning significant others, the nurse should carefully observe the patient for the following signs:

- Moaning or groaning at rest or with movement
- Failure to eat, drink, or respond to the presence of others
- Grimacing or strained facial expression
- Guarding or not moving parts of the body
- Resisting care or noncooperation with therapeutic interventions
- Rapid heartbeat, diaphoresis, or change in vital signs

Factors that may render an older person unable to report pain include delirium, language barriers, expressive aphasia, excessive fatigue and weakness, and profound depression. If a patient has a potential reason for pain at the end of life, the nurse should assume it is present until proven otherwise (American Pain Society, 1999).

Effects of Unrelieved Pain During the Dying Process

Unrelieved pain at the end of life can cause psychological distress to the patient and family and is often associated with negative outcomes such as suffering and spiritual distress.

Principles of Pain Relief During the Dying Process

Mild pain (patient rated as 1 to 3 on the 0 to 10 scale) should be treated with non-opioid medications with **adjuvant drugs** (antidepressants or muscle relaxers) if the patient has neuropathic pain. Moderate pain (4 to 6 on the pain scale) is treated with low doses of opioids; the use of non-opioids and adjuvants may be continued at this stage. If the pain is severe (7 to 10), higher opioid doses are used. Patients presenting with severe pain should be started at higher doses rather than risking prolonged periods of uncontrolled pain while medications are titrated up from lower doses. Medications should be titrated based on patient goals, requirements for supplemental analgesics, pain intensity, severity of undesirable or adverse drug effects, measures of functionality, sleep, emotional state, and patient's or caregiver's report of the impact of pain on quality of life (ELNEC, 2003).

Anticipate and treat adverse effects such as nausea and constipation. Most patients on opioids will require laxative/stool softener combinations.

Pharmacological Approach to Pain Management During the Dying Process

The following are types of drugs used to control pain at the end of life:

- *Non-opioids.* Common drugs in this category include acetaminophen and NSAIDs. These drugs are very effective for the treatment of mild to moderate pain. They may be used alone or in combination with other medications to enhance their effect. <u>Cautions:</u> Acetaminophen use should be limited to 4 g daily or less in patients with normal liver function to avoid liver damage. It is essential to use with caution in those with liver disease or in heavy drinkers of alcohol. NSAIDs can cause gastric irritation by inhibition of prostaglandin formation.

- *Opioids.* These drugs block the receptors in the central nervous system and prevent the release of chemicals involved in pain transmission. Examples are codeine, morphine, hydromorphone, fentanyl, methadone, and oxycodone. Morphine is considered the gold standard by the World Health Organization for the relief of cancer pain. Adverse effects are rare, and the one most often cited is respiratory depression. This rarely occurs at the end of life. Most often when the respiratory rate is slowed, it is the result of the dying process and not the medication. Constipation and sedation are two troublesome symptoms that are often associated with opioid use.

- *Adjuvant analgesics.* These drugs are given for other reasons. Their effect may be to enhance the effectiveness of other classes of drugs, thus allowing effective treatment of pain at lower doses and less chance of side effects. Medications in this class include muscle relaxers, corticosteroids, anticonvulsants, antidepressants, and topical medications.

Routes of Administration

Usually the oral route of administration is preferred because it is the easiest and most comfortable for the patient. However, at times alternative routes of administration offer benefits over the oral route. Pain medication may be administered by the following routes:

- *Oral.* Tablets, liquids, and capsules are administered orally to control pain. Long-acting or sustained-release tablets can control pain for up to 24 hours. Patients who can swallow can use this method until very close to the time of death. Liquid medications can be mixed in juice, and capsules may be opened and the contents mixed with applesauce.
- *Oral mucosa.* Highly concentrated liquids such as morphine may be given by dropper into the oral or buccal mucosa. The medication can be delivered even when the patient can no longer swallow because the medication is absorbed from the mucosa and swallowing is not necessary. The medication may need to be administered more frequently because of a short half-life and duration of action.
- *Rectal.* Some medications come in suppository form, and the rectal route may be used when the patient can no longer swallow or has problems with nausea and vomiting. The rectal route is invasive. If the patient cannot move easily, the positioning required for suppository insertion may be difficult.
- *Transdermal.* The fentanyl patch may be placed on the skin every 72 hours for relief of pain. Because of changes in blood flow, metabolism, and fat distribution, some patients do not achieve or maintain stable drug levels and adequate pain relief. Peak onset may be delayed up to 24 hours necessitating coverage with short-acting agents during the initial day of treatment.

- *Topical.* Topical capsaicin and local anesthetics (EMLA) can be used for pain associated with herpes and its aftermath, for arthritis pain, and before invasive procedures such as insertion of intravenous medication or injections. Topical medications usually have little systemic absorption when applied as recommended in small amounts to confined areas.
- *Parenteral.* The intravenous, intramuscular, and subcutaneous routes are used when the patient cannot swallow. Usually pain is associated with these methods of administration. If the intravenous route is used, it is important to use the appropriate fluid delivery system and use the smallest amount of fluid possible to minimize excess secretions that require suctioning and cause difficulty breathing.
- *Epidural or intrathecal.* The administration of drugs into or around the spinal cord is reserved for those patients who cannot achieve pain control in any other manner. There is increased cost and risk of infection when these techniques are used.

Addiction need not be feared when treating end-of-life pain. However, the patient can build up a tolerance for drugs. Dying patients may need more pain medication than the normal range for the prescribed drug. Organic changes are occurring rapidly and systems are closing down, thus, absorption levels of drugs are diminishing also.

Nursing Care at the End of Life

Personal hygiene needs to remain a top priority when providing terminal care. Oral hygiene is crucial. Mouth care should be provided several times a day and whenever the mouth has a foul smell or is uncomfortable for the patient. Eye care is provided to promote comfort.

Artificial tears or ophthalmic saline solutions may be used to prevent drying of the eyes.

Anorexia and dehydration are common and normal with the terminal patient. A benefit of dehydration is decreased lung congestion, which prevents noisy or labored respirations. Oliguria (less than 15 cc of urine produced per hour) is another favorable outcome because the patient does not have to be positioned to use the bedpan or urinal frequently. If intravenous fluids are administered, it may be helpful to administer drugs with anticholinergic side effects (atropine) to prevent noisy respirations.

Skin integrity should be monitored carefully to prevent further complications. Edema, bruising, dryness, and venous pooling may appear. Positioning on the side or in a semiprone position may also alleviate noisy respirations, as well as afford a comfortable change of position.

Bowel and bladder incontinence are frequent occurrences at the end of life. It is extremely important to prevent decubitus ulcers from forming at this time since the healing process does not occur. Barrier creams and change of position may also help maintain skin integrity. Avoid the use of indwelling urinary catheters if at all possible because they often are associated with urinary tract infections that can be distressing and painful to the older patient.

Visual or auditory hallucinations at the end of life sometimes occur. These hallucinations are usually not frightening to the patient, but the family may be upset if they witness the event. The patient may refer to this as a dream or a strange occurrence.

Eventually, neurological changes occur and the patient slips from a lethargic state into an unconscious state, which may include periods of lucidness, then coma, and finally death. Family members frequently ask how much longer their loved one will live. It is prudent to assume that the patient can hear what is being said. It is believed the sense of hearing is intact in obtunded and comatose patients. Those present must not say anything they would not want the patient to hear.

Postmortem Care

When death occurs the nurse should use the stethoscope or manually check the patient's carotid pulses. Next, the nurse should check the eyes for pupillary light reflex. If there is none of the above, the patient can be pronounced dead. Note the time you observed the occurrence of death and chart appropriately, notify the attending physician of the death, and chart the time of notification as well as any directions. Notify family members of the death and express your condolences. Even if the family is expecting the death, the actual notification of the death comes as a shock and needs to be handled gently and with empathy. If the family is present, they should be allowed sufficient time to spend with the deceased before having the body removed.

If possible, before death occurs the limbs should be straightened and the head placed on a pillow. If the death is suspicious or occurs outside of a healthcare facility, the coroner may request the body be left undisturbed until an autopsy can be performed.

After the pronouncement, the nurse should glove, remove all tubes, replace soiled dressings, pad the anal area in case of drainage, and gently wash the body to remove any discharges. The nurse should grasp the eyelashes and gently pull the lids down. Dentures should be inserted. It is important not to tie or secure any body parts as this may cause skin indentations. The nurse should gather eyeglasses and prepare necessary paperwork for the removal of the body from the facility; call the funeral home, morgue, or other personnel for the removal of the body; and note the time in the chart as well as who was called and again chart when the body was released and to whom. It is advisable to also note if eyeglasses, dentures, or any personal artifacts were released with the body and to whom they were given. If the facility has a policy to identify the body with an identification tag, it must be secured properly.

Advance Directives

Some state laws mandate the use of living wills. Others mandate the designation of healthcare proxies. Living wills are documents in which older persons describe their wishes regarding treatment at the end of life. This document must be copied and shared with others to be effective. The physician, nurse, family members, and significant others should have copies of the living will and indicate their willingness to comply with the terms stated therein. A **healthcare proxy** is a designation of another person (and a backup if the primary proxy is not available) to make decisions for the older person. The older person should then discuss his or her wishes with the proxy to ensure appropriate end-of-life care. The healthcare proxy is only responsible for healthcare decisions should the older person be unable to make the decisions. Multiple copies of the proxy form should be made and kept by healthcare providers and family members (including the proxies) for easy access if needed.

Advance directives usually address wishes for end-of-life care including cardiopulmonary resuscitation (CPR), renal dialysis, use of ventilators, insertion of feeding tubes, total parenteral nutrition, chemotherapies, and other life-prolonging interventions. When questions regarding the initiation, ongoing use, and removal of life-sustaining technologies arise and there are no advance directives in place, ethical and emotional issues will arise.

Use of Feeding Tubes for Artificial Nutrition

Patients with life-limiting, progressive illness often experience a decline in appetite, loss of interest in eating and drinking, and weight loss. Some patients may experience dysphagia, which also decreases oral intake. At some point in the illness trajectory, most patients will be unable to take food and fluids by mouth or will refuse food, including their favorite foods. These changes can cause distress, especially for families and other caregivers, and raise questions about artificial nutrition and hydration.

Many families are fearful that their loved ones are hungry and are "starving to death." Contrary to expectations, however, most actively dying patients do not experience hunger even if they have inadequate caloric intake. Collaboration with other healthcare professionals like nutritionists and speech therapists is indicated to explore alternatives to artificial nutrition techniques.

Cardiopulmonary resuscitation (CPR) is administered to a person who is suffering cardiac or respiratory arrest. It is seen as a very acceptable form of intervention, and there are even portable defibrillators available to the public in malls and on airplanes. The decision to designate an older person with a do not resuscitate (DNR) order is usually made by the older person, his or her family, the nurse, physician, and others on the healthcare team. In most facilities, the physician or primary healthcare provider must write the DNR order in the chart for it to be a legal order. In many facilities if no order is written, by default CPR must be administered if the need arises. CPR offers no medical benefits to the patient who is terminally ill. It can be very upsetting for the nurse to provide CPR to the ill older adult, and the patient may suffer injury from anoxia, broken ribs, and aspiration.

Mercy Killing or Euthanasia

Mercy killing, or euthanasia, is presently not legal in any state, but there are frequent bills by legislators and much public debate concerning this issue. Oregon does allow physician-assisted suicide. Other states may approve of the physician helping the patient intentionally take his or her life. The American Nurses Association does not endorse the concept of or participation of nurses in the process of euthanasia, mercy killing, or assisted suicide (American Nurses Association, 1994).

There are rare occasions when a medication given for pain relief may have the unintended consequence of shortening the patient's life span. This is not considered mercy killing. The intent was the relief of pain, not to hasten death, as occurs with euthanasia.

Cultural Religious Issues

Some family members may hope to provide care to their loved one, but finances, inability to cope with the responsibility of caregiving, or family obligations may hinder the decision. All settings should provide culturally appropriate support, comfort, and privacy for the dying patient. Provisions should be made for family members to stay at the bedside if they so choose and if the patient is comfortable with the family being there.

Religion plays an important role in the forming of beliefs and practices that are paramount when death is imminent. Feelings of guilt, remorse, comfort, or peacefulness may all be related to religious beliefs. Religious customs are extremely important to many dying patients, and concerns may be intensified. Requests by family or patients to seek spiritual counseling should be met with respect. Many healthcare facilities have chaplains, clergy, social workers, and others to assist staff.

Preparing for Death

Hope should never be taken away from the dying patient and family. The will to live is extremely strong in many older patients, especially when confronting death and unfinished business in life. Older patients sometimes need reassurance from their families and caregivers that all is well and it is OK to let go.

Grief

Although death may be expected, it is usually met with shock by those left behind. Rationalizations (e.g., he lived a long life) may help ease the initial numbness of the actual death. Relief statements, such as the person is no longer in pain, may help the bereaved to cope with the immediate loss. The grieving process is considered difficult work that lasts for years, and it truly is hard to endure at times. Past death experiences, emotional health, religious beliefs, and support of friends and family all are factors that may help to ease the grief process.

The widow or widower experiences grief for many years. Phases of grief include:

First phase: numb shock. The widow cannot believe the spouse's death occurred.

Second phase: emotional turmoil. Alarm or panic-type reactions occur. Anger, guilt, or longing for the deceased take place.

Third phase. When the full effects of widowhood set in, so do regret, self-doubt, and at times, despair. Life's purpose becomes confusing and mood swings are prevalent.

Fourth phase: reorganization. Eventually takes place and coping strategies and positive outlooks emerge (Hegge & Fischer, 2000).

Caring for the Caregiver

To AVOID burn-out a periodic self-assessment might be beneficial to the nurse providing end-of-life care. Some questions may include:

- What have I done to meet my own needs today?
- Have I laughed today?
- Did I eat properly, rest enough, exercise, and play today?
- What have I felt today?
- Do I have something to look forward to?

Caring for oneself prevents anger, frustration, and anxiety. It makes it possible to continue to be a sensitive caregiver. It is important not to neglect personal needs.

PATIENT-FAMILY TEACHING GUIDELINES

The following are guidelines that the nurse may find useful when instructing older persons and their families about their choices at the end of life.

Choices at the End of Life

1. I am seriously ill. My physician has recommended a palliative care program. Does that mean I am dying?

   No, not at all. Palliative care is a program of care that can be delivered to any person who is seriously ill. Palliative care programs have been developed to provide for pain and symptom control, to help with patient-centered communication and decision making, and to coordinate care across settings. Aggressive care and palliative care can be delivered at the same time by your healthcare provider, thus ensuring your comfort during the treatment process.

2. How is palliative care delivered?

   The main approach is the management of pain and distressing symptoms like nausea, bowel function, sleep, and nutrition. A team of healthcare experts will address your needs, including physicians, nurses, social workers, nutritionists, pharmacists, chaplains, and others. Because a person with serious illness has a variety of needs, it takes a team of experts to deliver quality care.

3. Does my insurance cover palliative care?

   Many insurance programs do cover the delivery of palliative care, and more are beginning to examine the payment of this service as a benefit for patients and families. In the long run, it may actually decrease costs to the healthcare system because it has the potential to decrease hospitalization for many things that can be prevented by the palliative care focus such as pain, dehydration, infections, constipation, and other symptom problems.

4. What is the difference between hospice and palliative care?

Generally, hospice programs accept patients who are near the end of life and are no longer receiving aggressive disease interventions like chemotherapy and radiation. However, many hospice programs are expanding services and accepting patients who are not near the end of life but may benefit from the principles of palliative care, including the emphasis on pain and symptom control, while they are still receiving aggressive treatment for their illness. Most palliative care programs will help you and your family to receive the care you need in a variety of settings, including your home, the hospital, the nursing home, or a hospice if you need that kind of care.

CHAPTER 10

THE INTEGUMENT

NORMAL CHANGES OF AGING

With aging, the skin looses subcutaneous fat and becomes thinner and more prone to injury. Elastin decreases and the skin may sag and lose turgor. There is a gradual decline in both touch and pressure sensations, causing the older person to be at risk for injury such as burns and pressure sores. The hair of the older person looks gray or white due to a decrease in the number of functioning melanocytes and the replacement of pigmented strands of hair with nonpigmented ones. The texture and thickness of the hair also changes, becoming coarse and thin. Hormones decline, resulting in gradual loss of hair in the pubic and axillary areas and the appearance of facial hair on women and hair in the ears and nose of men. Nail growth slows, which results in thicker nails that are likely to split. There is a decrease in the size, number, and function of both eccrine and apocrine glands, resulting in an inability to control body temperature by the normal sweating mechanism.

COMMON ILLNESSES OF OLDER PERSONS

Skin Cancer

Skin cancer is the most common and the incidence increases with age. Both basal cell carcinoma and squamous cell carcinoma occur and present as pigmented spots that bleed easily. Skin cancers that primarily result from sun exposure are basal cell carcinoma, squamous cell carcinoma, and malignant melanoma (Schober-Flores, 2001).

Erythematous actinic keratosis is the most common type and appears as a sore, rough, scaly, erythematous papule or plaque. Other types of actinic keratosis include hypertrophic and cutaneous horn. They appear on sun-exposed areas such as the hands, face, nose, tips of the ears, and bald scalp (Leber, Perron, & Sinni-McKeehan, 1999).

Basal cell carcinoma occurs commonly in Caucasians and can extend below the skin to the bone, but metastasis is rare. Basal cell carcinoma can occur on any exposed skin surface but is frequently found on the head, neck, nose, and ears.

Squamous cell carcinoma originates in the higher levels of the epidermis. It appears as flesh colored to erythematous, indurated scaly plaques, or nodules and may have ulceration or erosions in the center. Metastasis can occur and is more common in lesions of the mucous membranes, such as the lips, and in individuals with a history of inflammatory disease, immune suppression, or exposure to chemicals and other hazardous substances (Schober-Flores, 2001).

Melanoma is the most serious of skin cancers. Lesions, appearing brown, black, or multicolored, may crust or bleed and are usually greater than 6 mm in diameter with irregular borders. The risk factors for melanoma include a family or past history of melanoma, light skin and hair, a history of severe sunburns, or numerous atypical moles.

Skin Tears

A skin tear is a traumatic separation of the epidermis from the dermis, occurring primarily on the extremities of older persons. Causes include friction alone, or by a combination of **shearing forces** and friction often occurring with simple activities such as dressing, transferring, turning, or lifting.

Prevention and Management of Skin Tears

- Do not use any pulling or sliding movements when assisting older persons with a change in their position.
- Protect the older person by padding any surfaces that come in contact with leg and arm movements such as side rails, wheelchair arm and leg supports, and table corners.
- Keep the environment free of obstacles and well lit.
- Keep skin moist with adequate fluids and skin moisturizing creams.
- Use paper tape and remove it cautiously, or substitute tape with gauze or stockinette.
- Encourage long sleeves and long pants to add a layer of protection over the skin.

The recommended clinical care of a skin tear would include the following (Baranoski, 2001):

1. Clean with normal saline or other nontoxic cleaner.
2. Pat or air dry.
3. Gently place the torn skin in its approximate normal position.
4. Apply dressing (saline, foam, gels) and change per protocol or product requirements.
5. Document the assessment and intervention.

PRESSURE OR DECUBITUS ULCERS

Definition and Stages of Pressure Ulcers

A pressure ulcer is defined as a lesion caused by unrelieved pressure that results in damage to underlying tissue. Pressure ulcer formation often occurs on the soft tissue over a bony prominence, although it can occur on any tissue that is exposed to external pressure for a length of time that is greater than capillary closing pressure.

The stages of pressure ulcers and the general guidelines for nursing management are presented below.

Table 10–1 Pressure Ulcer Stages and Management

Stage	Wound Cleaning/ Definition	Debridement	Change Dressing Choices	Frequency*
I	Nonblanch-able erythema of intact skin		Transparent film; adherent hydrocolloid	q 3–7 days prn
II	Partial-thickness skin loss involving epidermis, dermis, or both	Normal saline or approved cleaner	Transparent film, hydrogel, hydrocolloid	q 3–7 days prn 3 × week q 3–7 days prn
III	Full-thickness skin loss involving damage or necrosis of	Normal saline or approved cleaner If necrotic tissue present, debridement	1. wet-to-dry saline dressings; or	q 4–6 h prn q 3–7 days prn q 12 h prn

(continued)

Table 10–1 Pressure Ulcer Stages and Management *(continued)*

Stage	Wound Cleaning/ Definition	Debridement	Change Dressing Choices	Frequency[*]
	subcutaneous tissue that may extend down to, but not through, underlying fascia	must be done	hydrogel, moistened gauze or calcium alginate 2. Cover with gauze, or foam wafer 3. Use least irritating taping method	
IV	Full-thickness skin loss with extensive destruction, tissue necrosis, or damage to muscle, bone, or supporting structures	Same as stage III	Same as stage III	

Change frequency depends on amount and type of drainage present.
Read specific product instructions.
Source: AHCPR, 1994.

Factors related to the development of decubitus ulcers include:

Extrinsic factors such as shear, friction, moisture, and skin irritants.

Intrinsic factors related to aging skin such as changes in collagen, advanced age, poor nutrition, and use of corticosteroids.

Risk Assessment for Pressure Ulcers

The nursing care of the older person should begin with an assessment of the risk for pressure ulcers. The Hartford Institute for Geriatric Nursing (1999) recommends the use of the Braden Scale for Predicting Pressure Sore Risk.

This scale can be used for risk assessment in the following categories of older patients:

- All bed- or chair-bound patients, or those whose ability to reposition is impaired
- All at-risk patients on admission to healthcare facilities and regularly thereafter
- All older patients with decreased mobility, mental status, incontinence, and nutritional deficits

BEST PRACTICES

Braden Scale for predicting Pressure Sore Risk

The Braden Scale (Braden & Bergstrom, 1994) is a widely used tool that assesses mobility, activity, sensory perception, skin moisture, friction, shear, and nutritional status. Each dimension is rated from 1 to 4 on a Likert type scale, and the total score range is from 6 to 23. A score of 16 or less indicates a pressure sore risk and a need for a prevention plan. The Braden Scale has been subjected to several validation studies and is considered the most valid of the available risk assessment tools. Once a risk assessment is completed, and a deficit exists, the nursing care plan should reflect ongoing prevention as well as complete documentation of the older person's progress.

(continued)

Braden Scale for Predicting Pressure Sore Risk

Patient's Name _____   Evaluator's Name _____   Date of Assessment _____

SENSORY PERCEPTION ability to respond meaningfully to pressure-related discomfort	**1. Completely Limited** Unresponsive (does not moan, flinch, or grasp) to painful stimuli, due to diminished level of consciousness or sedation. OR limited ability to feel pain over most of body.	**2. Very Limited** Responds only to painful stimuli. Cannot communicate discomfort except by moaning or restlessness. OR has a sensory impairment which limits the ability to feel pain or discomfort over $\frac{1}{2}$ of body.	**3. Slightly Limited** Responds to verbal commands, but cannot always communicate discomfort or the need to be turned. OR has some sensory impairment which limits ability to feel pain or discomfort in 1 or 2 extremities.	**4. No impairment** Responds to verbal commands. Has no sensory deficit which would limit ability to feel or voice pain or discomfort.
MOISTURE degree to which skin is exposed to moisture	**1. Constantly Moist** Skin is kept moist almost constantly by perspiration, urine, etc.	**2. Very Moist** Skin is often, but not always moist. Linen must be changed at least once a shift.	**3. Occasionally Moist** Skin is occasionally moist, requiring an extra linen change approximately once a day.	**4. Rarely Moist** Skin is usually dry, linen only requires changing at routine intervals.

			Dampness is detected every time patient is moved or turned.
ACTIVITY degree of physical activity	**1. Bedfast** Confined to bed.	**2. Chairfast** Ability to walk severely limited or non-existent. Cannot bear own weight and/or must be assisted into chair or wheelchair.	**3. Walks Occasionally** Walks occasionally during day, but for very short distances, with or without assistance. Spends majority of each shift in bed or chair.	**4. Walks Frequently** Walks outside room at least twice a day and inside room at least once every two hours during waking hours.
MOBILITY ability to change and control body position	**1. Completely Immobile** Does not make even slight changes in body or extremity position without assistance.	**2. Very Limited** Makes occasional slight changes in body or extremity position but unable to make frequent or significant changes independently.	**3. Slightly Limited** Makes frequent though slight changes in body or extremity position independently.	**4. No Limitation** Makes major and frequent changes in position without assistance.

(continued)

Braden Scale for Predicting Pressure Sore Risk (continued)

Patient's Name _____ Evaluator's Name _____ Date of Assessment _____

	1. Very Poor	2. Probably Inadequate	3. Adequate	4. Excellent
NUTRITION usual food intake pattern	Never eats a complete meal. Rarely eats more than 1/2 of any food offered. Eats 2 servings or less of protein (meats or dairy products) per day. Takes fluids poorly. Does not take a liquid dietary supplement OR is NPO and/or maintained on clear liquids or IV's for more than 5 days.	Rarely eats a complete meal and generally eats only about $\frac{1}{2}$ of any food offered. Protein intake includes only 3 servings of meat or dairy products per day. Occasionally will take a dietary supplement OR receives less than optimum amount of liquid diet or tube feeding.	Eats over half of most meals. Eats a total of 4 servings of protein (meat, dairy products) per day. Occasionally will refuse a meal, but will usually take a supplement when offered. OR is on a tube feeding or TPN regimen which probably meets most of nutritional needs.	Eats most of every meal. Never refuses a meal. Usually eats a total of 4 or more servings of meat and dairy products. Occasionally eats between meals. Does not require supplementation.

FRICTION & SHEAR	1. **Problem**	2. **Potential Problem**	3. **No Apparent**
	Requires moderate to maximum assistance in moving. Complete lifting without sliding against sheets is impossible. Frequently slides down in bed or chair, requiring frequent repositioning with maximum assistance. Spasticity, contractures, or agitation leads to almost constant friction.	Moves feebly or requires minimum assistance. During a move skin probably slides to some extent against sheets, chair, restraints, or other devices. Maintains relatively good position In chair or bed most of the time but occasionally slides down.	Problem Moves in bed and in chair independently and has sufficient muscle strength to lift up completely during move. Maintains good position in bed or chair.

Total Score

161

Laboratory Values to Determine Risk for Pressure Ulcer

Serum albumin and serum transferrin, as well as lymphocyte count, are useful values that will help to determine nutritional status. A serum albumin level below 3.5 g/dl is considered low, and below 2.5 g/dl is a serious depletion in protein. Serum transferrin is considered a more accurate indicator of protein stores since it is more responsive to acute changes. A serum transferrin level below 200 mg/dl is considered low, and below 100 mg/dl is a serious depletion in protein. A total lymphocyte count below 1,500 mm^3 indicates loss of energy to skin. A moderate decrease is 800 to 1,200/mm^3. The synthesis of lymphocytes is depressed when protein-energy malnutrition exists, which contributes to the decreased ability of the white blood cells to fight infection.

Prevention and Modification of Pressure Ulcer Risk Factors

The older person who is at risk for a pressure ulcer should have a turning and activity schedule. Nurses and nurse assistants should consistently document their interventions in the flow sheet or progress notes. Mobility and activity considerations for preventing pressure ulcers include the following:

- Reposition q2h. Use a pull sheet to prevent shear and friction. If redness occurs, consider a 1½-hour turning schedule.
- Ensure proper positioning. Use pillows or wedges to prevent the skin from touching the bed on trochanter, heels, and ankles. Do not use rings or donuts.
- Avoid sitting. The sitting position, either in bed or in the chair, should be limited to 2 hours. Time in the

chair should be scheduled around meal times. The person in bed should not be left in the 90-degree position except during meals.

- Increase activity. Encourage older persons to change positions by making small body shifts. This will redistribute weight and increase perfusion. Range of motion exercises should be done every 8 hours, and the techniques should be taught to family and patients.
- Choose a mattress surface based on the assessment and diagnosis:
    - A low-air-loss bed or air-fluidized bed is indicated for any stage pressure sore, and for persons having grafts or surgery.
    - A water mattress is indicated for high-risk persons, and for stage I, II, and III pressure ulcers.
    - An alternating pressure mattress is indicated for high-risk persons and for stage I and II pressure ulcers.
    - A convoluted foam pad is indicated for short-term use (AHCPR, 1992).

High-risk older persons should not be placed in a 90-degree side-lying position. This position places intense weight on the trochanter. Older persons at risk should be turned from supine to the right or left 30-degree oblique position. This position relieves pressure on the bony prominences of the trochanter and lateral malleolus.

- Keep the skin clean and dry.
- Lubricate the skin with a moisturizer. Massage the area around the reddened area or bony prominence. Do not massage any reddened area. Then apply a thin layer of a petroleum-based product, followed by a baby powder cornstarch product, to reduce friction and moisture.

- Evaluate and manage incontinence. A bowel and bladder management program should be in place. If soiling occurs, skin should be cleansed per routine. Underpads should be used that absorb moisture and present a quick drying surface to the skin. Plastic-lined bed pads should not be in contact with the person's skin. Use minimal pads and cover them with a sheet or pillowcase.
- Monitor nutrition. Determine factors that might cause inadequate nutrition. Obtain laboratory data. Provide additional canned supplements, vitamin C, and zinc to promote skin healing.

The area at risk for pressure sores should be washed gently with tepid water, with or without minimal soap. Soap removes natural oils from the skin, and cleaning the soap off may cause additional friction damage.

Treatment of Pressure Ulcers

Cleansing the Wound

Topical antiseptics such as povidone-iodine, acetic acid, hydrogen peroxide, and Dakin's solution should not be used on a wound because these products have been found to be toxic to the wound fibroblasts and macrophages (Ovington, 2001). The safest, most cost-effective and most common cleansing agent for wounds is isotonic saline (0.9%). Wound cleansing can be done by (1) pouring a saline solution over the wound, (2) applying saline-soaked gauzes to clean the debris, or (3) squeezing a saline-filled bulb syringe over the wound. To irrigate for the purpose of cleansing, the nurse should use saline in a catheter tip syringe (60 cc) and apply gentle pressure (4 psi) (Thompson, 2000). Wounds with large adherent areas of necrotic tissue or yellow slough should be irrigated (debrided) with a higher pressure stream between 8 and 15 psi. Pressure should not exceed 15 psi, or tissue damage and edema could result (Krasner & Sibbald, 1999).

Dressings to Provide a Moist Wound Bed

To heal a pressure ulcer, a clean, moist environment must be maintained. A moist wound environment promotes cellular activity in all phases of wound healing, provides insulation, increases the rate of epithelial cell growth, and reduces pain. A dry wound environment has been found to result in further tissue death, or dry necrosis, beyond the cause of the wound (Ovington, 2001).

The frequency of dressing change will be determined by the manufacturer's recommendations for the product selected and the type and amount of exudate and drainage. The amount of wound moisture may change during the healing stages, so the wound may need added absorption during one period, and added moisture during another (Thompson, 2000).

Preventing and Treating Infection

Wound cleansing and debriding are instituted to prevent the development of infection. Examples of serious infections that can be complications of pressure ulcers are bacteremia, sepsis, osteomyelitis, and advancing cellulitis.

Use of Topical and Systemic Antibiotics

Certain local conditions would warrant the use of topical antibiotics:

- A clean pressure ulcer that has not shown signs of healing over a 2-week period
- A pressure ulcer that has increased local discharge but shows no local signs of infection

Wound Cultures to Determine Infection

Wound cultures and microscopic examination can identify infectious organisms. Wound cultures should be obtained by the aspiration method or a tissue biopsy. If there is eschar or exudate visible, it must be removed so that the healthy tissue is accessible. The wound is then washed with saline and dried gently with sterile gauze.

Systemic Antibiotics

If a pressure ulcer shows signs of infection, such as cellulitis, osteomyelitis, or septicemia, appropriate systemic antibiotics should be instituted. Common offending organisms of bacteremia and sepsis include *S. aureus,* gram-negative rods, and *Bacteroides fragilis.* A blood culture will allow the causative organisms to be identified, and antibiotics can be directed at the offending organisms. These are very serious complications of pressure ulcers, and immediate medical attention is advised.

Selected Antimicrobials

Penicillinase-resistant penicillins (methicillin, nafcillin, oxacillin) are indicated against staphylococcal and beta-hemolytic streptococci infections of soft tissue. These drugs have a high degree of safety, but the dose should be adjusted for older persons with renal impairment to prevent nephrotoxicity.

Aminoglycosides

Gentamicin, tobramycin, and streptomycin are rapidly bactericidal against staphylocci and gram-negative aerobic bacteria. The dose of these drugs should be reduced in the elderly person because of the risk of renal impairment. Risk of ototoxicity increases with age and is more likely in older persons with pre-existing hearing problems.

Delayed Healing

The following are signs of delayed healing:

- Wound size is increasing.
- Exudate, slough, or eschar is present.
- Tunnels, fistula, or undermining has developed.
- Epithelial edge is not smooth and continuous and does not move toward wound.

A wound that does not heal within 6 weeks is considered a chronic wound. Common problems that often lead to chronic wounds are diabetes, peripheral vascular disease, and pressure ulcers. Normal aging and chronic disease factors that are often present in older persons will affect their ability to heal.

Some of the considerations related to delayed or impaired wound healing for the older person include inadequate blood supply or nutrition, impaired immunity, and reinjury to the wound (Boynton, Jaworski, & Paustian, 1999; Demling & DeSanti, 2001).

Fingernail and Toenail Problems

Onychomycosis, a fungal infection of the toenail, most commonly occurs on the big toe. The toenail appears thick, discolored, and protruding from the nail bed (Fielo, 2001). This disorder is characterized by separation of the cuticle from the nail, which allows organisms to enter. The organisms may cause swelling, redness, and tenderness of the nail fold, accompanied by purulent drainage.

The treatment of onychomycosis will include relief of pain, patient education, and oral antifungal agents as appropriate. Consult the podiatrist periodically for reduction of the nail plate. Patient education includes frequent treatment to prevent the condition from spreading to the other parts of the foot. Oral antifungal agents may provide a cure (O'Dell, 1998).

Antifungal agents such as itraconazole are used in the treatment of onychomycosis of the toenails and fingernails. The topical preparation is applied to the affected area and has few side effects. The suggested dosage for treatment of onychomycosis of the toenails is itraconazole 200 mg po daily for 12 weeks. Adverse effects include renal and hepatic damage.

The treatment of chronic paronychia will include keeping affected nails dry and perhaps antibiotics. The older person should be advised to keep the affected nails out of water and to keep the area protected. Drainage is sometimes needed. Consult a podiatrist for treatment recommendations.

Laboratory and Testing Values

Total body photography, skin surface microscopy, machine vision, and skin biopsy are the current modalities that can be used to diagnose malignant melanoma. All older persons with suspicious lesions should be referred to a dermatologist for evaluation. A biopsy is indicated for any lesion that has been present for longer than a month.

Prescription Creams and Lotions for Dry Skin

Often corticosteroids are prescribed as topical treatment for dermatological problems in older people. These creams should be applied sparingly in thin layers to maximize therapeutic outcome and minimize the risk of side effects. Hydrocortisone 1% or 2.5% is a low-potency topical corticosteroid that can be applied for short-term treatment of inflamed dry skin. Long-term use may cause systemic absorption.

When assessing the skin of people of color, the nurse should become familiar with the characteristics of darker skin. Nurses and other healthcare professionals may find the assessment of darker skin to be more challenging because the traditional hallmarks of redness and color changes may be obscured by the darker skin tone. Box 10–1 illustrates guidelines for assessment of darker skin.

Cellulitis

Cellulitis is an acute bacterial infection of the skin and subcutaneous tissue that results in intense pain, heat, redness, and swelling. Cellulitis may be accompanied by lymphadenopathy and fever. An elevated temperature, although a common sign of infection, may not be present in the older person. The organisms most commonly responsible for cellulitis are hemolytic streptococci (group G streptococci and *Streptococcus pyogenes*), and *Staphyloccus aureus* (Baddour, 2000).

Management of Cellulitis

The treatment includes appropriate antibiotics, prevention of further infection, immobilization and elevation of the affected limb, pain relief, and possibly anticoagulant therapy.

Appropriate antibiotics are the priority of treatment. They are usually given intravenously until the infection begins to resolve, and then they are changed to an oral route. If the cellulitis is on the lower extremities, the foot of the bed should be elevated to decrease swelling and allow the leg to be fully supported. Pain should be

Box 10–1   The Integument: Considerations for People of Color

- Some dark-skinned persons have bluish lips or gums.
- Black persons have freckle-like pigmentation of gums, buccal cavity, and borders of the tongue.
- A dark-skinned person may lose reddish tones if pallor is present.
- Cyanosis is difficult to assess in a dark-skinned person. The nurse should check soles and heels for color.
- Erythema is an area of inflammation on the skin. On a dark-skinned person, the skin assumes a purplish color when inflammation is present. To assess erythema in a dark-skinned person, the nurse should palpate for warmth and check for hardness and smoothness.
- Ecchymotic lesions are large bruises. Purple or dark color usually can be seen.
- To determine if an area of concern is erythema or ecchymosis, the nurse should use a glass slide and press gently over the area. If the color changes and becomes lighter, it is an erythema. If no change occurs, it is an ecchymotic area.
- Dermatosis papulosa nigra is a type of seborrheic keratoses that occurs only in Blacks. It is characterized by the appearance of many dark, small papules on the face.

Source: Gilchrist & Chiu, 2000.

assessed with a 0 to 10 visual analog scale and medicated with appropriate analgesics. Sheets and blankets must not be allowed to rub against the area and cause friction and added pain.

PATIENT-FAMILY TEACHING GUIDELINES

What treatment is most effective for dry skin?
Personal practices to improve or relieve dry skin include the following:

- Bathe once a day, using superfatted soaps such as Dove or Caress. Avoid any drying agents such as alcohol.
- Dry with a soft towel, including between the toes.
- Apply emollients liberally to the skin immediately after bathing, while skin is moist. Reapply frequently.
- Use white petroleum for an effective emollient for dry skin treatment. It is inexpensive and does not contain irritating additives such as perfumes.
- Keep humidity as high as possible, especially during the winter months.
- Wear soft, nonirritating clothing next to the skin.
- Prescription creams may also be useful (see Pharmacological Interventions).

CHAPTER 11

MOUTH AND ORAL CAVITY

Oral assessment and care are important responsibilities of gerontological nurses caring for older adults. The mouth is the beginning of the digestive system and also serves as an airway for the respiratory system. The oral cavity consists of the lips, palate, cheeks, tongue, salivary glands, and teeth.

NORMAL CHANGES OF AGING

In healthy aging with proper oral hygiene, the teeth and gums appear normal.

Salivary function decreases over time and results in production of less saliva. The gums may recede, leaving teeth vulnerable to cavities below the gum line. The enamel on the surface of teeth may be worn away or abraded, leaving teeth open to staining, damage, and cavities. With tooth loss and malocclusion, the older person may avoid eating healthy foods high in fiber such as fruits and vegetables, causing further problems related to poor nutrition.

COMMON DISEASES OF AGING RELATING TO THE MOUTH AND ORAL CAVITY

Oral diseases and conditions are common to those older people who grew up without the benefit of community water fluoridation and other fluoride products.

About 30% of adults 65 and older no longer have any natural teeth and are **edentulous** (without teeth) (Centers for Disease Control, 2001). **Periodontal disease** (gum disease) or dental **caries** (cavities) most often cause tooth loss. The severity of periodontal disease increases with age.

Older adults who belong to racial or ethnic minorities or who have a low level of education are more likely to report dental pain than older adults who are White or better educated (Centers for Disease Control, 2001). Medicare does not provide coverage for routine dental care. Medicaid funds dental care in some states, but reimbursement rates are so low that it is often difficult to locate a dentist who will accept Medicaid patients.

Oral and pharyngeal cancers result in about 8,000 deaths annually. These cancers, primarily diagnosed in older people, carry a poor prognosis.

Most older Americans take prescription and over-the-counter medications that can decrease salivary flow and result in **xerostomia** or dry mouth. For example, antihistamines, diuretics, antipsychotics, and antidepressants can reduce salivary flow. This can be especially problematic for institutionalized elderly adults, who take an average of eight medications a day and often drink very little fluid.

Barriers to Mouth Care

Although many older people regularly seek and receive dental care, older adults' use of dental services is the lowest of all adults (Walton, Miller, & Tordecilla, 2002). Frail or institutionalized older adults may not have the physical or financial resources to travel to the dentist. Barriers to mouth care include lack of training and knowledge about the importance of oral hygiene, lack of perceived need for oral care, heavy workloads, and resistance by older persons with dementia (Matear, 2000).

Negative Effects of Poor Oral Care

Poor oral care can have serious adverse effects on the physical and psychosocial function and health of the older person. Consequences of poor oral care include the following:

- Social isolation and depression
- Systemic illness such as aspiration pneumonia and perhaps heart disease
- Periodontal disease, which can negatively affect glycemic control in persons with diabetes
- Malnutrition, vitamin deficiencies
- Pain, halitosis, tooth loss, dental caries, periodontal disease
- Denture stomatitis

(Coleman, 2002; Connell, McConnell, & Francis, 2002; Yoneyama et al., 2002)

NURSING ASSESSMENT OF ORAL PROBLEMS

Patients should be carefully questioned regarding their oral health history, including date of last dental examination, presence and function of dentures, missing or loose teeth, bleeding gums, dry mouth, presence of sores or lesions, medications, usual oral hygiene routine, altered sense of taste, chewing or swallowing difficulties, and presence of bad breath or halitosis.

A complete oral cavity assessment includes examination of the lips, teeth, interior of the buccal mucosa, anterior and base of the tongue, gums, soft and hard palate, and back of the throat. Careful notation of any cracks, lesions, ulcers, swelling, induration, gingival bleeding, hypertrophy, or dental caries should be made in the patient's record. **Leukoplakia,** or a white patchy coating on the surface of the oral mucosa, should be referred to a dentist or oral surgeon for further evaluation and biopsy.

Wearing gloves, the nurse should lift the tongue with a 4×4 inch dressing to examine the posterior surface. Extra light will be required to complete visualization. Observe any tremor, coating, or deviation of the tongue.

The lymph nodes of the head and neck should be carefully palpated and any tenderness or enlargement noted. The condition and number of natural teeth should also be noted. Loose or broken teeth should be referred for dental evaluation because the patient is at risk for losing and swallowing the tooth during a meal. Likewise, dentures should be examined for fit and condition. Cracks, poor fit, and missing or broken teeth should be noted.

COMMON ORAL PROBLEMS

Xerostomia

The most common oral problem occurring in the older adult is xerostomia (Ship, Pillemer, & Baum, 2002; Walton et al., 2001). Dry mouth can result from mouth breathing, dehydration due to diuretic use, oxygen therapy, oral and systemic diseases, and head and neck radiation. The most common cause appears to be drug induced. The most common offenders are tricyclic antidepressants, sedatives, tranquilizers, antihistamines, antihypertensives (alpha- and beta-blockers), diuretics, calcium channel blockers, ACE inhibitors, cytotoxic agents, antiparkinsonian agents, chemotherapy drugs, and antiseizure drugs (Ship et al., 2002).

Nursing interventions to improve xerostomia include the following:

- Urging regular dental evaluation
- Low-sugar diet
- Mouth rinses
- Sugar-free chewing gum, hard candies, and mints
- Artificial saliva and mouth lubricants (Salivart, Xero-Lube)
- Bedside humidifiers
- Dietary modifications including avoidance of foods known to be difficult to chew or swallow and careful use of fluids while eating

Oral Candidiasis

Oral candidiasis is a frequent complication of dry mouth and is treated with oral antifungal agents. Persons who have diabetes and have high or elevated glucose levels are at risk for candidiasis (thrush) because the oral flora is altered and the organism *Candida albicans* is encouraged to overgrow.

The usual treatment is rinsing with topical antifungal agents (nystatin) four times a day for 2 weeks. The nurse should carefully observe older patients to make sure they adequately "swish" the solution for about 2 minutes but do not swallow the solution. If an oral troche (a medicated lozenge to soothe the throat) is used, it must be held in the mouth and allowed to slowly dissolve. Patients with dentures should remove their dentures before rinsing to ensure that the medication reaches all areas of the oral mucosa.

A small soft toothbrush is considered the most effective mechanical method to control dental plaque. Teeth or gums should be brushed twice daily for about 3 to 4 minutes. Toothbrushes perform substantially better than foam swabs in the ability to remove plaque from the teeth and gingival margins and from the areas between teeth (Pearson & Hutton, 2002). Swabs are useful to cleanse and moisten oral mucosa and prevent damage to delicate tissue and may be effectively used when caring for the dying, but a moist toothbrush is more effective in reducing bacterial plaque and cleaning the oral cavity (Coleman, 2002).

Lemon and glycerine swabs are not only ineffective but also in fact harmful and should not be used (Coleman, 2002).

Mouth rinses are available and can serve the purposes of cleansing, moisturizing, or killing germs. Chlorhexidine (Peridex) is used widely to treat gingival and periodontal disease and other oral infections. It can improve oral hygiene in populations with special needs in whom mechanical plaque removal is difficult, such as those with Alzheimer's disease or those who do not possess the dexterity or strength for manual plaque removal.

Oral Pain

Oral pain is an advanced problem in a tooth or the gingival tissues. Although pain may resolve with time, an untreated problem can result in a tooth abscess or serious infection. Patients with a dental abscess will often have swollen or enlarged lymph nodes under the ear or jaw. Clusters of vesicles of "punched out looking" ulcers on the lips and mucosa can indicate the presence of herpes simplex or zoster. Treatment with an antiviral topical ointment or suspension is indicated after referral and assessment by the primary care provider.

Gingivitis and Periodontal Disease

Inflammation of the gums associated with redness, swelling, and a tendency to bleed are the common presenting signs of gingivitis. **Gingivitis** is a precursor to chronic periodontitis. The gums become red and swollen and bleed easily. Daily flossing and twice-daily brushing with fluoride toothpaste often helps reduce the symptoms of gingivitis. An oral hygienist is needed to remove plaque and tartar with special instruments.

Risk factors for gingivitis include:

- *Smoking.* Smoking cigarettes greatly increases the risk of periodontal disease and lowers the chances of success of dental treatments.
- *Diabetes.* Persons with diabetes are at higher risk of all forms of periodontal disease.
- *Medications.* Many drugs can reduce saliva production, and thus the protective effect of saliva on the teeth and gums is lost.
- *Poor nutrition.* A poor diet, especially one low in calcium, can lower resistance to gum disease. Eating and drinking foods and drinks high in sugars can damage teeth.
- *Stress.* Older people under stress have more difficulty fighting infection, including gingivitis.
- *Illness.* Diseases like HIV/AIDS and cancer can make fighting any infection more difficult.
- *Genetic susceptibility.* Although not directly inherited, gum disease seems more common in some families.

Patients with bright red or magenta-colored gums or those complaining of gum bleeding with toothbrushing or eating should be referred to the dentist or periodontist for evaluation. The dentist will recommend medications such as antimicrobial mouth rinses, antibiotic gels, and perhaps surgery with bone and tissue grafts to replace lost bone and protect the vitality of the teeth.

These treatments are difficult and expensive; therefore, prevention and early intervention is important.

Urge all older patients to engage in self-care activities to prevent gum disease, including daily flossing, twice-daily brushing with fluoride toothpaste, twice-yearly dental cleaning and evaluation, eating a well-balanced diet, and avoiding tobacco products.

Stomatitis

Stomatitis is the inflammation of the mouth that is frequently caused by chemotherapy agents and is a common problem among older patients undergoing cancer treatment. Anticancer drugs cause cell destruction throughout the body, and the cells of the mouth can become damaged leading to erosion, ulceration, inflammation, and secondary infections. Eating and drinking can be painful, and nutritional problems may occur as a result of stomatitis.

Treatments include meticulous oral hygiene, frequent use of a mild saline mouthwash, and avoiding extremes of hot, cold, or very spicy food and liquids. In extreme cases, a swish-and-spit solution of kaolin and pectin, diphenhydramine hydrochloride, and lidocaine may provide relief before mealtime.

Oral Cancer

Benign and malignant tumors can occur in the mouth and pharynx. Oral cancer that metastasizes will usually travel via the lymph nodes in the neck. Squamous cell carcinoma is the most frequent cancer of the oral cavity and occurs most often in older persons. The 5-year survival rate for treated oral cancer is about 50%, with mortality the highest for cancers of the tongue and lowest for cancers of the lips (National Cancer Institute, 2002).

Symptoms of oral cancer include the following:

- A sore on the lip or mouth that does not heal
- A lump on the lip or in the mouth
- A white or red patch on the gum, tongue, or buccal mucosa
- Unusual bleeding, pain, or numbness in the mouth
- A feeling that something is always caught in the throat
- Difficulty or pain with chewing or swallowing
- Swelling of the jaw that changes the fit and comfort of dentures
- Changes in the voice
- Pain in the ear (National Cancer Institute, 2002)

Diagnosis of oral cancer involves checking histopathology of suspicious cells after biopsy and x-ray techniques like computerized axial tomography scans or magnetic resonance imaging. Treatment involves surgery, radiation therapy, and chemotherapy.

Risk factors for the development of oral cancer include:

- *Tobacco use.* Smoking cigarettes, pipes, and cigars accounts for 90% of oral cancers. Cigar, pipe, and chewing tobacco users have the same risk as cigarette smokers.
- *Chronic and heavy alcohol use.* The risks are even greater for older people who smoke and use alcohol.
- *Sun exposure to the lips.* Wearing a brimmed hat and lip balm with sunscreen reduce the risk. Pipe smokers are especially prone to lip cancer.
- *History of leukoplakia.* Older people with white patches in the mouth should be closely monitored.
- *Erythroplakia.* People in their 60s and 70s may develop red or magenta patches in the mouth.

Nursing Strategies for Providing Oral Care to Patients with Cognitive Impairments

Some strategies that may be used and adapted in the nursing home setting when providing mouth care for difficult residents with a cognitive impairment include:

- *Task breakdown.* Time is taken to slowly break down the task into small steps. For instance, "Now I will place some toothpaste on the toothbrush. Does this look like enough to you?" The resident should be involved in each step of the process.
- *Distraction.* Playing music or looking at family pictures may provide some distraction while the caregiver carries out oral care.
- *Hand over hand.* The caregiver places a hand over the resident's hand and guides the activity.
- *Chaining.* The caregiver starts the activity and then asks the resident to complete it. For instance, the nurse may move the toothbrush back and forth a few times and then say, "Now you do it, Mrs. Jones. I may not be doing it exactly how you like it."
- *Protection.* Nurses should never insert their fingers into the mouth of a resident who bites or resists care. Human bites can be painful and infection prone. In extreme circumstances, several tongue blades may be taped together and inserted into the resident's open mouth, providing some small measure of protection should the resident decide to clamp down (modified from Chalmers, 2000).

As always, timing is key to approaching residents with cognitive impairments. Choose the time of day when the resident is most calm and accepting of care. Should the resident vehemently refuse oral care, it is best to walk away and reapproach the resident at a later time.

It is seldom effective to try to force the resident to open the mouth and accept oral care.

Sometimes the presence of a family member can be reassuring and calming to the resident. A staff member who seems to have a good rapport with the resident should take responsibility for the provision of oral care. Effective and ineffective nursing interventions should be carefully noted in the nursing care plan so that a consistent approach can be used and the resident will come to associate oral care with the pleasant feeling of having a clean mouth.

PATIENT-FAMILY TEACHING GUIDELINES

Education Guide to Oral Health

Being older does not necessarily mean wearing dentures and being toothless. Older patients should be urged to take these steps to protect their oral health and preserve their teeth.

1. What can I do to protect my teeth now that I am older?

   Suggestions for good oral health include:
   - Drink fluoridated water and use fluoridated toothpaste; fluoride provides protection against dental decay at all ages.
   - Practice good oral hygiene. Brush teeth carefully twice a day and floss daily to reduce dental plaque and prevent periodontal disease. Use an egg timer to ensure that brushing is carried out for at least 3 minutes.
   - Get professional oral healthcare, even if you have no natural teeth. Professional care helps to maintain the overall health of the teeth and mouth, and provides for early detection

of precancerous or cancerous lesions. For patients with teeth, see the dentist and dental hygienist twice a year for evaluation, cleaning, and scaling. For the patient without teeth, see the dentist yearly for an oral cancer check.

2. Are there substances I should avoid in my daily habits?

- Avoid tobacco. In addition to the general health risks of tobacco use, smokers have 7 times the risk of developing periodontal disease compared to nonsmokers. Tobacco used in any form—cigarettes, cigars, pipes, and smokeless (chewing) tobacco—increases the risk for periodontal disease, oral and throat cancers, and oral fungal infections.
- Limit alcohol. Excessive alcohol consumption is a risk factor for oral and throat cancers. Alcohol and tobacco use together greatly increase the risk.
- Get dental care before, after, and during cancer treatment with chemotherapy and radiation. Careful attention is needed to treat and prevent damage that can destroy teeth and oral tissues.
- Caregivers should attend to the daily oral hygiene of older people who cannot care for themselves. This includes older people with cognitive impairments and physical frailty. It is important to note effective techniques and provide a consistent approach.

Geriatric Oral Health Assessment Index (GOHAI)

The Hartford Institute for Geriatric Nursing Try This assessment series recommends the Geriatric Oral Health Assessment Index (GOHAI) for use in the clinical setting (Atchison, 1997). The GOHAI has been tested and used extensively primarily in the community and acute care setting; however, it is appropriate for the long-term care facility as well. This is a 12-item scale. A score of 57 to 60 is considered a high score, 51 to 56 a medium score, and below 50 a low score. Individuals with a high score or troublesome symptoms should be referred for a dental examination and follow-up (Hartford Institute of Geriatric Nursing, 1999).

(continued)

The Geriatric Oral Health Assessment Index

Indicate, in the past three months, how often you feel the way described in each of the following statements. Circle one answer for each.

	1	2	3	4	5
1. How often did you limit the kind or amounts of food you eat because of problems with your teeth or dentures?	Always	Often	Sometimes	Seldom	Never
2. How often did you have trouble biting or chewing any kinds of food such as firm meat or apples?	Always	Often	Sometimes	Seldom	Never
3. How often were you able to swallow comfortably?*	Always	Often	Sometimes	Seldom	Never
4. How often have your teeth or dentures prevented you from speaking the way you wanted?	Always	Often	Sometimes	Seldom	Never
5. How often were you able to eat anything without feeling discomfort?*	Always	Often	Sometimes	Seldom	Never
6. How often did you limit contacts with people because of the condition of your teeth or dentures?	Always	Often	Sometimes	Seldom	Never
7. How often were you pleased or happy with the looks of your teeth and gums or dentures?*	Always	Often	Sometimes	Seldom	Never

(continued)

185

	1	2	3	4	5
8. How often did you use medication to relieve pain or discomfort from around your mouth?	Always	Often	Sometimes	Seldom	Never
9. How often were you worried or concerned about the problems with your teeth, gums, or dentures?	Always	Often	Sometimes	Seldom	Never
10. How often did you feel nervous or self-conscious because of problems with your teeth, gums, or dentures?	Always	Often	Sometimes	Seldom	Never
11. How often did you feel uncomfortable eating in front of people because of problems with your teeth or dentures?	Always	Often	Sometimes	Seldom	Never
12. How often were your teeth or gums sensitive to hot, cold, or sweets?	Always	Often	Sometimes	Seldom	Never

Total Score: _____

* Items 3, 5, 7 are reverse scored with a "1" for never and a "5" for always. All other items are a "1" for always.

Adapted from Atchison, K. A. (1997). The Geriatric Oral Health Assessment Index. In Slade, G. D. (Ed.), Measuring Oral Health and Quality of Life. Chapel Hill: University of North Carolina, Dental Ecology 1977. Kurlowicz, L. *Try This: Best Practices in Care for Older Adults* (2002). New York: New York University, The Steinhardt School of Education, Division of Nursing, The John A. Hartford Foundation Institute for Geriatric Nursing.

CHAPTER 12

SENSATION: HEARING, VISION, TASTE, TOUCH, AND SMELL

Changes in vision, hearing, smell, taste, and touch occur naturally throughout the aging process. Older persons with sensory dysfunction may suffer functional impairment, injury, social isolation, and depression.

VISION

Visual impairment is defined as visual acuity of 20/40 or worse while wearing corrective lenses, and legal blindness or severe visual impairment is 20/200 or more as measured by a Snellen wall chart at 20 feet. Visual impairment and blindness in the older person is the result of four main causes: **cataracts,** age-related **macular degeneration, glaucoma,** and **diabetic retinopathy.**

The healthy older adult should schedule a complete eye examination every other year. During this examination, visual acuity should be evaluated, pupils should be dilated with examination of the retina, and intraocular pressure should be tested. Older persons with diabetes should have this complete visual evaluation yearly (Reuben et al., 2002).

In addition to annual or biennial examinations, the gerontological nurse should urge all older persons who complain of a visual problem to seek a visual evaluation if they experience any of the following problems:

- Red eye
- Excessive tearing or discharge
- Headache or feeling of eyestrain when reading or doing close work
- Foreign body sensation in the eye
- New-onset double vision or rapid deterioration of visual acuity
- New-onset haziness, flashing lights, or moving spots
- Loss of central or peripheral vision
- Trauma or eye injury

Telescopic lenses, books in braille, computer scanners and readers, tinted glasses to reduce glare, large-print books and magazines, guide dogs, and canes are often rejected because of the stigma attached to them. Older persons who are registered with the Commission for the Blind can borrow books on tape with a tape player, telephones with large numbers, and high-intensity lighting, without cost, if they can furnish a letter from a physician noting that they are legally blind.

Normal Age-Related Changes

External changes of the eye related to age include graying and thinning of the eyebrows and eyelashes. Wrinkling of the skin surrounding the eyes occurs as a result of subcutaneous tissue atrophy. Arcus senilis, grayish yellow rings around the peripheral cornea, develop due to lipid deposits; however, this condition is unrelated to hypercholesterolemia or lipid abnormalities, except in rare cases.

The lenses thicken and harden with age and appear yellowish and opaque. Thickening of the lenses occurs with loss of pliability. This loss of pliability in the lens contributes to **presbyopia** or the decrease in near vision, which generally occurs around the age of 40. Visual acuity tends to diminish gradually after 50 years of age and then more rapidly after the age of 70.

Pupils continue to react to light by dilating and constricting; however, this process occurs more slowly with increased age. Accommodation, or the ability to focus on objects at varying distances, declines with age. A delay in pupillary reaction makes it difficult for older adults to adapt to light changes, putting them at greater risk for falls. Overall pupil diameter is also decreased, which reduces the amount of light reaching the retina, and more light is required to see clearly (Smith, 1998).

Light sensitivity, or the ability to adapt to varying degrees of light, declines with age. With increased age, there is a need for increased light, increased time for dark adaptation and longer time to recover from glare (Burke, 2002).

Nursing Implications Related to Caring for Patients with Vision Problems

Recommendations include the following:

- Provide adequate lighting in high-traffic areas.
- Recommend motion sensors to turn on lights when an older person walks into a room.
- Look for areas where lighting is inconsistent. Dark or shadowy areas can obscure objects.
- Use proper lampshades to prevent glare.
- Use contrast when painting so that the older person can easily discriminate between walls, floors, and other structural elements of the environment.
- Avoid reflective floors.
- When designing signs, use bright colors such as red, orange, and yellow. Avoid soft blues, grays, and light

greens because the contrast between colors will be poor.

- Use supplementary lamps near work and reading areas.
- Use red-colored tape or paint on the edges of stairs and in entryways to provide warning and signal the need to step up or down.
- Avoid complicated rug patterns that may overwhelm the eye and obscure steps and ledges.

The leading cause of accidental death in persons over the age of 65 is a motor vehicle accident; in those older than 75, it is the second leading cause after falls (Li & Smith, 2003). Therefore, it is very important for elderly adults to have their vision and driving ability screened regularly. In the United States, driving is sometimes seen as a right, and many older people are hesitant to relinquish their driver's licenses because they fear loss of independence.

It is important to be aware of the potential for visual disturbance as a side effect of the following drugs:

- *Hydroxychloroquine (Plaquenil)*—retinopathy, blurred vision, and difficulty focusing
- *Tamoxifen (Nolvadex)*—decreased visual acuity and blurred vision
- *Thioridazine (Mellaril)*—blurred vision, impaired night vision, and color discrimination problems
- *Levodopa*—blurred vision
- *Propranolol*—dry eyes, visual disturbances

Source: Wilson, Shannon, & Stang, 2002.

Visual Problems

Age-related macular degeneration (ARMD) is a degenerative disorder of the macula, which affects both central vision (scotoma) and visual acuity. They often experience blurry vision, central scotomas (blind spots within the visual field), and metamorphopsia in which images are distorted to look smaller (micropsia) or larger (macropsia) than they actually are. Another symptom typical of ARMD is that straight lines appear crooked or wavy. A person with macular degeneration will experience a dark spot in the center of the field of vision and must learn to rely upon and interpret peripheral vision in order to function.

Risk factors for ARMD include the following:

- Age above 50
- Cigarette smoking
- Family history of ARMD
- Increased exposure to ultraviolet light
- Caucasian race and light-colored eyes
- Hypertension or cardiovascular disease
- Lack of dietary intake of antioxidants and zinc

(Fine, Berger, Maguire, & Ho, 2000; Uphold & Graham, 2003)

Treatment and prevention of ARMD with steroid injections, plasmapheresis, and radiation therapy is still under investigation. Currently, there are no treatments for the dry form of ARMD; however, the wet form may benefit from laser treatments to stop neovascularization. Laser therapy may result in secondary vision loss due to collateral damage; however, use of photosensitive dye may decrease damage to the normal retina. Surgery may be another option for some patients, but benefits have been limited (Weston, Aliabadi, & White, 2000).

Cataracts

Cataracts are opacities or yellowing of the lenses. Cataracts cloud the lens, decrease the amount of light able to reach the retina, and inhibit vision. Cataracts are the leading cause of blindness in the world. Ultraviolet light exposure may be a contributing factor to cataract formation.

Patients with cataracts may experience blurry vision, glare, halos around objects, double vision, lack of color contrast or faded colors, and poor night vision. They may need more light or illumination when reading, and repeated alterations of their corrective lens prescriptions (Solomon & Donnenfeld, 2003).

Risk factors for the development of cataracts include the following:

- Increased age
- Smoking and alcohol
- Diabetes, hyperlipidemia
- Trauma to the eye
- Exposure to the sun and UVB rays
- Corticosteroid medications

Surgical removal of the affected lens is generally the treatment of choice because there are no medications to treat this problem (Lee & Beaver, 2003). Corrective lenses that filter out glare may be effective in managing symptoms in the early phases, but do not stop progression of vision loss. Surgical recommendations are made when vision problems interfere with daily activities such as reading and driving. Cataract surgery is recommended in the following circumstances:

- Visual acuity is 20/50 or less with symptoms of loss of functional ability.
- Visual acuity is 20/40 or better with disabling glare or frequent exposure to low light situations, diplopia, disparity between eyes, or occupational need.
- Cataract removal will treat another lens-induced disease such as glaucoma.

- Cataract exists with other diseases of the retina, such as diabetic retinopathy, requiring unrestricted monitoring.

(National Guideline Clearinghouse, 2001)

Glaucoma

Glaucoma is associated with optic nerve damage due to an increase in intraocular pressure (IOP), which can ultimately lead to vision loss. When the IOP is greater than 21 mmHg, the optic nerve has the potential for atrophy and vision loss. The two types of glaucoma are open-angle glaucoma and angle-closure glaucoma (Weston et al., 2000).

Open-angle glaucoma occurs when the flow of aqueous humor through the trabecular meshwork is slowed and eventually builds up.

In angle-closure glaucoma, which is not as common, the angle of the iris obstructs drainage of the aqueous humor through the trabecular meshwork. It may occur suddenly as a result of infection or trauma; symptoms include unilateral headache, visual blurring, nausea, vomiting, and photophobia. Acute-closure glaucoma is an ophthalmic emergency requiring immediate attention by an ophthalmologist to preserve vision (Weston et al., 2000).

Risk factors for glaucoma include the following:

- Increased intraocular pressure
- Older than 60 years of age
- Family history of glaucoma
- Personal history of myopia, diabetes, hypertension, migraines
- African American ancestry (Whitaker, Whitaker, & Dill, 1998)

The American Academy of Ophthalmology (2003) recommends that patients over the age of 65 be examined and screened for glaucoma at least every 1 to 2 years.

Management of glaucoma involves lowering the IOP to stop damage to the optic nerve and prevent further vision loss. Therapy involves medications (oral or topical) to decrease IOP, and/or laser surgery to increase the flow of aqueous humor, by creating a new drainage exit (Weston et al., 2000). Follow-up care with the ophthalmologist is essential to monitor the adequacy of treatment and to ensure that the IOP remains below 20 mmHg. Open-angle glaucoma is usually managed with one or several of the following medications: beta-blockers, miotics, alpha-adrenergic agonists, prostaglandin analogues, and carbonic anhydrase inhibitors. Beta-blockers remain the first-line therapy for glaucoma because they decrease the rate of intraocular fluid production (Weston et al., 2000).

Potential adverse effects of ophthalmic solutions include the following:

- *Beta-blockers (Betagan, Timoptic, Ocupress) (bottles with blue or yellow caps)*. Bradycardia, congestive heart failure, syncope, bronchospasm, depression, confusion, sexual dysfunction.
- *Adrenergics (Lopidine, Alphagan, Epinal) (bottles with purple caps)*. Palpitation, hypertension, tremor, sweating.
- *Miotics/cholinesterase inhibitors (pilocarpine, Humorsol) (bottles with green caps)*. Bronchospasm, salivation, nausea, vomiting, diarrhea, abdominal pain, lacrimation.
- *Carbonic anhydrase inhibitors (Trusopt, Azopt) (bottles with orange caps)*. Fatigue, renal failure,

hypokalemia, diarrhea, depression, exacerbation of chronic obstructive pulmonary disease.

- *Prostaglandin analogues (Xalatan, Lumigan).* Changes in eye color and periorbital tissues, itching.

(Epocrates.com, 2003; Reuben et al., 2002)

When administering eyedrops it is important for the nurse to first wash his or her hands, ask the patient to tip the head backward and look upward, then slightly pull the lower lid down to make a small pouch. The nurse should try not to drop the medication directly onto the eye but rather into the eyelid pouch to prevent a violent blink reflex and excessive tearing. Do not contaminate the dropper by touching it to the eye, and wait several minutes before administering an additional dose of the same medication or a second medication to allow time for complete absorption and prevent additional medication from simply running out of the eye. The nurse should provide the patient with a facial tissue to blot any medication or tears that may run down the cheek, and when finished, wash the hands carefully again.

Diabetic Retinopathy

Diabetic retinopathy is a microvascular disease of the eye occurring in both type 1 and type 2 diabetes.

Prevention of diabetic retinopathy is dependent on tight glycemic control in addition to managing hypertension and hyperlipidemia. Goals of treatment for patients with diabetes include maintaining an average preprandial blood glucose of 80 to 120 mg/dl, an average bedtime capillary blood glucose of 100 to 140 mg/dl, and an Hemoglobin (HA_{1c}) of less than 7. Patients should be referred for ophthalmic examination after diagnosis of diabetes, and recommendations for follow-up will be made at that time (Lee & Beaver, 2003). Patients with diabetic retinopathy experience gradual vision loss with generalized blurring and areas of focal vision loss.

Treatment involves laser therapy for both types of retinopathy. Laser therapy can repair leaking micro-aneurysms, reducing the amount of ocular edema. Neo-vascularization may also be halted through the use of laser therapy, decreasing the risk of retinal detachment, hemorrhage, and neovascular glaucoma.

HEARING

Hearing loss related to normal aging is the most common cause, but other risk factors include the following:

- Long-term exposure to excessive noise
- Impacted **cerumen** (earwax)
- Ototoxic medications
- Tumors
- Diseases that affect sensorineural hearing
- Smoking
- History of middle ear infection
- Chemical exposure (e.g., long duration of exposure to trichloroethylene)

Age-Related Changes

In the older adult, cerumen tends to be drier and harder and tends to accumulate in the ear canal due to de-creased activity of the apocrine glands. Hearing may become impaired if cerumen accumulates to impact the canal. Dryness of the canal can also cause pruritus, and the epithelial lining of the ear canal may be easily irri-tated and injured if anything is inserted into the ear, in-creasing the risk of infection (Hazzard, Blass, Ettinger, Halter, & Ouslander, 1999).

About one third of all hearing impairments are at least partially attributable to damage from exposure to loud sounds. Sounds that are sufficiently loud to damage sensitive inner ear structures can produce hearing loss that is not reversible. Virtually all of the structures of the ear can be damaged, in particular the organ of Corti, the delicate sensory structure of the auditory portion of the inner ear (cochlea), which may be torn apart.

Types of Hearing Loss

A thorough history and physical examination is important to help determine the cause of the hearing loss. It may be conductive, due to the external aspect of the ear, or sensorineural from inner ear problems.

Conductive hearing loss is related to a problem in the external or middle ear canal, tympanic membrane, bones in the outer and middle ear, or the ossicles (Marcincuk & Roland, 2002). This type of hearing loss may be a result of an external ear infection (otitis externa), impacted cerumen, middle ear infection (otitis media), benign tumors or carcinoma, perforation of the tympanic membrane, foreign bodies, or otosclerosis (a disease affecting the mobility of the middle ear bones) (Marcincuk & Roland, 2002).

An occlusion of cerumen can greatly affect hearing, as sound is unable to reach the inner ear (Marcincuk & Roland, 2002). Examination of the ear canal for cerumen impaction is recommended as part of routine preventive healthcare screening for older adults. The person with cerumen impaction may complain of a feeling of fullness or itching in the ear canal. In addition to hearing loss, cerumen may also cause tinnitus, ear pain, or vertigo.

Contraindications for cerumen removal include perforated tympanic membrane, ear trauma, tumors, and cholesteatoma. Use extreme caution in patients with diabetes due to the increased risk for infection.

Two common methods for removal of cerumen from the ear canal are:

- *Curette.* A small instrument with a scoop on the end is inserted into the ear canal while the helix is lifted posteriorly and laterally. The tip of the curette is placed over the top of the impacted cerumen and pulled forward. It is helpful to use both hands and wear a headlamp to provide bright light to visualize the canal as much as possible. The advantage of this method is that no water is needed and therefore there is a lower risk of infection. The disadvantage is that the procedure requires a greater degree of skill, and the risk of injury to the tympanic membrane or ear canal is greater.

- *Lavage or irrigation.* Some nurses like to soften the cerumen for up to 3 days before attempting irrigation with mineral oil or Debrox eardrops up to three times daily. Irrigation is the simpler and more straightforward approach to cerumen removal. However, because it is a blind procedure, the risk exists that water and infectious agents could be pushed through a perforated tympanic membrane into the middle ear space.

Contraindications to ear lavage or irrigation include history of ear surgery and history of otitis externa (swimmer's ear). It is safer to make a referral to an ear, nose, and throat specialist.

To irrigate, the following equipment is needed: a clean bulb syringe, a clean container of warm water or saline solution, an emesis basin, an otoscope, and lots of towels.

The tip of a bulb-irrigation syringe is placed into the external canal. Water should be warmed to 37°C. The nurse can make sure the water is not too hot by testing it on the inside of a wrist. A plastic cape can be used to protect the patient's clothing. Place gentle pressure on the syringe and aim the water stream posteriorly to wash the impacted cerumen away from the tympanic membrane. It is important to avoid getting air into the syringe as it will sound deafening to the patient and will terrify a patient with a cognitive impairment. Pulling the helix of the ear upward and outward will straighten the ear canal. Use the otoscope to check progress and stop the irrigation when you can visualize the tympanic membrane. If the patient experiences discomfort, the nurse should stop. Large pieces of cerumen will be apparent in the emesis basin. Following irrigation, swab, and dry the canal carefully to reduce the risk of infection. Some nurses use a water jet dental device, but this is risky because the water pressure cannot be controlled and damage to the tympanic membrane may occur.

Because of the risk of tympanic membrane perforation or damage to the lining of the ear canal, the curette method should be performed only by an advanced practice nurse, physician, or gerontological nurse with specialized training and experience. Neither the curette nor irrigation method should be attempted if a perforated tympanic membrane is present or suspected.

Use only sterilized equipment to avoid spreading bacteria and possibly infection from one patient to another during ear irrigation for cerumen impaction.

Sensorineural hearing loss is a manifestation of problems within the inner ear. Sound is transmitted to the inner ear, but problems with the cochlea and auditory nerve (eighth cranial nerve) create sound distortion. Causes of this type of hearing loss include **presbycusis** (loss of hearing due to age-related changes in the inner ear), damage due to excessive noise exposure,

Meniere's disease, tumors, and infections (Danner & Harris, 2003).

The American Speech-Language-Hearing Association recommends that asymptomatic adults should be screened every 10 years until the age of 50, and every 3 years thereafter with an audiometric battery test (Jackler, 2003). Evaluation of hearing loss is dependent on a thorough history and physical examination. Inspect the auricle for lumps, lesions, and deformities. Examine the ear canal with an otoscope. If the tympanic membrane is not obstructed it will appear as a smooth, pearly gray object at the end of the ear canal. Carefully document all findings. A red bulging membrane is a sign of a middle ear infection and requires immediate referral to a physician or advanced practice nurse.

Assessing Hearing Loss

Patients whose hearing does not resolve after treatment of an ear infection, removal of cerumen, or discontinuation of ototoxic medications; patients with sudden unexplained hearing loss; and those with abnormal unilateral Rinne or Weber tests should be referred to an audiologist (Bogardus, Yueh, & Shekelle, 2003).

Hearing Aids

Hearing aids amplify sounds and deliver them directly into the ear. Improvements have made them smaller and more discreet. Gerontological nurses should be aware of the cleaning, inserting, and troubleshooting involved with hearing aids. The first priority is to identify patients wearing hearing aids on admission to the hospital or nursing home and make an appropriate notation on each patient's nursing care plan. It is helpful to note the type, model number, and serial number of the hearing aid in case it should become lost. The working condition of the hearing aid is then assessed. Assessment parameters include:

- *Integrity of the ear mold.* Are there cracks or rough areas? Is there a good fit?
- *Battery.* Use a battery tester if one is available. Is the battery inserted correctly with clean contacts?
- *Dials.* Are they clean? Easily rotated? Does the patient report variation of volume when the volume dial is moved?
- *Switches.* Do they easily turn on and off? Is there excessive static or feedback?
- *Tubing for behind the ear aids.* Are there cracks? Is there good connection to the earpiece?

(Modified from Palumbo, 2000)

Each evening at bedtime, the hearing aid should be removed and cleansed with warm water or saline and a cotton pad. Harsh soaps or alcohol should not be used, as they will degrade the plastic. Any cerumen should be carefully removed from the earpiece while still soft. The battery should be disengaged from the contacts and the hearing aid stored securely in its case in a safe place. Frequent inventory and labeling will assist the staff to keep track of these expensive and difficult-to-replace items.

The U.S. Food and Drug Administration (FDA) has approved implantable hearing devices (cochlear implants) for older adults with moderate to severe sensorineural hearing loss. The device allows many people who were previously unable to do so to speak on the telephone, thus improving safety and quality of life.

Assistive Listening Devices

Many theaters are equipped with assistive listening devices that amplify the performers' voices by the use of small microphones and then transmit them to headphones or earpieces that are worn in the ear. A telecommunications device for the deaf (TDD) is an assistive device that allows telephone conversation for a deaf person via a keyboard that transmits signals over the telephone wires to another person with a TDD receiver. The use of computers and e-mail has greatly assisted many deaf people to communicate with the hearing world.

Common Hearing Problems in Older Persons

Tinnitus (ringing in the ears) can occur with or without hearing loss and is associated with increased age. Causes of tinnitus are medications, infections, neurological conditions, and disorders related to hearing loss (Lockwood, Salvi, & Burkard, 2002).

A thorough history including a complete description of the sound is extremely important to assist in determining the cause. The underlying condition that may be causing the tinnitus must first be addressed.

No drugs have yet been approved by the FDA to treat tinnitus specifically; however, benzodiazepines and tricyclic antidepressants have been shown to be effective (Danner & Harris, 2003). Approved therapies include tinnitus retraining therapy, relaxation, biofeedback, and masking devices to cover up the sounds (Lockwood et al., 2002).

Box 12–1 provides tips for communicating with older persons who have hearing impairments.

If a patient on one or more of the following drugs reports a change in hearing, be suspicious of a drug side effect:

- Aminoglycoside antibiotics (gentamicin)—ototoxic
- Antineoplastics (cisplatin)—ototoxic
- Loop diuretics (furosemide)—ototoxic

Box 12–1 Nursing Interventions to Use When Speaking with a Hearing Impaired Individual

- Eliminate extraneous noise in the room. For example, turn the television or radio down or off.
- Stand 2 to 3 feet from the patient.
- Have the patient's attention before speaking. Touch lightly on the arm or shoulder if needed.
- Try to lower the pitch of your voice.
- Pause at the end of each phrase or sentence.
- If the patient has a hearing aid, provide assistance with the device, plus glasses if needed.
- Assess the illumination in the room and make sure that the patient can see you. Face the patient at all times during the conversation.
- The patient may read lips, so it is important not to cover your mouth or chew gum. Do not speak into the chart or converse with someone over your shoulder. The patient will misinterpret your message.
- Speak slowly and clearly in a normal tone of voice—do not shout.
- If the patient does not understand your message, rephrase it rather than repeating the same words.
- Gestures, if appropriate, may help.
- Use written communication if the patient is able to see and read.
- Ask the patient for an oral or written response to determine if the communication was successful.

Source: Reuben, D., Herr, K. Pacala, J. Potter, J., Pollock, B., & Selma, T. (2002). "*Geriatrics at Your Fingertips.*" *Copyright © 2002* Blackwell Publishing. Reprinted with permission.

- Baclofen—tinnitus
- Propranolol (Inderal)—tinnitus and hearing loss

(Source: Jackler, 2003; Wilson et al., 2002; Epocrates. com, 2003)

TASTE

A diminished sense of taste, **hypogeusia,** is a normal sensory change usually occurring after the age of 70. Many nerves are responsible for transmitting taste information to the brain, including cranial nerves VII, IX, and X. Taste buds are continually bathed in secretions from the salivary glands, and excessive dryness can distort taste sensation.

Additional factors that may influence alterations in taste include oral condition, olfactory function, medications, diseases, surgical interventions, poorly fittting dentures and environmental exposure (McCague, 1999).

Medications can alter taste sensation by affecting peripheral receptors and chemosensory pathways (Schiffman, 1997). Drugs known to alter taste include antibiotics, antidepressants, lipid lowering agents, and NSAIDS.

Nursing Assessment of the Older Patient with Taste Disturbances

A thorough assessment of the head and neck should be performed to rule out obvious deformity, injury, infection, or obstruction. Mucous membranes should be assessed for dryness, ulceration, or presence of candidiasis. If the patient wears dentures, they should be removed in order to thoroughly inspect the gums.

There are no pharmacological treatments to improve taste; however, seasonings and additives to enhance flavor and aroma may amplify taste. Encouraging patients to alternate and eat the different foods on their plate rather than sticking to one food may decrease sensory exhaustion.

Xerostomia, or dry mouth, occurs with salivary gland dysfunction. Conditions that may induce xerostomia include systemic diseases (diabetes, HIV, Alzheimer's disease), radiation, medications (anticholinergic drugs), and Sjögren's syndrome. The leading cause of dry mouth in the geriatric population is a result of medication.

Implications of dry mouth include altered taste, difficulty swallowing (dysphagia), periodontal disease (dental caries, gingivitis, oral lesions), speech difficulties, dry lips, halitosis, and sleeping problems (Ship et al., 2002). Speech and eating difficulties may be embarrassing and discourage individuals from wanting to socialize, ostracizing themselves from loved ones (Ship et al., 2002).

Management of xerostomia involves good oral care, regular dental examinations, and a diet low in sugar. Over-the-counter artificial saliva, oral lubricants, and drinking fluids with meals may help relieve symptoms and dysphagia. Using a humidifier adds moisture to the air and can help with xerostomia that may interfere with sleep. Pilocarpine (Salagen) and cevimeline (Evoxac) are both secretagogues approved by the FDA to relieve symptoms associated with xerostomia (Ship et al., 2002).

SMELL

Olfactory dysfunction is more common than taste dysfunction. The three most common causes of loss of smell are nasal and sinus disease, upper respiratory infection, and head trauma (Bromley, 2000).

Similar to taste disturbances, poor dentition can inhibit olfactory perception if food is not chewed properly because most flavors are perceived retronasally. Dentures covering the soft palate can also block aroma from reaching these receptors (McCague, 1999).

Nursing Assessment of the Older Patient with Disturbances of Smell

Patients with obvious deficits in smell who cannot identify familiar smells like coffee and vanilla should be referred to their primary care provider, an otolaryngologist, and a neurologist of a specialized smell or taste center, usually housed in a large medical center.

PHYSICAL SENSATION

As people age, tactile sensation diminishes, in addition to the ability to detect temperature extremes (Watson, 2000). Loss of physical sensation may be harmful for older adults because it increases their risk for injury. Inability to feel the heat of bath or shower water may lead to harmful burns. Injuries or infections may go unnoticed in the lower extremities, delaying needed treatment. Certain medical diagnoses such as diabetes mellitus are associated with peripheral neuropathies that can further decrease touch sensation.

Sedating medications can decrease touch sensation by clouding the sensorium and inducing lethargy. Patients taking opioids require additional supervision and monitoring to ensure that foot ulcers or other injuries do not occur without apparent notice.

Nursing Assessment of the Older Person with Diminished Tactile Impairment

Touch is usually assessed using a wisp of cotton. Patients are asked to close their eyes and nod or say "yes" when they are touched on the face, upper back, and extremities. A cotton swab can also be used with the wooden end pressed lightly against the skin for a sensation of "sharp" and the cotton end for the sensation of "dull." The patient's ability to discriminate between one and two points can also be assessed using the wooden ends of a cotton swab. Deficits in touch may be referred for further evaluation to the patient's primary care provider or a neurologist.

For patients with impaired sense of touch, nursing interventions could focus on continuous monitoring of the intactness of the skin, assessment of safety risks, and the development of a safety plan with instructions to minimize injury. Water heaters should be turned down to 110°F to prevent scalding. Protective padding of upper and lower extremities can prevent bruising and protect skin integrity. Older patients with diabetes mellitus should place a mirror on the wall close to the floor, remove their shoes, and examine the bottom of their feet daily for blisters, redness, or ulcerations. The use of a good strong light will ease the process and compensate for visual impairment.

Advise all older persons to use heating pads on the "low" setting only. Serious burns can result from use of the higher settings.

PATIENT-FAMILY TEACHING GUIDELINES

The following are guidelines that the nurse may find useful when instructing older persons and their families about vision problems (adapted from National Institute on Aging, 2004).

1. How can I protect my eyes as I get older?

   With aging, vision problems become more common. Some are serious and some are easily treated. The best way to protect your eyes is to:

   - Have regular eye examinations every 1 to 2 years.
   - Find out if you are at high risk for vision loss (diagnosis of diabetes, family history of eye disease, hypertension).

(continued)

- Wear sunglasses and a wide brim hat. This will protect your eyes from the sun and prevent cataracts.
- See an eye professional at once if you have loss or dimness of eyesight, eye pain, double vision, swelling, or redness of the eyes.

2. What are some common eye complaints experienced by older people?

   Some common complaints include:

   Floaters
   - These are tiny spots that float across your eyes. They are usually normal but if you see floaters with spots or flashes, call your eye care professional right away.

   Tearing
   - This can result from light sensitivity or dry eye as your body tries to compensate by producing excess tears.

   Eyelid problems
   - Pain, itching, tearing, drooping, or irritation can be corrected with eyedrops or minor surgery.

   Conjunctivitis
   - Also called pink eye, this condition results from allergies or infection. It is easily treated with eyedrops.

   Presbyopia
   - This is the loss of ability to see close objects or small print. Reading glasses can usually correct the problem.

3. What can I do to function better if I have low vision?

   Low-vision adaptations can help you to carry out your normal routines. See a low-vision expert for help choosing the right product because they are not all covered by insurance and can be expensive. Most clinics will let you try out some devices to improve your function at home for a week or so before you make the decision to buy them. Simple things you can do at home include:

- Write with bold felt-tip markers.
- Put colored tape on the edge of steps to prevent falls.
- Use contrast whenever possible, like light furniture on dark floors, red dishes on a light-colored table, and so on.
- Use motion lights that turn on by themselves when you walk into a room and timers that turn on lights at dusk.
- Use telephones, clocks, and watches with large numbers.
- Have several pairs of magnifying glasses around the house so that you can set the microwave, adjust the TV, and read the mail easily.
- Use appropriate assistive devices and environmental interventions to improve safety, functional ability, and quality of life.

4. I think I am getting a little hard of hearing. Is this common at my age?

Yes, about one third of Americans over 60 have hearing problems. It is important to get testing and find out the severity of your problem. See your doctor if:

- You cannot hear on the phone.
- It is hard to keep up with a conversation when several people are talking.
- You need to turn the TV up so loud others complain.
- You have trouble hearing women and children talking.

(continued)

5. What causes hearing loss?

   Many things such as earwax, noise exposure over a long period of time, viral or bacterial infections, heredity, certain medications, and other factors cause hearing loss. The only way to know is to see a doctor for examination and testing.

6. How can I help myself to overcome my hearing loss?

   Some tips include:
   - Look at people's faces when they speak.
   - Ask people to speak slowly and clearly.
   - Read facial expressions like grins or frowns.
   - Be patient and ask people to repeat if you do not hear the first time.
   - Use a hearing aid if you need it.

7. I have a decreased sense of touch and smell. What should I be concerned about?

   The main issue is safety. Our sense of touch and smell alert us to dangers in the environment like smoke from a fire or spoiled food in the refrigerator. It is a good idea to see an ear, nose, and throat doctor for further testing if you have problems with smell, and an internist or neurologist for problems with touch. Some of these problems can be treated and your safety improved.

Box 12–2 Home Safety Inventory— Older Person

Safety Consideration	Yes	No
Lighting adequate on stairs?	[ ]	[ ]
Stair rails present and in good repair?	[ ]	[ ]
Nonskid surfaces on stairs?	[ ]	[ ]
Throw rugs present safety hazard?	[ ]	[ ]
Crowded living area presents safety hazard?	[ ]	[ ]
Tub rails installed?	[ ]	[ ]
Tub has nonslip surface?	[ ]	[ ]
Space heaters present safety hazard?	[ ]	[ ]
Adequate provision made for refrigeration of food?	[ ]	[ ]
Medications kept in appropriately labeled containers with readable print?	[ ]	[ ]
Toxic substances have labels with readable print and are stored well away from food?	[ ]	[ ]
Home is adequately ventilated and heated?	[ ]	[ ]
Neighborhood is safe?	[ ]	[ ]
Fire and police notified of older person in home?	[ ]	[ ]

Source: Clark, M. J. C. (2002). *Community health nursing: Caring for populations* (4th ed.). Upper Saddle River, NJ: Prentice Hall.

CHAPTER 13

THE CARDIOVASCULAR SYSTEM

STRUCTURE AND FUNCTION

The heart is a four-chambered organ slightly left of the sternum. The two upper chambers of the heart are the atria. The two lower chambers of the heart are the ventricles. The ventricles generate power to pump blood through the body systems to which they are connected. The cardiac cycle is the sequence and timing of contraction and relaxation in the heart.

The amount of blood pumped from the left ventricle with each beat is the **stroke volume.** The amount pumped per minute is the **cardiac output.** This value is reflective of overall functioning of the heart. It can be calculated using the following formula:

cardiac output = heart rate × stroke volume

With aging and the diagnosis of cardiovascular disease, it is important to know how efficiently the heart is able to pump blood throughout the body. The blood pumped from the left ventricle at the end of diastole with each beat is not the full volume of the blood in the ventricle. The proportion that is pumped is the ejection fraction. Its formula is:

ejection fraction = stroke volume/end diastolic
volume of left ventricle

The higher the ejection fraction, the more efficiently the heart is able to provide adequate circulation to the body systems.

The Electrocardiogram

The electrocardiogram (ECG) can offer valuable information about the cardiac function and electrical regulation of the heart. The ideal ECG deflections represent depolarization and repolarization of cardiac muscle tissue in a regular pattern and rhythm. The waves of interest include the P, QRS, and T waves. The P wave represents atrial depolarization. The PR interval represents delay in conduction at the AV node. The QRS complex represents ventricular depolarization. The T wave represents ventricular repolarization. A diagram of a normal ECG is illustrated in Figure 13–1.

Cardiac Circulation

The two coronary arteries arise from the aorta just above the aortic valve. The left coronary artery branches to become the left anterior descending and the circumflex artery. The right coronary artery supplies the right side of the heart. The coronary arteries travel on the outside of the heart, and the branches penetrate to the deeper layers of muscle. Atherosclerotic changes in the coronary arteries and the plaque accumulation of coronary artery disease can result in myocardial ischemia, myocardial infarction, and sudden death.

The heart is surrounded by the pericardium, a double-walled sac filled with a small amount of fluid. Increased fluid in the pericardium is called *cardiac tamponade* and can result in cardiac compression and death.

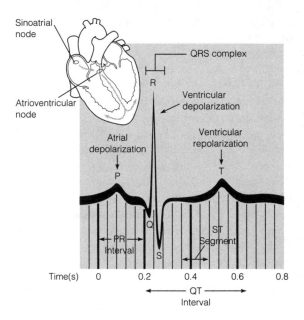

Figure 13–1 ■ Normal electrocardiogram.

NORMAL CHANGES WITH AGING

Many older women will complain of vague symptoms when having a myocardial infarction, including fatigue, sleep disturbances, and epigastric pain. Heart valves become stiff with aging as the result of fibrosis and calcification. In addition, changes in the valve rings can contribute to stenosis or incompetence. (Reuben et al., 2004).

Resting heart rate is relatively unchanged with normal aging. In the absence of disease, cardiac output is not much changed. The older heart cannot respond to stressful stimuli as well as the younger heart. Fibrosis of the AV node can lead to AV block with no other cardiac pathology. The AV node refractory period is also increased with aging. The electrocardiogram shows no specific changes with age, although some lengthening of the PR, QRS, and QT interval has been described. The stress of illness can precipitate conduction difficulties for the older person (Craven, 2000). New-onset atrial fibrillation and other arrythmias may signal the onset of serious underlying illness such as hyperthyroidism, electrolyte disturbances, or myocardial infarction.

The vascular system undergoes a range of changes with aging. Blood pressure elevation frequently occurs with aging, although it is not considered a normal variant. Isolated systolic hypertension (systolic >140 mmHg) is frequently seen in the older person.

Renal function declines with age, and the kidneys decrease in size and weight. With aging, decreased levels of renin and aldosterone are found in the plasma. This leads to an increased sensitivity to dietary sodium consumption. Decreased ability to clear sodium from the blood can lead to body water overload. This increased preload can tax the myocardium.

COMMON ILLNESSES WITH OLDER PERSONS

Hypertension

JNC 7 (Joint National Committee on Prevention, Detection, Evaluation, and Treatment of High Blood Pressure, 2003) has defined hypertension in stages (see Table 13–1). When the systolic and diastolic of a particular reading fall in different categories, the higher category should be identified. Isolated systolic hypertension is common in the older person. It is defined as systolic blood pressure greater than 140 mmHg.

Table 13–1 Classification of Blood Pressure

Category	Systolic Pressure (mmHg)	Diastolic Pressure (mmHg)
Optimal	<120	<80
Prehypertension	120–139	80–89
Hypertension		
Stage 1	140–159	90–99
Stage 2	≥160	≥100

Source: Adapted from Joint National Committee, 2003.

Highlights from the JNC 7 report include the following:

- In persons older than 50 years, systolic blood pressure greater than 140 mmHg is a much more important cardiovascular disease (CVD) risk factor than diastolic blood pressure.
- The risk of CVD beginning at 115/75 mmHg doubles with each increment of 20/10 mmHg; individuals who are normotensive at age 55 have a 90% lifetime risk for developing hypertension.
- Individuals with a systolic blood pressure of 120 to 139 mmHg or a diastolic blood pressure of 80 to 89 mmHg should be considered as prehypertensive and require health-promoting lifestyle modifications to prevent CVD.
- Thiazide-type diuretics should be used in drug treatment for most patients with uncomplicated hypertension, either alone or combined with drugs from other classes. Certain high-risk conditions are compelling indications for the initial use of other anti-hypertensive drug classes (angiotensin-converting

enzyme inhibitors, angiotensin receptor blockers, beta-blockers, calcium channel blockers).

- Most patients with hypertension will require two or more antihypertensive medications to achieve goal blood pressure (<140/90 mmHg, or <130/80 mmHg for patients with diabetes or chronic kidney disease).
- If blood pressure is more than 20/10 mmHg above goal blood pressure, consideration should be given to initiating therapy with two agents, one of which usually should be a thiazide-type diuretic.
- The most effective therapy prescribed by the most careful clinician will control hypertension only if patients are motivated. Motivation improves when patients have positive experiences with, and trust in, the clinician.
- Empathy builds trust and is a potent motivator (Joint National Committee, 2003).

Non-Hispanic Black men and women at almost every age group have higher blood pressures than other racial cohorts (National Heart, Lung, and Blood Institute, 2004). It is not known if the cause of this higher incidence is genetic or environmental.

Because changes of aging cause the baroreceptors to be less efficient, it is essential to check postural blood pressures in older patients to prevent postural hypotension and falls.

Untreated hypertension results in several physical changes in the body including arterial narrowing and stiffness, left ventricular hypertrophy, damage to the kidney resulting in proteinuria, hemorrhages and exudates in the retina leading to vision loss, and stroke. Stroke is the number one cause of disability and the number three cause of death in the United States (Cunningham, 2000a).

Assessment of the patient with hypertension includes accurate blood pressure monitoring. The nurse should record pressures in both upper extremities and in the positions of lying, sitting, and standing. Assessment should also include looking for evidence of target organ damage with ophthalmic examination and urinalysis for proteinuria. For blood pressure that develops suddenly or is refractory to treatment, secondary hypertension should be considered and immediate medical referral and evaluation is indicated.

Management of hypertension includes: life style changes, weight loss, and following the Dietary Approaches to Stop Hypertension (DASH) diet. Beginning an exercise program, stopping smoking, and reducing alcohol intake are also effective measures to lower blood pressure (Cunningham, 2000a).

The nurse's role in caring for older patients with hypertension is to screen for high blood pressure in a variety of community settings and to promote healthy lifestyles through low-fat and low-sodium diets, exercise, smoking cessation, and controlled alcohol consumption. Another important role is to teach older patients who are diagnosed with hypertension about the importance of staying on medications even though they do not feel any different, or perhaps feel worse because of side effects. Monitoring the effect of medication and determining barriers to healthy living are important in supporting the patient in self-management.

Hypotension

Hypotension (low blood pressure) is a frequent side effect of many cardiovascular conditions and many medications. Diagnosis of orthostatic hypertension can be made by having the patient maintain a supine position for at least 5 minutes. The nurse should check the blood pressure while the patient is supine, and 1 and 3 minutes after sitting or standing. If the pressure drops as much as 20 mmHg systolic or 10 mmHg diastolic, postural hypotension exists (Stone & Wyman, 1999).

Medications that can cause postural hypotension include alpha-adrenergic blockers, centrally acting antihypertensive agents, psychotropic drugs and tranquilizers, high-dose antibiotics, and nonsteroidal anti-inflammatory drugs (NSAIDs). Patients who experience hypotension can be taught to rise slowly from a lying or sitting position, to use a cane or walker if unsteady, and to drink water, unless restricted, to maintain blood volume (Reuben et al., 2004).

Hyperlipidemia

Elevated cholesterol has been shown to be a risk factor for the development of cardiovascular disorders. LDLs have been shown to be the type of lipid associated with increased risk for mortality or morbidity. HDLs have been shown to have a beneficial effect on overall vascular health, probably because they help to mobilize cholesterol from the blood vessels and carry it back to the liver for processing.

The Heart Protection Study (HPS) has also shown that controlling LDL with simvastatin assists in the prevention of coronary heart disease. Patients taking statins should be taught to report muscle aches and symptoms to their healthcare provider as this may be a signal of the development of a dangerous side effect.

Other medications useful in reducing serum cholesterol are most often used to augment the effect of the statins and include bile acid sequestrants, fibrates, and nicotinic acid.

Table 13-2 Medications Used For the Management of Hypertension

Medication Group	Sample Drugs	Reason to Choose	Side Effects/Precautions
Diuretics	Hydrochlorothiazide (HydroDIURIL) Furosemide (Lasix) Bumetanide (Bumex) Spironolactone (Aldactone) Triamterene (Dyrenium)	Good first-line agent, inexpensive, useful with heart failure	Can increase cholesterol and glucose, uric acid, decrease potassium hyperkalemia
Adrenergic inhibitors Beta-blockers	Acebutolol (Sectral) Atenolol (Tenormin) Betaxolol (Kerlone) Metoprolol (Lopressor, Toprol-XL) Nadolol (Corgard) Penbutolol sulfate (Levatol) Propranolol HCl (Inderal) Timolol HCl (Blocadren)	Coexisting coronary artery disease, angina, arrhythmias, post-myocardial infarction	Asthma exacerbation, bradycardia, reduced peripheral circulation, fatigue, decreased exercise tolerance

Drug Class	Agents	Indications	Side Effects
Adrenergic inhibitors Alpha-blockers	Doxazosin mesylate (Cardura) Prazosin HCl (Minipress) Terazosin HCl (Hytrin)	Dyslipidemia, benign prostatic hypertrophy	Postural hypotension bronchospasm
Adrenergic inhibitors Combined alpha- and beta-blockers	Carvedilol (Coreg)	Heart failure	Postural hypotension
Adrenergic inhibitors Centrally acting inhibitors	Clonidine HCl (Catapres) Guanfacine HCl (Tenex) Methyldopa (Aldomet)		Sedation, dry mouth bradycardia
ACE inhibitors	Benazepril HCl (Lotensin) Captopril (Capoten) Enalapril maleate (Vasotec) Fosinopril Na (Monopril) Lisinopril (Prinivil, Zestril) Moexipril (Univasc) Quinapril HCl (Accupril) Ramipril (Altace) Trandolapril (Mavik)	Diabetes mellitus, heart failure, renal insufficiency	Dry cough angioedema, hyperkalemia

(continued)

Table 13-2 Medications Used For the Management of Hypertension (continued)

Medication Group	Sample Drugs	Reason to Choose	Side Effects/Precautions
Angiotensin receptor blockers	Losartan K (Cozaar) Valsartan (Diovan) Irbesartan (Avapro)	Heart failure	Angioedema, hyperkalemia
Calcium channel blockers Nonhydropyridines	Diltiazem HCl (Cardizem SR) Verapamil (Isoptin, Calan, Verelan Covera)	Angina Atrial tachycardia	Slows conduction, decreased cardiac output
Dihydropyridines	Amlodipine besylate (Norvasc) Felodipine (Plendil) Isradipine (DynaCirc) Nicardipine (Cardene SR) Nifedipine (Procardia XL, Adalat CC) Nisoldipine (Sular)	Isolated systolic hypertension	Ankle edema, flushing, headache
Vasodilators	Hydralazine HCl (Apresoline) Minoxidil (Loniten)		Headache, tachycardia fluid retention

Source: Data from Cunningham, 2000a, pp. 796, 798–799.

Note: Information pertinent to full group presented first. Specific information on line right of drug name.

Angina

Patients with stable angina report chest pain that is relieved with rest. It is precipitated by activities that increase the workload on the heart. Angina is frequently managed with sublingual nitroglycerin, which causes vasodilation and increases blood flow to the heart. Patients who need multiple doses of nitrates every day can be placed on long-term nitrate therapy. Symptoms that are not relieved with rest or medication can indicate progression of the angina or myocardial infarction. This requires immediate medical intervention. Unstable angina occurs when angina is not relieved with rest or medication. It indicates a progression of the coronary artery disease.

Prinzmetal's angina or atypical angina is less common and is characterized by chest pain experienced at rest. The pain is not relieved with nitroglycerin, but does not usually progress to myocardial infarction. It is thought to be caused by transient coronary artery constriction.

The development of coronary heart disease is related to identifiable risk factors, some of which are modifiable. Nurses can help older patients with angina by supporting lifestyle change and by teaching proper medication usage.

Myocardial Infarction

Clot development within a coronary artery can cause blockage in blood flow resulting in myocardial cell death or myocardial infarction (MI). Ischemia is reversible, but cell death is not.

The diagnosis of MIs involves good history and physical assessment as well as laboratory and electrocardiographic analysis. Focus on the presence of chest pain and accompanying symptoms including nausea or vomiting, weakness, shortness of breath, diaphoresis, confusion, or syncope.

Electrocardiographic changes associated with MI include ST segment elevation in the leads associated with the area of the infarct. New bundle branch blocks can be seen with widened QRS complexes. The presence of a Q wave (a 1-mm negative deflection before the QRS complex) indicates infarcted tissue. Q waves persist after recovery from MI, so one cannot assume that a Q wave represents a new or recent event (Del Bene & Vaughan, 2000).

Laboratory findings consistent with MI include creatine kinase (CK) and the specific enzyme found in heart muscle (CK-MB) elevation 4 to 6 hours after tissue necrosis. Troponin levels rise 6 to 8 hours after infarct. Lactate dehydrogenase is elevated later with a peak at 36 hours after infarct. This is important to remember because patients frequently fail to report significant events when they occur and only mention the problem later or after they feel bad for a day or two (Del Bene & Vaughan, 2000).

Immediate complications of MI include arrhythmia and blockages of electrical conduction, heart failure with possible pulmonary edema, and extension of an infarct. Long-term complications from MI include ventricular aneurysms and pericarditis, an inflammation of the pericardial space resulting in pain.

New medications that can dissolve clots in evolution can prevent permanent loss of myocardial cells if they are used within the first several hours of the myocardial event. These clot-busting drugs can result in sudden and excessive bleeding. Patients with risk factors for MI should be taught to report any change in symptom pattern promptly so that they can receive appropriate therapy. Many cardiologists advise older patients with symptoms of heart attack to chew one aspirin while waiting for the ambulance to arrive.

Some patients benefit from coronary angioplasty procedures, which can be done when unstable angina develops or at the time of MI. This procedure is relatively noninvasive. By threading a balloon-tipped catheter into the coronary artery, the blockage of the artery can be opened. Stents or mechanical supports to keep the artery open can be placed during angioplasty.

If an MI does occur, patients are usually admitted to the hospital for monitoring of hemodynamic status and for arrhythmias. Patients will receive oxygen therapy, pain control, and antiarrhythmic drugs as needed. The nurse's role is to monitor for changes in the patient's condition and treat complications from MI using protocols or to refer to the cardiologist for treatment. After the initial insult is survived, a cardiac rehabilitation program can be designed to offer gradual, supervised increase in activity and to support other healthy lifestyle changes.

Many medications that are important during the evolving MI event and following recovery are useful in other cardiovascular conditions. These medications include beta-blockers, ACE inhibitors and aspirin or warfarin. However, patients at risk for falling may not be appropriate for warfarin therapy because anticoagulated patients who fall can sustain life-threatening bleeds.

Valvular Heart Disease

The most common valve disorder in the older person is aortic stenosis. Angina can be experienced because blood has difficulty perfusing a thickened myocardium. Syncope can occur because of reduced blood flow to the brain. Orthostatic changes in blood pressure can also reflect a low cardiac output. Increased ventricular and atrial arrhythmias can also occur.

The diagnosis of aortic stenosis is begun during the history and physical examination. Progressive shortness of breath should indicate that aortic stenosis is a possible diagnosis. On physical examination, the murmur of aortic stenosis can be detected as a systolic ejection murmur heard most prominently in the second intercostal space. As the condition progresses, the murmur may decrease as less blood is being pumped forward. Jugular venous pressure is normal unless heart failure has developed. The echocardiogram is a good way to evaluate all heart valve function. This test allows the visualization of the valves as they open and close.

Definitive therapy for aortic stenosis requires mechanical or surgical intervention. Aortic valve replacement is required for true correction of aortic stenosis.

Nursing considerations in the care of patients with aortic stenosis are to maintain an index of suspicion with patients who have signs of congestive heart failure, particularly without MI. Nurses should explain the progression of the condition to patients and answer their questions. Monitoring the progression of the disease is important because many patients minimize their symptoms.

Congestive Heart Failure

Heart failure was once thought to be due entirely to pump failure and was diagnosed with an ejection fraction less than 40%. Recent research has described another facet of heart failure due to diastolic dysfunction. During diastole, the ventricle cannot relax and open enough to allow returning blood to fill it. This is called noncompliance and can be due to a thickened muscle or septal wall (Caboral & Mitchell, 2003).

The most common risk factors for heart failure include coronary artery disease and hypertension. Other risk factors include family history, cardiotoxic drugs (some cancer chemotherapy drugs), smoking, obesity, alcohol abuse, and diabetes mellitus. Reducing modifiable risk factors is important at all stages of heart failure, and the nurse can do much to support patients in making lifestyle changes.

Most heart failure symptoms include breathlessness or dyspnea. This can take the form of orthopnea, which is an inability to breathe comfortably while lying flat. Crackles detected on lung auscultation are a sign of left-sided heart failure. Physical signs of right-sided heart failure include edema in the extremities, dilated neck veins, and congested liver.

Laboratory and diagnostic tests used to evaluate heart failure include electrocardiogram, which may reveal ST-T wave changes indicating myocardial ischemia, atrial fibrillation, or Q waves from previous MIs. Echocardiogram can reveal chamber size and valve function and can provide an estimated stroke volume, ejection fraction, and cardiac output. Blood tests include the complete blood count to evaluate anemia, which can aggravate heart failure; tests for elevated serum creatinine, which may indicate renal insufficiency; and thyroid function tests. Hyper- or hypothyroid conditions can aggravate heart failure (Laurent-Bopp, 2000).

Ways of classifying heart failure patients to guide therapy have been proposed by the New York Heart Association. A more recent classification system has been proposed by the American College of Cardiology and the American Heart Association to focus on prevention as well as on treatment (Hunt et al., 2001).Table 13–3 summarizes both sets of classification systems for heart failure patients. The newer guidelines emphasize the

Table 13–3   Functional and Therapeutic Classification Systems

New York Heart Association Functional Classification (1964)	American College of Cardiology/American Heart Association Task Force (2002)	Recommendations
	Stage A: Asymptomatic and no evidence of structural problems but high risk for developing heart failure.	• Manage: -Hypertension. -Lipid disorders. -Diabetes mellitus. • Teach: -Smoking cessation. -Exercise promotion. -Moderate EtOH. • ACE inhibitor if indicated.
Class I: Evidence of cardiac disease but no limitation in physical activity.	Stage B: Evidence of structural disease but no symptoms of heart failure.	• All Stage A therapies. • ACE inhibitor unless contraindicated. • Beta-blocker unless contraindicated.

Class	Stage	Therapies
Class II: Evidence of cardiac disease with slight limitation in physical activity. Comfortable at rest. Ordinary activity results in fatigue, palpitations, dyspnea, or angina.	Stage C: Evidence of structural disease with current or prior symptoms of heart failure.	• All stage A and B therapies. • Sodium-restricted diet. • Diuretics, digoxin. • Avoid antiarrhythmic agents, most calcium channel blockers, NSAIDs. • Consider aldosterone antagonists, angiotensin receptor blockers, hydralazine, and nitrates.
Class III: Evidence of cardiac disease with marked activity limitation, comfortable at rest. Less than ordinary activity causes symptoms. Class IV: Evidence of cardiac disease, symptomatic at rest, any activity causes discomfort.	Stage D: Heart failure refractory to stage C treatment outlined above, requiring specialized interventions.	• All therapies as above. • Mechanical assist devices, biventricular pacemakers, left ventricular assist device. • Continuous inotropic IV therapy. • Hospice care.

Source: Functional and Therapeutic Classification Systems, adapted from Caboral, M., & Mitchell, J. (2003). New Guidelines for Heart Failure Focus on Prevention, The Nurse Practitioner, 28 (1) 13, pp. 22–23. Copyright © Lippincott Williams & Wilkins. Reprinted with permission.

progressive nature of heart failure and guide the gradual increase in therapies as the disease advances.

Patients need to weigh themselves daily to monitor body water. Follow the same scale, same clothing, and same time of day rule. If their weight increases by 2 lb in a day, they should call their provider to report the change.

Arrhythmias and Conduction Disorders

Atrial fibrillation is the most common sustained arrhythmia and is characterized by rapid and disorganized atrial activity. The ECG shows no P wave. The incidence of atrial fibrillation increases with age. Common causes include hypertension, valvular stenosis that causes stretching of the atria, and ischemic heart disease. Thyroid disorders can also precipitate atrial fibrillation. One complication of atrial fibrillation is embolic cerebrovascular accidents. This is the result of the failure of the atria to fully empty with an organized atrial contraction. Clots that form in the blood and stagnate in the atria can break loose and follow the circulation to any part of the body. The incidence of stroke is five times baseline for people with atrial fibrillation. Anticoagulant therapy is indicated for any patient with atrial fibrillation for more than 24 hours.

Short-term anticoagulation is usually begun with heparin. The blood test that determines the level of anticoagulant activity is the activated partial thromboplastin time. For long-term therapy, warfarin (Coumadin) is usually prescribed. It can take several days for Coumadin levels to reach a steady state, and patients are usually maintained on heparin until this occurs. The laboratory test that assesses the blood-thinning effects of Coumadin is the International Normalized Ratio (INR).

Overall treatment goals for atrial fibrillation are to correct hemodynamic instability, control ventricular rate, and restore sinus rhythm if possible. Several medication groups are frequently used for atrial fibrillation. Conversion to sinus rhythm can be achieved by using antiarrhythmic drugs. Ventricular response can be slowed with calcium channel blockers (particularly verapamil) and with digoxin.

If drug therapy is not successful, electrophysiologic studies can be performed to determine whether one particular area of the atria is initiating the irregular rhythm. If an area is located, it can be ablated using radio frequency waves. This can prevent the recurrence of new atrial fibrillation.

Conduction disturbances can occur with age as well. First-degree heart block is blockage of the impulse at the AV node, resulting in prolonged PR interval. First-degree block can progress so that no atrial impulses are transmitted and only the underlying ventricular rate (30 beats per minute) maintains circulation. This is called complete heart block. Heart blocks that result in decreased cardiac output will need to be treated with an internal pacemaker insertion. Patients usually tolerate this procedure well. The nurse will need to monitor functioning of the pacemaker by checking pulse rates and looking for pacemaker activity on the ECG.

Peripheral Vascular Disease

Arterial Disease

Arterial disease is usually the result of atherosclerosis, which is a diffuse process causing changes in many places in the arterial system. Pain occurs at rest as the disease progresses.

A good history can indicate the extent and location of the blockage, but arteriograms need to be performed to determine the extent of the blockage. To evaluate circulation of the leg, the ankle brachial index (ABI)—equal to the systolic pressure of the ankle divided by the systolic pressure of the brachial artery—is useful. In the normal extremity, the ABI is close to 1.0. Decreased arterial flow to the leg is indicated by values less than 1.0. Intermittent claudication is often seen with ABIs of .5 to .7. Rest pain, arterial ulcers, or gangrene can occur with ABIs of .3 or less (Fahey, 1999).

New classes of drugs can improve peripheral circulation. Antithrombotic agents, prostaglandins, and calcium channel blockers are frequently prescribed. Surgical bypass of the occluded artery is often required to preserve circulation to the leg and prevent amputation. Meticulous care of surgical sites and ischemic extremities can preserve tissue, prevent infection, and preserve function (Fahey & McCarthy, 1999).

Venous Disease

Thrombophlebitis sometimes results in damage to the valves of the deep veins. Obesity and occupations that require prolonged standing or sitting can also lead to venous insufficiency. Over time, a thickening of the tissues around the ankles develops along with a brownish discoloration due to red blood cells that are pressed outside the capillaries. As the cells break down, hemosiderin (a breakdown product of hemoglobin) deposits collect. Eventually, chronic venous insufficiency can lead to nonhealing ulcers. The chronic ulcers caused by venous insufficiency tend to develop over the medial malleolus, the ankle area. The ulcers are different from arterial ulcers in that they are wide and have irregular borders.

Treatment for chronic venous insufficiency often involves wearing external compression hose every day.

Because venous insufficiency can co-occur with arterial insufficiency, the ankle brachial index should be measured before external compression is begun. Non-healing ulcers can be effectively treated with multi-layer compression bandages such as the Unna's boot. Occasionally, skin grafts must be performed.

Nursing Assessment

Comprehensive histories include demographic information, chief complaint, history of the present illness, past history, a review of systems, family history, social history, and a functional health pattern assessment. The nurse should collect vital demographic information including the patient's date of birth. The source of history other than the patient should be noted. For the older person, a family member or caretaker frequently becomes an important source of information. Sometimes a decrease in function is more obvious to an outside observer than to the patient.

The nurse should carefully note the chief complaint in the patient's own words. For patients with multiple complaints, a numbered problem list can help to focus assessment and treatment planning.

Next the nurse should assess the history of the present illness, again using the patient's own words. Pain and fatigue can be assessed using numeric scales, although these may be harder for the older person to quantify. The thermometer scale might be more easily understood for some patients.

The next step is to assess the older person's past health history. This section includes health problems other than the present illness; it includes hospital admissions and surgical procedures. The current medication list is a clue to medical problems. The medication list should include prescription and over-the-counter medications and vitamins and supplements. Allergies should be noted in this section.

Assessing family history is important to identify risk factors for cardiovascular disorders. For the older person, asking age and cause of death of parents and health status of siblings and children can offer evidence on genetic risk factors. Such conditions as coronary events, cerebrovascular accidents, peripheral vascular disease, aneurysms, diabetes, alcoholism, and depression all have family patterns of incidence and can affect cardiovascular status.

Next the nurse assesses the older person's personal or social history. This area contains much information that the nurse will need to plan appropriate care, including current living situation, resources, and supports.

Finally, the nurse conducts a complete review of systems. For older patients with cardiovascular problems, the nurse should focus on the presence or absence of chest pain, shortness of breath, syncope, palpitations, edema, nocturnal dyspnea, nocturia, pain in the extremities, cough, and fatigue. It is important to ask if the patient has been less active than previously or seems more easily fatigued.

Pharmacology and Nursing Implications

Medications can be both a support and a stress. Because medications cause changes in body systems, the older person takes time to adjust to changes. The general rule of starting with low doses and increasing them slowly is a good practice. The nurse should be alert to side or toxic effects even when the older person is taking medications in the normal adult dosage range.

Non-pharmacological Treatments

One of the most useful methods to help patients adjust to cardiovascular problems is the concept of rehabilitation. Cardiac rehabilitation can be used for patients with angina, recent MI, heart failure, recent revascularization, or other risk factors for heart disease. Most rehabilitation programs include information on exercise and are available while patients exercise in case arrhythmias develop. They also include information on diet and stress management. The support of rehabilitation programs can encourage patients to engage in healthy lifestyle patterns.

Nursing Interventions

Activity and exercise support is an intervention that provides for supervised increase in activity. Patients should be monitored for changes in vital signs and sudden fatigue. Along with exercise, planning is important for rest.

Diet therapy will involve teaching and may also involve consultation with dietitians. It is best to start with the patient's preferred diet and suggest small changes that are acceptable to the patient.

Smoking cessation is important for cardiovascular patients, and it can be used to prevent cardiovascular problems. Behavioral approaches and medications can assist with smoking cessation.

Medication management is important because so many medications are useful in treating cardiovascular concerns. Older persons need to be able to open their medication bottles. They should take medications as ordered and report side effects.

Caregiver support is important in any chronic condition. Family members need to understand medications and their effect and they need to know what signs or symptoms should be reported to the nurse or doctor. Adult day health programs can offer respite for the caregiver and support for the patient.

Advance directives should be discussed with the patient and family members. Does the patient want aggressive treatment for the condition and understand the burdens of that treatment? Has the patient discussed treatment preferences with a healthcare proxy or with the physician? These are topics best addressed during a stable time. The nurse can assist patients in clarifying their values and wishes and can support them in preparing written advance directives.

Community resources are important in chronic conditions. The American Heart Association has many programs that support healthy living. Many senior centers have cardiovascular programs available. The nurse can become familiar with resources in the community and can refer patients appropriately.

The patient-family teaching guidelines in the following feature will assist the nurse to assume the role of teacher and coach. Educating patients and families is critical so that nurses can interpret scientific data and individualize the nursing care plan.

PATIENT-FAMILY TEACHING GUIDELINES

The following are guidelines that the nurse may find useful when instructing older persons and their families about hypertension.

High Blood Pressure or Hypertension

1. What is high blood pressure?

   High blood pressure is a condition of higher than normal pressures inside the blood vessels. It can cause:
   - Changes in the thickness of the blood vessels.
   - Increased risk of heart attack and stroke.
   - Damage to kidneys.

2. What causes high blood pressure?

   The cause of most high blood pressure is frequently not known, but is most likely an imbalance in:
   - the body's ability to control body water.
   - the body's ability to control sodium levels.
   - neuroendocrine controls of blood pressure.

3. What can a person do to decrease blood pressure to a healthy level?

   It is important to make healthy choices such as the following:
   - Maintaining a normal body weight
   - Decreasing intake of high-fat and high-sodium foods
   - Exercising regularly
   - Stopping smoking
   - Limiting alcohol intake
   - Taking prescribed medications
   - Having blood pressure checked regularly

   (continued)

4. What is heart failure?

   Heart failure happens when the heart is not able to pump enough blood to the body to allow a person to do the things he or she wants or needs to do. People who have heart failure often experience these symptoms:

   - Fatigue
   - Shortness of breath
   - Inability to be comfortable lying flat in bed
   - Shortness of breath at night
   - Needing to use the bathroom frequently at night
   - Swollen ankles

   Heart failure patients frequently need to be hospitalized to balance fluid in their body and ease their breathing.

5. What causes heart failure?

   Heart failure is caused by damage to the heart muscle. This can occur from heart attacks (myocardial infarctions) or from long-standing high blood pressure. In some cases, heart valve problems can lead to heart failure. Either the heart cannot pump as well as it should or the workload that the heart is pumping against is increased.

6. What can a person do to live with heart failure?

   Heart failure patients can improve the quality of their life and reduce hospitalizations by:

   - Taking medications as prescribed. If there is any trouble with the medications, either in obtaining them or from side effects, the doctor or nurse should be told.
   - Avoiding high-sodium and salty foods.
   - Balancing activity and rest.
   - Weighing themselves daily to determine if they are holding fluid.
   - Reporting any change in how they feel to a doctor or nurse.

CHAPTER 14

THE RESPIRATORY SYSTEM

ANATOMY AND PHYSIOLOGY

The respiratory system is composed of the lungs, the airways leading to the lungs, the blood vessels serving the lungs, and the chest wall. The right lung has three lobes (upper, middle, and lower). To leave space for the heart, the left lung has two lobes (upper and lower). The lobes consist of segments and lobules. The lung is delicate enough to allow the exchange of oxygen and carbon dioxide, yet strong and resilient enough to maintain its shape. Two support systems, the airways for ventilation and the circulatory system for perfusion, are coordinated by special muscles and nerves. This coordinated system enables the lung to perform its primary function of rapidly exchanging oxygen from inhaled air with the carbon dioxide in the blood.

The lungs have two major functions: one is respiratory and the other is nonrespiratory. Respiratory functions include gas exchange or the transfer of oxygen from the air into the blood and the removal of carbon dioxide from the blood.

The respiratory centers respond to changes in blood levels of oxygen, carbon dioxide, and blood pH. The nonrespiratory functions of the lungs are mechanical, biochemical, and physiological. The lungs defend against airborne irritants and bacterial, viral, and other infectious agents by entrapping and **lysing** foreign invaders. Finally, the lungs manufacture a variety of essential hormones and other chemicals that direct and carry out biochemical reactions (NHLBI, 2002a).

NORMAL CHANGES OF AGING

The following changes occur in lung structure and function with normal aging:

- Stiffening of elastin and the collagen connective tissue supporting the lungs
- Altered alveolar shape resulting in increased alveolar diameter
- Decreased alveolar surface area available for gas exchange
- Increased chest wall stiffness

RESPIRATORY DISEASES COMMON IN OLDER PEOPLE

Asthma

Asthma is a respiratory disease characterized by usually reversible airflow obstruction, airway inflammation, increased mucous secretion, and increased airway responsiveness (contraction of airway smooth muscles) to a variety of stimuli. With asthma, inflamed airways are characterized as "twitchy" and overreact to common irritants like viruses, cigarette smoke, cold air, and allergens. These triggers can activate an inflammatory response including mobilization of mast cells, eosinophils, macrophages, and T lymphocytes. With these inflammatory changes, airway smooth muscle contracts, swells, and produces excessive mucous secretions making it difficult to breathe. The common symptoms of an asthma attack include the following:

- Coughing
- Wheezing

- Shortness of breath
- Chest tightness

(Nurses Asthma Education Partnership Project, 2003)

The diagnosis of asthma is based on the clinical history, physical examination, and laboratory studies. Nocturnal dyspnea is common and often occurs between 4 a.m. and 6 a.m.

Diagnostic Studies

Testing includes the results of pulmonary function tests, chest radiography, electrocardiography, and a complete blood count with differential to confirm the diagnosis of asthma in the older person. The electrocardiogram will help identify the presence of cardiac disease and the risk associated with certain medications that may be used to treat the older patient with asthma and cardiac disease (e.g., theophylline).

Pulmonary function tests are the most reliable way to diagnose asthma and differentiate it from other illnesses like COPD. Spirometry is used to measure the volume of air expired in 1 second from maximum inspiration (FEV_1) and the total amount of air expired as rapidly as possible (forced vital capacity, FVC). The diagnosis of asthma is confirmed by:

- Demonstrated airflow obstruction of FEV_1 less than 80% of predicted and an FEV_1/FVC ratio of less than 70%.
- Evidence that airflow obstruction is reversible (greater than 12% and 200 ml in FEV_1, after the administration of a bronchodilator or over time after a course of corticosteroids).
- Peak expiratory flow (PEF) measurements indicating the maximum flow (expressed in liters per second)

that can be generated during a forced expiratory maneuver with fully inflated lungs as measured using a peak flow meter. PEF measurements before and after bronchodilator administration may be useful in confirming the asthma diagnosis. A pattern of greater than 20% variation in PEF from late afternoon to arising the next morning confirms the presence of variable airflow obstructions, often indicative of asthma.

(American Thoracic Society, 2002).

Once diagnostic testing is completed, asthma is classified as to severity so that the appropriate treatment and monitoring may be initiated. Table 14–1 presents the four categories of asthma severity before treatment based on duration of symptoms, presence and severity of nocturnal symptoms, and results of spirometry testing.

Based upon the classification of severity, medications are prescribed using the following goals of therapy for asthma control:

- Minimal or no chronic symptoms day or night
- Minimal or no exacerbations
- No limitations on functional ability and ability to perform activities of daily living
- Maintenance of normal or nearly normal pulmonary function
- Minimal use of "rescue" short-acting inhaled beta$_2$-agonist (less than once daily or one canister per month)
- Minimal or no adverse effects from medication

(Nurses Asthma Education Partnership Project, 2003)

Medications required to maintain long-term control are prescribed according to the level of severity of

Table 14–1 Classification of Asthma Severity: Clinical Features Before Treatment

	Days With Symptoms	Nights With Symptoms	PEF or FEV$_1$*	PEF Variability
Step 4 Severe Persistent	Continual	Frequent	≤ 60%	> 30%
Step 3 Moderate Persistent	Daily	≥ 5/month	> 60%– < 80%	> 30%
Step 2 Mild Persistent	3–6/week	3–4/month	≥ 80%	20–30%
Step 1 Mild Intermittent	≤ 2/week	≤ 2/month	≥ 80%	< 20%

*Percent predicted values for forced expiratory volume in 1 second (FEV$_1$) and percent of personal best for peak expiratory flow (PEF) (relevant for children 6 years old or older who can use these devices).

Notes:

- Patients should be assigned to the most severe step in which *any* feature occurs. Clinical features for individual patients may overlap across steps.
- An individual's classification may change over time.
- Patients at any level of severity of chronic asthma can have mild, moderate, or severe exacerbations of asthma. Some patients with intermittent asthma experience severe and life-threatening exacerbations separated by long periods of normal lung function and no symptoms.
- Patients with two or more asthma exacerbations per week (i.e., progressively worsening symptoms that may last hours or days) tend to have moderate-to-severe persistent asthma.

Source: NHLBI, 2002.

asthma using the four-step classification system. It is recommended that the treatment protocol be reviewed on a regular basis, about every 6 months, to review the medication technique, to monitor for adherence and environmental control, and to step up or down a level according to progression and manifestation of symptoms and PEF variability. Increased use of short-acting beta$_2$-agonists on a daily basis or more than three to four times in one day would indicate the need to seek physician advice and possibly step up to the next level to achieve better control. Referral to an asthma specialist for consultation or comanagement with the primary care provider is recommended if there is difficulty maintaining control or if the older patient requires step 3 or step 4 care. Table 14–2 indicates preferred daily medications by asthma classification.

Common side effects of asthma medications are listed in Table 14–3. As with all drugs, the benefits of the medication must be weighed against the risk of adverse effects.

Several medications now come prepared as dry powder inhalers and contain no propellant. The dry powder is inhaled into the upper airway when done properly.

Older patients using inhaled steroids should rinse their mouths with warm water and expectorate after medication administration to prevent the overgrowth of candidiasis or thrush, prevent gum disease, and deter tooth decay.

Certain medications should be avoided when treating patients with asthma because adverse reactions can exacerbate asthmatic problems. These drugs include:

- *Beta-blockers.* Commonly used to treat hypertension in older people, beta-blockers (propranolol) can induce bronchospasm. Even ophthalmologic solutions like timolol should be avoided if possible. Hypoxemia can result from bronchospasm and lead to serious consequences.

Table 14-2 Stepwise Approach for Managing Asthma in Adults and Children Older Than 5 Years of Age: Treatment

Classify Severity: Clinical Features Before Treatment or Adequate Control

	Symptoms/Day Symptoms/Night	PEF or FEV, PEF Variability	Daily Medications
Step 4 Severe Persistent	Continual Frequent	$\leq 60\%$ $> 30\%$	• **Preferred treatment:** —High-dose inhaled corticosteroids AND —Long-acting inhaled beta$_2$-agonists AND, if needed, —Corticosteroid tablets or syrup long term (2 mg/kg/day, generally do not exceed 60 mg per day). (Make repeat attempts to reduce systemic corticosteroids and maintain control with high-dose inhaled corticosteroids.)
Step 3 Moderate Persistent	Daily > 1 night/week	$> 60\% - < 80\%$ $> 30\%$	• **Preferred treatment:** —Low-to-medium dose inhaled corticosteroids and long-acting inhaled beta$_2$-agonists.

(continued)

245

Table 14–2 Stepwise Approach for Managing Asthma in Adults and Children Older Than 5 Years of Age: Treatment (*continued*)

Classify Severity: Clinical Features Before Treatment or Adequate Control

Symptoms/Day Symptoms/Night	PEF or FEV, PEF Variability	Daily Medications
		• Alternative treatment (listed alphabetically): —Increase inhaled corticosteroids within medium-dose range OR —Low-to-medium dose inhaled corticosteroids and either leukotriene modifier or theophylline. If needed (particularly in patients with recurring severe exacerbations): • **Preferred treatment:** —Increase inhaled corticosteroids within medium-dose range and add long-acting inhaled beta$_2$-agonists.

- Alternative treatment:
  - Increase inhaled corticosteroids within medium-dose range and add either leukotriene modifier or theophylline.

Step 2
Mild
Persistent

> 2/week but < 1×/day   ≥ 80%
> 2 nights/month   20–30%

- **Preferred treatment:**
  - Low-dose inhaled corticosteroids.
  - Alternative treatment (listed alphabetically): cromolyn, leukotriene modifier, nedocromil, OR sustained release theophylline to serum concentration of 5–15 mcg/mL.

Step 1
Mild
Intermittent

≤ 2 days/week   ≥ 80%
≤ 2 nights/month   < 20%

- No daily medication needed.
- Severe exacerbations may occur, separated by long periods of normal lung function and no symptoms. A course of systemic corticosteroids is recommended.

Quick Relief
All Patients

- Short-acting bronchodilator: 2–4 puffs short-acting inhaled $beta_2$-agonists as needed for symptoms.
- Intensity of treatment will depend on severity of exacerbation; up to 3 treatments at 20-minute intervals or a single nebulizer treatment as needed. Course of systemic corticosteroids may be needed.
- Use of short-acting $beta_2$-agonists > 2 times a week in intermittent asthma (daily, or increasing use in persistent asthma) may indicate the needed to initiate (increase) long-term control therapy.

(continued)

Table 14-2 Stepwise Approach for Managing Asthma in Adults and Children Older Than 5 Years of Age: Treatment *(continued)*

Classify Severity: Clinical Features Before Treatment or Adequate Control

Symptoms/Day Symptoms/Night	PEF or FEV, PEF Variability	Daily Medications
↓ **Step down** Review treatment every 1 to 6 months; a gradual stepwise reduction in treatment may be possible. ↑ **Step up** If control is not maintained, consider step up. First, review patient medication technique, adherence, and environmental control.		**Note** • The stepwise approach is meant to assist, not replace, the clinical decision making required to meet individual patient needs. • Classify severity: assign patient to most severe step in which any feature occurs (PEF is % of personal best; FEV$_1$ is % predicted). • Gain control as quickly as possible (consider a short course of systemic corticosteroids); then step down to the least medication necessary to maintain control. • Provide education on self-management and controlling environmental factors that make asthma worse (e.g., allergens and irritants). • Refer to an asthma specialist if there are difficulties controlling asthma or if step 4 care is required. Referral may be considered if step 3 care is required.

Goals of Therapy: Asthma Control

- Minimal or no chronic symptoms day or night
- Minimal or no exacerbations
- No limitations on activities; no school/work missed
- Maintain (near) normal pulmonary function
- Minimal use of short-acting inhaled beta$_2$-agonist (< 1x per day, < 1 canister/month)
- Minimal or no adverse effects from medications

Source: Nurses: Partners in Asthma Care 1998.

Table 14-3 Asthma Medications and Potential Adverse Effects

Class of Therapeutic Agent	Drug	Potential Adverse Clinical Effects
Anti-inflammatory	Oral corticosteroids	↑ Blood pressure, edema, congestive heart failure due to Na^+ retention
		Hypokalemia, alkalosis, and resulting arrhythmias due to K^+ and H^+ excretion
		Worsening diabetes mellitus, cataracts, polyuria with dehydration due to elevated blood glucose
		Thinning of the skin, reduced muscle mass with myopathy, osteoporosis, ↑ blood urea nitrogen without change in renal blood flow due to protein catabolism
		Hypoadrenalism due to decreased ACTH
		Cataracts
		Altered cognitive function, depression
		Joint effusions and articular pain with corticosteroid withdrawal
		Osteoporosis due to decreased calcium absorption

(continued)

Table 14–3 Asthma Medications and Potential Adverse Effects *(continued)*

Class of Therapeutic Agent	Drug	Potential Adverse Clinical Effects
	Inhaled corticosteroids	Glaucoma due to decreased absorption of aqueous humor
		Aggravation of existing peptic ulcer disease
	(High doses, e.g., > 1.6 mg/day)	Cough; dysphonia, loss of taste, laryngomalacia, oral candidiasis
		Effects on ACTH secretion with hypoadrenalism may be related to the effects on calcium absorption with acceleration of osteoporosis
		Development of cataracts
	Cromolyn sodium	No significant adverse effect known
	Nedocromil	No significant adverse effect known
Bronchodilator	Short-acting beta$_2$-agonists	Myocardial ischemia due to $\uparrow$ myocardial oxygen consumption and mild increase in hypoxemia
		Complex ventricular arrhythmia due to $\uparrow$ myocardial irritability

	Cardiac arrhythmias and muscle weakness related to hypokalemia
	Hypotension or hypertension
	Tremor
	With excessive use, $\downarrow$ bronchodilator effect and $\uparrow$ airway hyperresponsiveness related to downregulation to beta receptors
Long-acting beta$_2$-agonists	Same as for short-acting beta$_2$-agonists
Theophylline	Cardiac arrhythmias, effect is related to $\uparrow$ catecholamine release and is additive with beta$_2$-agonists
	Nausea and vomiting from gastric irritation, gastroesophageal reflux
	Insomnia, seizures related to central nervous system stimulant
	Cardiac arrhythmia due to inotropic and chronotropic effects
	Serum levels increased by heart failure, liver disease, beta-blocker therapy, selected H$_2$ blocker therapy, quinolone therapy, macrolide therapy, ketoconazole therapy
Ipratropium bromide	Mucosal dryness

Source: Nurses: Partners in Asthma Care, 1998.

- *Nonsteroidal anti-inflammatory drugs (NSAIDs).* Sudden, potentially life-threatening bronchospasm has been associated with NSAID and aspirin use in older patients.
- *Diuretics.* Hypokalemia can develop for patients taking thiazide (non–potassium sparing) diuretics. Hypokalemia can be associated with cardiac arrythmias, especially for those taking digitalis.
- *Antihistamines.* The QT interval can be prolonged in older patients taking beta$_2$-agonists or diuretics. The sedative effect of some antihistamines is also of concern.
- *Angiotensin-converting enzyme (ACE) inhibitors.* Widely used as antihypertensives, ACE inhibitors can produce cough in some patients. This may exacerbate asthma symptoms, causing asthma medications to be increased or diagnostic category moved a step upward.
- *Antidepressants.* Corticosteroids can worsen underlying depression in the older person and interact with monoamine oxidase (MAO) inhibitors and tricyclic antidepressants.

It is crucial that the patient be instructed in the use of a peak flow meter to measure how well air moves in and out of the lungs. By taking medications before the onset of symptoms, the asthma attack may be lessened in severity or stopped completely. Further, the peak flow meter can alert the patient and the physician by:

- Illustrating the response of various conditions like exercise, exposure to cold weather, and psychological stress.
- Monitoring the effect of medications.
- Indicating when medication changes are needed.
- Indicating that emergency care is needed.

The peak flow meter should be used:

- Every day for the first 2 weeks after diagnosis or with change in treatment.
- Mornings after awakening and between noon and 2 p.m.
- Before and after taking beta$_2$-agonists to document effect.
- When symptoms occur such as wheezing or tightness in the chest.
- When the patient feels he or she is coming down with a cold or respiratory infection.

Patients should keep a peak flow diary and carefully record readings. Good control indicates a feeling of respiratory well-being for the patient and absence of asthma symptoms. Peak flow readings can be classified into three categories:

1. Green zone (80% to 100% of personal best) indicating *good control*. No asthma symptoms are present and medication should be taken as usual.
2. Yellow zone (50% to 79% of personal best) indicating *caution*. An asthma attack may be starting and the patient may not be under control. Medication changes may be needed.
3. Red zone (below 50% of personal best) indicating *danger*. The patient should take a short-acting beta$_2$-agonist immediately and notify the physician.

Older patients with asthma should be instructed that because of their sensitive airways, they may need to avoid allergens and triggers to asthma attacks. The common offenders include animals, dust mites, tobacco and wood smoke, strong odors and sprays, respiratory infections, cold weather, molds and pollen, and exercise.

Nursing Assessment

It is recommended that each visit follow a three-part process. These three parts can occur more than once in any given session:

1. Assess the older patient's needs, expectations, and progress.
2. Introduce or review an action the older patient should take.
3. Obtain an agreement to take specific actions and schedule a follow-up visit to discuss the patient's progress.

Physical assessment of the older patient with asthma should include observation of the overall shape and movement of the thorax during respiration. Check for wheezing, chest excursion, and tactile fremitus.

Chronic Obstructive Pulmonary Disease

Chronic obstructive pulmonary disease is a term used for two closely related diseases of the respiratory system: chronic bronchitis and emphysema. Chronic bronchitis is defined as cough and sputum production present on most days for a minimum of 3 months for at least 2 successive years or for 6 months during 1 year. In chronic bronchitis, there may be narrowing of the large and small airways, making it more difficult to move air in and out of the lungs. In emphysema, there is permanent destruction of the alveoli, the tiny elastic air sacs of the lung, because of irreversible destruction of elastin, a protein in the lung that is important for maintaining the strength of the alveolar walls. Most patients with these diseases have a long history of heavy cigarette smoking.

Pathophysiology

As COPD progresses, the amount of oxygen in the blood decreases, causing blood vessels in the lungs to further constrict. The right ventricle enlarges and thickens, which can result in abnormal rhythms called *cor pulmonale.*

The body tries to boost the amount of oxygen carried in the blood by making extra red blood cells. This condition is *secondary polycythemia* and these cells can clog up small blood vessels and thicken the blood. This results in the formation of a bluish color in the skin, lips, and nail beds called *cyanosis.* Too little oxygen can also affect the brain, resulting in headache, irritability, impaired cognition, and sleep problems.

Symptoms

The earliest presenting symptom of COPD is early morning cough with the production of clear sputum. The sputum will turn to yellow or green should the older person develop a respiratory infection. Shortness of breath on exertion with severe episodes of **dyspnea** can occur during even modest activity like walking.

Diagnosis

At present, it is impossible to diagnose COPD before irreversible lung damage occurs. Spirometry is the preferred diagnostic method for testing pulmonary function. The three volume measures most relevant to COPD are:

1. Forced vital capacity (amount of air exhaled in 1 second) declines rapidly.

2. Residual volume (the amount of air remaining in the lungs after forced vital capacity is measured) increases.
3. Total lung capacity. Combination of the forced vital capacity and residual volume.

Treatment

The goals of treatment are to reduce disability, prevent acute exacerbations, reduce hospitalization, and avoid premature mortality.

Home oxygen therapy has been shown to increase the survival rate of patients with advanced COPD who have hypoxemia, low blood oxygen levels. This treatment can improve a patient's exercise tolerance and ability to perform on cognitive and physical tests, reflecting improvement in the function of the brain and increased muscle coordination. Oxygen also improves cardiac function and prevents the development of cor pulmonale. Continuous oxygen therapy is recommended for patients with low oxygen levels at rest, during exercise, and while sleeping (NHLBI, 2002b). It is imperative that the older patient not smoke anywhere near oxygen or oxygen equipment because of the danger of explosion.

Medications used to treat patients with COPD are similar to those used to treat patients with asthma and include bronchodilators, corticosteroids, antibiotics, and expectorants.

Additional Treatment Options

Bullectomy or lung reduction surgery has shown some limited success in selected patients. Portions of the lung that are nonfunctional and filled with stagnant air are removed to make room for the more healthy parts of the lung to expand. However, this is major surgery and many patients with COPD are poor surgical risks and prone to life-threatening surgical complications. Lung transplantation has also been used with some COPD patients. The 1-year survival in patients with transplanted lungs is over 70%.

Pulmonary rehabilitation is useful in patients with COPD. Relaxation techniques may also reduce the perception of ventilatory effort and dyspnea. Breathing exercises and techniques such as pursed lip breathing can improve functional status.

Clearing the air passages of mucus with postural drainage, chest percussion, tracheal suctioning, and controlled coughing may be effective in older patients who cannot clear their own airways of troublesome secretions.

Smoking Cessation

The most important thing a patient with COPD can do is to quit smoking. Older patients and their families may think that if lung damage has occurred, it is too late and therefore not worth the effort. The gerontological nurse can function as educator and change agent for the older smoker.

Transdermal nicotine patches, nicotine gum, and Bupropion (Zyban) are helpful adjuncts to behavioral interventions.

Additional suggestions for patients with COPD include avoiding exposure to dust and fumes, air pollution, and secondhand smoke; receive a yearly flu shot and pneumococcal vaccine at age 65; avoid excessive heat, cold, and high altitudes; drink lots of fluids; maintain a healthy lifestyle; and engage in routine spirometry testing.

Tuberculosis

The number of active cases in the United States began to rise because of weakened immunity in those with diabetes, cancer, and HIV/AIDS, increased numbers of foreign-born persons in the United States from regions where TB is indigenous, increased poverty, IV drug use and homelessness, increasingly resistant strains of TB, and increased numbers of persons living in institutions.

Transmission

TB is primarily an airborne disease that is spread by droplets when an infected person coughs, sneezes, speaks, sings, or laughs. Only people with active disease are contagious. It usually takes repeated exposure to someone with active TB before a person becomes infected. People with TB who have been treated with appropriate drugs for at least 2 weeks are no longer contagious and are incapable of spreading the disease (National Institute of Allergy and Infectious Diseases, 2002). Adequate ventilation is the most important measure to prevent transmission.

Diagnosis

About 2 to 8 weeks after infection with *M. tuberculosis,* a person's immune system responds by walling off infected cells. From then on the body maintains a standoff with the infection, sometimes for years. Most people undergo complete healing of their initial infection, and the bacteria eventually die off. A positive TB skin test and old scars on a chest x-ray may provide the only evidence of past infection. If, however, resistance is low because of aging, infection, malnutrition, or other reason, the bacteria may break out of hiding and cause active TB (National Institute of Allergy and Infectious Diseases, 2002).

The hallmarks of TB diagnosis are the skin test and the chest x-ray. People who should be skin tested include:

- Those known to have spent time with someone with active TB.
- Those with HIV or malignancy.
- Those who think they may have the disease.
- Those from parts of the world where TB is common (Latin America, the Caribbean, Africa, Asia, eastern Europe, and Russia).
- Those who use intravenous drugs and alcohol to excess.
- Those living in institutions where TB is common (homeless shelters, migrant farm camps, prison, nursing homes).

The purified protein derivative (PPD) skin test involves the injection of 5 TU (Bioequivalent) per dose (0.1 mL) under the skin in the forearm. It should not be given subcutaneously, but rather subdermally. It should barely raise a wheal. If an area of induration results (raised, reddened area) around 72 hours after the PPD has been injected, it should be measured and recorded. Referral for follow-up is indicated if the area of induration is greater than 15 mm in a low-risk adult; greater than 10 mm in a health care worker, recent immigrant, person with chronic illness or comorbidities, or an IV drug user; greater than 5 mm in a person who has HIV/AIDS, takes corticosteroids, or has had recent contact with an active TB patient.

When PPD testing in an older adult, the two-step approach is recommended. If the initial PPD is negative, testing is repeated after waiting 1 to 2 weeks. The second PPD provides a more accurate reading because the older person's immune system may be sluggish and not adequately react to the first exposure. It is unclear how the PPD results should be interpreted for those who have received the BCG, the antituberculosis vaccine. Some advocate the same guidelines for interpretation as those who have not received BCG while others do not advocate testing. Patients who have received BCG should be closely followed up with symptom checklists and chest x-rays if they are in high-risk categories. Patients with positive symptoms are referred to physicians for further testing including a chest x-ray and sputum analysis to check for acid-fast bacillus.

Treatment

Treatment of active TB involves the medications including isoniazid (INH), rifampin (or rifampin plus), and/or pyrazinamide. With appropriate antibiotic treatment, TB can be cured in more than 90% of patients. Serious side effects of isoniazid include loss of appetite, nausea, vomiting, jaundice, fever for more than 3 days, abdominal pain, and tingling in the fingers and toes (Centers for Disease Control, 2003). Patients taking isoniazid are urged not to drink alcoholic beverages, including wine, beer, and liquor.

When the antibiotic treatment is interrupted because of unpleasant side effects or financial reasons, the TB bacteria may become resistant and be more difficult to eradicate when treatment is started again. Treatment of multidrug-resistant TB requires the use of special drugs that have more serious side effects.

Prevention

TB is largely a preventable disease. Once persons infected with *M. tuberculosis* are identified, they are treated with isoniazid to prevent active disease. This drug can cause hepatitis in a small percentage of patients and is especially a risk for those over 35. Liver function tests should be routinely monitored in the older patient to prevent liver complications.

Hospitals and clinics should take special precautions and isolate patients with active TB. Special filters and ultraviolet light can sterilize the air. Patients with TB should be in special rooms with controlled ventilation and reverse airflow. Healthcare workers should be tested with PPD every year.

Lung Cancer

Cigarette smoking and exposure to environmental or occupational toxins (air pollution, asbestos, or lead exposure) may have a synergistic effect and speed the production of lung cancer. Growth rate and metastasis rate vary by tumor type.

Symptoms

Chronic cough, **hemoptysis** (coughing up of blood or production of bloody sputum), chest pain, shortness of breath, fatigue, weight loss, and frequent lung infections such as pneumonia and bronchitis that do not resolve with antibiotic treatment could all be warning signs to refer the older person to the primary care provider for further testing. The chest x-ray is usually the first examination the physician will order. Suspicious masses seen on the chest x-ray may signal the need for a computerized axial tomography (CAT) scan or a magnetic resonance imaging (MRI) scan. Both the CAT scan and MRI can provide additional information about soft tissue masses. Further tests may include pulmonary function tests; bronchoscopy with the collection of lung tissue, cells, or fluids for analysis under the microscope; and biochemical and cellular studies of respiratory fluids removed from the lungs by lavage. Other important tests may include measures of arterial blood gas tensions (Pao_2 and $Paco_2$) (NHLBI, 2002b).

Older patients with lung cancer may undergo surgical removal of the tumor or the lung if they are good surgical candidates and are not diagnosed with comorbid conditions. Chemotherapy, ionizing radiation to the thorax, and palliative care are less aggressive approaches used for older patients with comorbid conditions.

Respiratory Infections

Sinusitis is inflammation of the mucosal lining of the paranasal sinuses that can lead to mucous stasis, obstruction, and subsequent infection. Sinusitis should not be confused with rhinitis, a condition characterized by inflammation of the mucous membranes of the nose, usually accompanied by nasal discharge. Sinusitis can also be caused by allergens, air pollution, and irritants such as the use of inhaled recreational drugs. Sinusitis can also be induced by dental abscess, irritation of nasogastric tubes, and immune deficiency syndromes.

Acute sinusitis may be diagnosed by the presence of dull pain over the maxillary sinuses that is worsened by bending over. Congestion, green nasal discharge, periorbital edema, and fever may also be present.

Treatment of sinusitis usually involves nasal decongestants (phenylephrine 0.25%), one or two sprays every 4 hours in each nostril for up to 5 days; saline spray to lubricate and moisten the nares; and acetaminophen for discomfort. Humidified air may provide some relief. For acute sinusitis, some clinicians advocate treatment with antimicrobials such as Augmentin 500 mg every 12 hours for 2 weeks. As the sinuses are poorly perfused, longer treatment may be necessary to ensure that all areas of infection receive adequate concentrations of antibiotics and that the responsible bacteria are truly eradicated.

The use of antibiotics to treat upper respiratory infections and simple pharyngitis is not recommended because it encourages antibiotic resistance. Most upper respiratory infections will resolve spontaneously within 7 to 10 days. However, infections of the lower respiratory tract such as bronchitis and pneumonia are more serious in the older person and require aggressive evaluation and treatment.

The following risk factors are thought to increase susceptibility to respiratory infection in the older lung and to affect the outcome of pneumonia including history of nosocomial pneumonia (last 1 year), diagnosed lung disease, nursing home residence, smoking, alcohol use, heart failure, malnutrition, enteral tube feeding, immunosuppression, neurologic disease (dementi), heart failure, and oxygen use. Aspiration is a major risk factor for the development of pneumonia and stroke, dementia, and dysphagia. Gastric tube placements are major risk factors for aspiration. Sedative and narcotic use is associated with decreased levels of consciousness, lethargy, and nighttime aspiration. Viral infections, in particular influenza A, are a risk factor for secondary bacterial pneumonia (Reichmuth & Meyer, 2003).

Pathogens

Common pathogens include: *Streptococcus pneumoniae, Haemophilus influenzae, Staphylococcus aureus, Legionella, Mycoplasma pneumoniae, H. influenzae,* and *Moraxella catarrhalis.* Influenza is four times more common in persons over 70 years of age than in younger adults. In most years, persons over 65 account for about 90% of influenza-associated deaths in the United States. Epidemics, sometimes associated with high mortality, are a problem in institutional settings. Virus can be spread by airborne droplets, caregivers, and exposure to contaminated respiratory equipment.

Symptoms of Pneumonia

The classic symptoms of pneumonia are cough, fever, and sputum production. Fever may be absent because many older people have a lower basal temperature and will not exhibit a fever response in the face of infection. Bacterial pneumonias are commonly preceded by a viruslike prodrome of headache, myalgia, and lethargy. Other symptoms may include abrupt onset of shaking chills (rigors). Nonbacterial pneumonia may be accompanied by substernal chest pain and dyspnea. New-onset tachycardia and tachypnea are important clues to illness with both viral and bacterial pneumonia. Changes in function, appetite, continence, and other subtle symptoms may be the first signs of the onset of illness.

Nursing Assessment of Pneumonia

The assessment should include checking vital signs, inspecting the thorax, and auscultating the lungs. The skin should be examined for cyanosis. Crackles that do not clear with coughing may be suggestive of pneumonia. Signs of consolidation (bronchial breath sounds, dullness to percussion, and egophony) are common findings with late-stage pneumonia.

The primary care provider will probably request a chest x-ray; however, it may be negative in early stages of the disease. Physical findings will probably precede the appearance of an infiltrate by about 24 hours. After resolution of the pneumonia, the chest x-ray will not appear normal for about 6 weeks. Sputum for analysis is difficult to obtain from an older person as it requires a vigorous cough reflex. Pulse oximetry of arterial blood gases provides valuable information about the patient's status. Hypoxemia is associated with poor outcome. Older patients with severe hypoxemia should be referred to the acute care setting for immediate evaluation. A blood chemistry analysis may reveal marked leukocytosis, indicating white blood cells are being produced to try to fight off the infection.

Hospitalization for pneumonia should be considered when:

- Comorbidities are present (lung disease, alcoholism, malnutrition, congestive heart failure).
- Respiratory rate exceeds 30 breaths per minute.
- Hemoptysis is present.
- Diastolic blood pressure is less than 60 mmHg or systolic blood pressure is less than 90 mmHg.
- Temperature exceeds 38.3°C or 101°F.
- PaO_2 is less than 60 mmHg on room air.
- Chest x-ray shows more than one lobe involvement, presence of a cavity, or presence of a pleural effusion.
- There is evidence of sepsis.
- Patient is unable to take oral fluids.

(American Thoracic Society, 2002).

Treatment of Pneumonia

The treatment recommendations for older outpatients with community-acquired pneumonia are an oral macrolide (erythromycin, azithromycin, or clarithromycin) or an oral beta-lactam (cefuroxime, amoxicillin, or amoxicillin-clavulanate). Patients allergic to a macrolide or a beta-lactam may take a fluoroquinolone (Reuben et al., 2002). For critically ill hospitalized older patients, an intravenous third-generation cephalosporin in combination with a macrolide is recommended.

Additional supportive treatments include chest percussion to clear secretions, inhaled beta-adrenergic agonists to dilate constricted airways, oxygen if needed, and rehydration. Although treatment of pneumonia is the same for all patients regardless of age, the older person requires more careful monitoring. Agents with nephrotoxic potential, like the aminoglycosides, should be used with caution. Hypersensitivity reactions are more frequent in older patients, and risk of antibiotic-associated diarrhea or colitis is common with ampicillin or clindamycin. Drug interactions may also occur between antibiotics and other therapeutic agents commonly used in older persons such as warfarin. Intravenous fluids should be administered slowly in patients with congestive heart failure to prevent overhydration and pulmonary edema.

Prevention

Vaccination with pneumoccal vaccine is recommended for all persons 65 years of age and older and all adults with immunosuppression or chronic illnesses. When an older person's immunization status is unknown, the pneumococcal vaccine should be administered (Morbidity and Mortality Weekly Report, 2003). Revaccination has minimal side effects, with the most common being a localized reaction at the injection site.

The influenza vaccine should also be received yearly in persons who are at risk for pneumonia. The pneumococcal and influenza vaccines may be administered at the same time.

Older patients with pneumonia should be urged to rest and restrict activities to allow themselves time to heal and completely recover. Many will begin to recover after 5 to 7 days of antibiotic therapy. Additional patient education points include the following:

- Stop smoking (permanently if possible, mandatory during acute treatment).
- Take 10 deep breaths an hour to aerate lungs and loosen secretions.
- Drink plenty of fluids to keep secretions moist.
- Take antibiotics as prescribed and finish all medication.
- Report any adverse reactions immediately such as diarrhea, gastrointestinal irritation, rash or hives, and difficulty breathing.
- Avoid contact with others who are ill, infants, and frail older persons.
- Avoid coughing in public and practice good hand washing.
- Receive the pneumococcal vaccine as soon as possible after recovery and get a flu shot yearly to minimize the risk of further infection.

Acute Bronchitis

Acute bronchitis is an acute inflammation of the bronchi. It is usually a self-limiting viral illness. The signs and symptoms are similar to those of pneumonia and include productive cough, chills, lethargy, and low-grade fever. Chest x-ray will be negative, showing no active disease or infiltrates. Chest pain may be produced by muscle strain from prolonged and excessive coughing. Treatment consists of rest, humidification of the air, use of cough suppressants, and acetaminophen for aches.

Persons with COPD will usually be treated for bronchitis with antibiotics because their bronchitis may easily progress to pneumonia. This condition is sometimes called acute exacerbation of chronic bronchitis. Some physicians instruct their COPD patients to phone immediately upon noticing a change in sputum color from clear to white or green.

Pulmonary Embolism

Pulmonary embolism is an occlusion of a portion of the pulmonary vascular bed by an embolus consisting of a thrombus, an air bubble, or a fragment of tissue or lipids. When the blockage occurs, gas exchange can no longer take place in this section of the lung. The result is shortness of breath, heart failure, or death. Pulmonary emboli in older persons most often originate from deep-vein thrombosis in the calf.

Risk factors for formation of pulmonary embolus include clotting disorders, immobility, dehydration, recent surgery, atherosclerotic changes in the circulatory system, atrial fibrillation, and obesity. As many as 65% of patients with lower extremity trauma or surgery will develop deep-vein thrombosis (American Thoracic Society, 2004). Typical symptoms of pulmonary embolus include tachypnea, dyspnea, chest pain, hypoxia, decreased cardiac output, systemic hypotension, and possible shock.

Nursing Assessment

Patients with leg swelling, duskiness, and a positive Homans' sign (calf pain on dorsiflexion of the foot) are at risk for pulmory embolus. In persons with suspected deep-vein thrombosis, the calf of the affected leg should be carefully measured and the size noted and compared to the other leg. Asymmetry of more than 1 cm increases the likelihood of deep-vein thrombosis from 27% to 56% in an at-risk individual (McCance & Huether, 2001). Positive ultrasound studies of the leg warrant the initiation of anticoagulation therapy for prevention of pulmonary embolus (Reuben et al., 2002). Hypoxemia and hyperventilation are suggestive of the diagnosis of pulmonary embolus. A perfusion scan, in which lungs are scanned after injection of a radioactive dye into the venous circulation, can indicate obstruction of pulmonary circulation.

Treatment

Treatment consists of intravenous administration of heparin and other anticoagulant therapy. For large, life-threatening pulmonary obstructions, a fibrinolytic agent such as streptokinase is sometimes used; however, streptokinase cannot be administered within 7 to 10 days after surgery (Reuben et al., 2002). Warfarin therapy may be continued for 3 to 6 months after discharge to prevent the formation of another pulmonary embolus.

Preventive interventions include minimizing venous stasis by leg elevation, urging passive and active range of motion exercises in the immobile older person, encouraging early postoperative ambulation, and placing elastic compression stockings and pneumatic calf compression boots on the postoperative patient. Low-dose anticoagulation therapy with heparin is sometimes beneficial to prevent clots in postoperative patients until they become mobile. Prevention is key because less anticoagulant is needed to prevent a clot than to dissolve one already formed.

Severe Acute Respiratory Syndrome (SARS)

The primary symptoms of SARS are lethargy, muscle aches, dry cough, difficulty breathing, and persistent fever over 38°C or 100.4°F (Centers for Disease Control, 2003). Older people with these symptoms who have traveled to a high-risk country or have been exposed to someone who has, should seek medical attention immediately.

Preventive measures include wearing a face mask when in public areas of high-risk countries, strict isolation of infected persons, and careful hand washing. The virus is hardy and has been shown to survive on various surfaces for 24 hours. The mortality rate from SARS is highest in persons over 50. Intensive efforts to find an accurate diagnostic test and effective treatment or cure are under way at the time of this writing.

PATIENT-FAMILY TEACHING GUIDELINES

Lung Disease

The following are guidelines that the nurse may find useful when instructing older persons and their families about lung disease.

1. How can I prevent lung disease?

   Because respiratory problems are so often caused or aggravated by environmental exposure to toxins and pollutants, try to avoid these substances if at all possible. Some points to consider are:

   • Do not smoke cigarettes or other tobacco products.

- Do not visit or work in areas where dangerous substances or irritants are in the air (oven cleaner, glues, spray paints, etc.).
- Do not go outside or exercise when smog is present or air pollution warnings are in effect.
- Try to avoid contact with ill people and places where illness rates are high.

2. If I already have lung disease, is there anything I can do to stop it?

Yes. If you smoke, stop immediately! Also carry out all the suggestions listed in question 1. If you are prescribed medication by your doctor, take it exactly as directed. Report any worsening of your condition or new symptoms to your doctor. Have your disease monitored with spirometry testing as often as recommended by your doctor and get to know your numbers.

3. Is there anything else I should do to make the most of living with lung disease?

Yes. Exercise to keep your muscles fit and strong, eat a healthy diet, control your weight, get a flu shot every fall, get the pneumonia shot at age 65 and then every 6 years afterward, and visit the dentist regularly. Good oral hygiene can decrease respiratory infections and keep you healthy.

CHAPTER 15

THE GENITOURINARY AND RENAL SYSTEMS

NORMAL CHANGES OF AGING

With age, the size of the kidney and the number of glomeruli decline. Blood flow to the kidney decreases as a result of atrophy in the supplying blood vessels, particularly in the renal cortex. More urine is formed at night, potentially interrupting sleep patterns. In addition, because older adults excrete lower levels of glucose in the urine, testing for glycosuria is not an accurate method of monitoring blood glucose levels.

Because of renal excretion changes, be particularly vigilant for signs of toxicity when older patients are taking antibiotics, digoxin, diuretics, beta-blockers, statin lipid-lowering agents, ACE inhibitors, and oral antidiabetic agents (Schwartz, 1999).

The ability to respond to a fluid overload by increasing urine production is also decreased in the older adult. The changed ability to concentrate urine also makes the elderly adult more susceptible to dehydration, a problem that is further complicated by a deficit in the thirst response. Therefore, the elderly person will not feel thirsty even when significantly dehydrated (Beck, 1999).

The bladder becomes more fibrous, with subsequent decreased capacity and increased postvoiding residuals

(Bravo, 2000). The **detrusor muscles,** three layers of muscle that cover the bladder, become less contractile but also somewhat unstable. This means the older adult is subject to both inability to completely empty the bladder and involuntary contractions of the bladder (McCance & Huether, 2001). There is age-related weakening of the voluntary pelvic floor muscles that are important to controlling the release of urine from the urethra. These changes make older adults more likely to have difficulty delaying urination and predispose them to urinary incontinence and urinary tract infection. Even though there are anatomical and physiological changes that make incontinence more probable with increased age, urinary incontinence is *not* a normal part of aging.

The urethral changes in women are mostly related to the loss of estrogen following menopause (Bravo, 2000). In men, there is no muscle thinning, but the enlargement of the prostate may constrict the urethra (Saxon & Etten, 2002).

Due to estrogen-mediated changes in the perineal area of postmenopausal women, the urinary meatus may be difficult to visualize. When attempting urinary catheterization, you may wish to consider placing the older woman in a side-lying position, and visualize the perineum by lifting the buttock. If you are right-handed, assist the woman to lie on her left side, with her back toward you. If you are left-handed, assist the woman to her right side. By lifting the buttock, you should be able to visualize the urinary meatus on or near the anterior vaginal wall.

For both men and women, the major age-related change in sexual response is timing. It takes longer to become sexually aroused, longer to complete intercourse, and longer before sexual arousal can occur again (Butler & Lewis, 2003).

In general, the older man's libido may decrease but does not disappear. Older men achieve an erection that is less firm than in younger men, and ejaculation may take longer to occur in women. Estrogen levels fall off dramatically and remain at very low levels causing the vaginal tissues to thin and become less elastic, and the vagina to shorten (Duffy, 1998). There is less vaginal lubrication, potentially making intercourse more painful.

Older women also experience changes in their sexual responses. It takes longer for the older woman to become sexually aroused and produce vaginal lubrication. During orgasm, the uterus will contract less frequently, but the contractions remain vigorous, and orgasm is as intense as in younger women.

COMMON GENITOURINARY CONCERNS IN OLDER ADULTS

Acute and Chronic Renal Failure

Acute renal failure is found in approximately one fifth of older adults (Bailey & Sands, 2003). Prerenal causes are common in older adults and lead to poor perfusion of the kidney. Renal causes may be secondary to chronic diseases such as hypertension and diabetes mellitus. The most prevalent postrenal cause is prostatic hypertrophy.

Postural hypotension is a common finding in prerenal acute renal failure (Bailey & Sands, 2003), and the nurse is in a position to monitor. BUN and serum creatinine levels increase, and dependent edema may be present. Ultrasound may demonstrate changes in the size of the kidney, or presence of calculi, in renal and postrenal causes. Dehydration in the older adult is a causative factor in acute renal failure; therefore, fluid restrictions should be modest (Jassal et al., 1998).

Chronic renal failure is caused by irreversible damage to the kidney and is much more common in older adults than in younger adults (Beers & Berkow, 2000). Diabetes mellitus, benign prostatic hyperplasia, hypertension, and long-term use of NSAIDs all contribute to the higher prevalence of chronic renal failure in older adults. The symptoms and signs are similar to those exhibited by younger persons, and include decreased glomerular filtration rate, hyperphosphatemia, hypocalcemia, hyperkalemia, metabolic acidosis, hypertension, and anemia. As the disease progresses, the older adult may experience pruritus, general lack of well-being, generalized edema, altered cognition, anorexia, nausea, and weight loss. As with acute renal failure, prompt consultation by a nephrologist is critical to improving the older adult's quality of life and long-term survival (Bailey & Sands, 2003).

The treatments for chronic renal failure should be modified for the older adult. The restrictions on fluid intake and dietary protein should be less stringent, since most older adults have already decreased their protein and sodium intakes (Jassal et al., 1998). Constipation, a concern for many older adults, may exacerbate the hyperkalemia that accompanies chronic renal failure.

The definitive treatment for chronic renal failure is renal replacement therapy, either through dialysis or through renal transplant (Bailey & Sands, 2003).

Urinary Tract Infection

A **urinary tract infection (UTI)** is the presence of bacteria in the urethra, bladder, or kidney, although the majority of UTIs in older adults are asymptomatic (Nicolle, 2003). Some authors term this condition *asymptomatic UTI,* whereas others apply the term *UTI* only to those older adults with symptoms, and use *bacteriuria* to define the presence of bacteria in the urine with no concomitant symptoms (Nicolle, 2003). UTIs in catheterized older adults tend to be polymicrobial and difficult to eradicate. Before using an indwelling catheter, the potential benefits to the older adult must be carefully weighed against the serious risks posed.

A change in behavior may be the only indicator of a UTI (McCue, 1999). If, however, an older adult has not previously experienced **urinary urgency,** the shortened period of time between the urge to void and actual urination, or **urinary frequency,** more than seven voids per 24-hour period, these symptoms should be thoroughly investigated.

Asymptomatic UTI does not require treatment. In fact, treatment does not improve the morbidity or mortality in affected older persons (Krogh & Bruskewitz, 1998; McCue, 1999; Nicolle, 2003; Steers, 1999). Routine urinalysis for older adults without symptoms is neither appropriate nor cost-effective. In the presence of symptoms, however, treatment decisions should be based on urine culture and sensitivity test. UTI in an older person with an indwelling catheter is considered to be complicated and may include a variety of microorganisms, such as *Escherichia coli, Proteus mirabilis, Klebsiella pneumoniae, Citrobacter* spp., *Providencia* spp., and *Pseudomonas aeruginosa* (Nicolle, 2003). The only way to accurately identify the causative organism, and thus treat the infection effectively, is to obtain a urine culture (McCue, 1999). Many experts recommend straight catheterization for collecting an uncontaminated specimen from older women who are unable to cooperate.

Urinary Incontinences (UI)

Stress incontinence is defined as the involuntary loss of urine when the intra-abdominal pressure is increased, such as during coughing or laughing. Either the pelvic floor muscles or the internal urethral sphincter is not strong enough to counter the pressure on the bladder, and urine is released. **Urge incontinence** occurs when the detrusor muscles contract forcefully and unexpectedly, and the internal sphincter is unable to retain urine in the bladder. **Overflow incontinence** is sometimes known as mechanical incontinence because a blockage of the urethra may be the cause of the bladder overfilling and stretching the bladder muscles beyond the point of contractility. Overflow may also occur if the muscles are unable to contract properly because of lack of innervation, as in spinal cord injury or in diabetes mellitus. Finally, **functional incontinence** is defined as incontinence related to causes external to the urinary apparatus, such that the older adult is unable to get to a toilet to void. Older persons with dementia may experience functional incontinence because they are unable to find the toilet.

Assessment should include the six areas of health history related to UI, mental status evaluation, functional evaluation, environmental assessment, social supports, bladder records, and physical examination (Jarvis, 2004). The mnemonic DIAPPERS can help the nurse identify the cause of new-onset urinary incontinence (Resnick & Yalla, 1985; Reuben et al., 2004).

- **D**elirium
- **I**nfection (urinary or systemic)
- **A**trophic urethritis/vaginitis (irritation, inflammation)

- **P**harmaceuticals (diuretics, psychotropics, ACE inhibitors)
- **P**sychological (depression, dementia, agitation)
- **E**ndocrine (diabetes mellitus)
- **R**estricted mobility/restraints (gait disorders, CVA, environmental obstacles)
- **S**tool impaction

Health history questions related to UI should include:

- Is there a concurrent medical condition, such as UTI, cerebrovascular accident (CVA), or diabetes mellitus that may be affecting continence status?
- Has UI occurred before, and under what conditions?
- What is the pattern of UI? The nurse should ask questions that will help categorize the type of UI (see Table 15–1).
- What medications are currently being used?
- What amount, type, and timing of fluid intake are present? It is important to assess fluids that may irritate the bladder, or increase urine production such as caffeine-containing coffee or tea, carbonated beverages, alcohol, citrus juices, and diet drinks containing aspartame.
- How does the UI affect the older person's quality of life?

(Kennedy-Malone, Fletcher, & Plank, 2000; Lekan-Rutledge & Colling, 2003; Ouslander, 2000; Bottomley, 2000)

In addition to these health history questions, a mental status examination and functional assessment must be completed to evaluate the effect these areas might have on continence. A careful assessment of the environment and the older person's clothing are also indicated.

New-onset urinary incontinence should be aggressively investigated by the gerontological nurse. The earlier the cause is identified, the sooner nursing

Table 15-1 Types of Urinary Incontinence

Type	Etiology	Examples	Group Most Affected
Stress	Weakened external sphincter/pelvic floor, increased intra-abdominal pressure	Urine loss during sneezing, laughing, exercise	Women under age 60 Men after prostate surgery
Urge	Detrusor instability, internal sphincter weakness	Overactive bladder	Older adults of both sexes, older men somewhat more affected
Overflow	Bladder muscles overextended and have poor tone, overflow of retained urine	Enlarged prostate causes obstruction of the urethra, urine backs up in bladder; diabetic nephropathy affects the contractility of the detrusor muscles	Persons with diabetes mellitus Men with enlarged prostates Persons taking calcium channel blockers, anticholinergics, and adrenergics
Functional	Physical or psychological factors impair ability to get to the toilet	An older adult unable to transfer from wheelchair to toilet is unable to obtain needed assistance	Frail elderly adults Nursing home residents Persons with dementias

Source: Assad, 2000; Hartford Institute for Geriatric Nursing, 2001; Malone-Lee, 1998; Ouslander, 2000.

interventions can be instituted to correct the problem and improve the patient's situation.

Bladder records or diaries are a critical tool in evaluating and managing UI.

The nurse should perform a physical assessment including an abdominal examination, particularly looking for distended bowel or bladder; rectal examination, evaluating for impacted stool; and genital examination, observing for skin condition and presence of organ prolapse (Kane, Ouslander, & Abrass, 2004).

Treatments for UI are categorized into five groups: lifestyle modification, scheduled voiding regimens, pelvic floor muscle strengthening, anti-incontinence devices, and supportive interventions (Wyman, 2003). Medications form a sixth category. A combination of interventions from several categories is usually referred to as a toileting program (Lekan-Rutledge & Colling, 2003). The older adult must be a partner in choosing the interventions (Palmer, 2000).

Timed voiding has been demonstrated to be effective for older women with stress incontinence and for some older men after prostatectomy (Wyman, 2003). A schedule is established for toileting, usually every 2 hours, but as long as 3 hours may be acceptable. Bladder training is similar to timed voiding, but the intervals between trips to the toilet are gradually lengthened, training the bladder to hold slightly increased amounts of urine. Prompted voiding also uses some of the techniques of timed voiding, but rather than assisting the older adult to the toilet every 2 hours, the nurse reminds the older adult every 2 hours to go to the toilet. An older adult who is taking diuretics should be helped to identify the onset and peak action of the diuretic, and then aided in developing a toileting schedule to maximize continence.

Pelvic floor exercises, or **Kegel exercises,** are another UI intervention frequently employed by nurses. The technique works well for urge and stress incontinence. It requires that the older adult be motivated to perform the exercises and be cognitively intact enough to learn them (Wyman, 2003). The older adult is instructed to tighten the muscles of the perineum, without also tensing the muscles of the abdomen, thigh, or buttock (Assad, 2000). A recommended pattern is 15 repetitions of rapid contractions, one to three sets, daily (Assad, 2000).

Several medications are available to assist the person with stress or urge UI. Urge UI medications are generally anticholinergic and inappropriate for persons with narrow-angle glaucoma or urinary retention, or antiadrenergics that may potentiate other antihypertensives (Smith & Ouslander, 2000). Stress incontinence in women may be treated with estrogen applications, and in both men and women with pseudoephedrine, which is contraindicated in people with hypertension (Smith & Ouslander, 2000). Medications should be used as an adjunct to other therapies. Addition of Detrol© to a behavioral UI therapy in nursing home residents may be helpful in maintaining continence.

Many older adults who experience UI use disposable incontinence pads or protective undergarments. Excellent skin care remains a nursing priority because urine can be very damaging to the skin. Pads or undergarments must be changed frequently and after every episode of incontinence. They should be disposed of in ways that minimize environmental impact, especially the patient's immediate surroundings. Used incontinence products can have an unpleasant odor, and care should be taken to keep the older adult's room or home aesthetically pleasing.

Benign Prostatic Hyperplasia (BPH)

The symptoms of BPH include difficulty starting a stream of urine, weak stream, straining to urinate, longer time needed to urinate, and a feeling of incomplete bladder emptying (Letran & Brawer, 1999). As the prostate continues to grow, urinary retention may occur. Symptoms of bladder irritation secondary to the enlarged prostate include urinary urgency, frequency, and **nocturia.** Some men experience urge incontinence as a result of BPH.

Urinary retention in men with BPH can be precipitated by several classes of medications, including those with anticholinergic properties and over-the-counter medications for the common cold.

Treatment for BPH includes managing urge incontinence (discussed earlier) and decreasing the other urinary symptoms. Alpha-adrenergic blocking medications such as tamsulosin and doxazosin mesylate may be prescribed. Saw palmetto is an over-the-counter herbal preparation that appears to be effective in improving BPH symptoms and has relatively few side effects (Chow, 2001). As with any herbal preparation, saw palmetto is not regulated by any organized group. When urinary retention becomes refractory to other treatments, or renal insufficiency due to bladder outlet obstruction develops, surgical intervention may be recommended (Letran & Brawer, 1999).

The most commonly performed surgery for BPH is transurethral resection of the prostate. Older men who have the surgery are at risk for erectile dysfunction, retrograde ejaculation, hemorrhage, and infection, although most have dramatic improvement in their presurgery symptoms (Chow, 2001; Letran & Brawer, 1999).

Hormone Replacement Therapy Concerns

Current recommendations are that HRT be used only as a last resort for the relief of vasomotor symptoms related to menopause (Nelson, Humphrey, Nygren, Teutsch, & Allan, 2002). The potential for harm from HRT should be thoroughly discussed with the older woman before she initiates the therapy.

Atrophic vaginitis may result in urogenital infection, ulceration, and uncomfortable sexual intercourse. The treatment of choice is topical estrogen as a cream that is applied to the affected tissues (Messinger-Rapport & Thacker, 2001). Topical creams have not demonstrated the link to adverse effects that systemic HRT has (Strandberg, Ylikorkala, & Tikkanen, 2003).

Genitourinary Malignancies
Cancer of the Urinary Bladder

Some symptoms of bladder cancer are similar to those of other urinary tract diseases: microhematuria, urinary frequency, urgency, and dysuria (Beers & Berkow, 2000). Pyuria, the presence of pus in the urine, may also be a symptom of bladder cancer. In the absence of UTI, an older adult with either gross or microhematuria should be referred for cystoscopy. In many cases, this procedure can be carried out in a physician's office.

Available treatments range from depositing chemotherapeutic agents into the bladder to removal of the bladder and surrounding organs. These surgeries present challenges to the older adult's body image, and the nurse must work with the patient to address these challenges. Specific concerns include the psychomotor skills of managing the urinary reservoir, ongoing fear of cancer, and "the bag" (Beitz & Zuzelo, 2003).

Prostate Cancer

The most commonly used screening tests for prostate cancer are digital rectal examination (DRE) combined with prostate-specific antigen (PSA) testing (Gambert, 2001). A normal PSA level is below 4 ng/ml. Values over 10 ng/ml are strongly indicative of prostate cancer, while values between 4 ng/ml and 10 ng/ml are difficult to interpret. During the DRE, the practitioner is able to palpate the prostate, feeling for nodules suspicious for cancer. If either of these screens demonstrates abnormalities, a transrectal ultrasound is usually recommended.

Once prostate cancer is diagnosed, the older man has a variety of treatment options including *radical prostatectomy* (removing the prostate through a perineal or retropubic incision), *radiation therapy, surveillance* (watchful waiting). If the cancer is more advanced, external radiation or hormonal treatment may be recommended (Balducci, Pow-Sang, Friedland, & Diaz, 1997). The older patient should be offered a thorough discussion of all options with a urologist.

Gynecological Malignancies

Ovarian, uterine, and breast cancer are more prevalent in older women than in younger women (Ries et al., 2002). Cervical cancer, although more prevalent in young and midlife women, remains a concern. Vulvar cancer, signaled by a palpable nodule on the labia and prurituis, is not common in any age group (Brown & Cooper, 1998).

The symptoms of ovarian cancer are vague, including diffuse abdominal discomfort and gastrointestinal distress (Beers & Berkow, 2000). The vagueness of the symptoms may account, in part, for the poor prognosis because women are rarely diagnosable when the tumor is confined to the ovary. More obvious symptoms, such as ascites or a palpable mass, are not frequently present until lymph nodes are involved or metastases are found.

Treatment options for the older woman with ovarian cancer include surgery to remove the uterus, ovaries, fallopian tubes, and omentum (Balducci et al., 1997). Chemotherapeutic agents may also be used, but recurrent disease is common (Brown & Cooper, 1998).

Cancer of the body of the uterus or endometrium is the most common gynecological cancer in older women (Ries et al., 2002). Risk factors include celibacy, late menopause, obesity, hypertension, and diabetes mellitus (Brown & Cooper, 1998). HRT, particularly estrogen, has also been implicated in the development of endometrial cancer (Nelson et al., 2002). The most common symptom is uterine bleeding after menopause, which occurs early in the disease, making early diagnosis and treatment possible. The diagnosis is usually made by endometrial biopsy, and treatment includes hysterectomy, oophorectomy, and salpingectomy. Chemotherapy after surgery is common. Prognosis is much better if the treatment is begun earlier in the course of the disease.

The risk factors of cervical cancer include infection with human papillomavirus, early onset of sexual activity, history of abnormal Pap smears, HIV-positive status, and many sexual partners (Brown & Cooper, 1998; National Cancer Institute, 2003). Current recommendations are that women who are over age 65, who have had a regular history of normal Pap smears, and who are not at high risk because of other factors (see above) should *not* receive routine Pap smears (U.S. Preventive Services Task Force, 2003). Older women who have had a total hysterectomy (cervix removed) for nonmalignant reasons do not need to be screened with Pap smears.

Strong evidence exists that yearly mammography for all women over the age of 40 decreases mortality from breast cancer and should be encouraged (U.S. Preventive Services Task Force, 2003). Teaching an older woman breast self-examination, however, may be socially unacceptable to her. Women who do not examine their breasts on a regular basis cannot enjoy the same preventive value as women who perform this examination regularly.

The treatment for breast cancer depends on the stage of the tumor when detected. Small, contained tumors may be treated with modified radical mastectomy, or lumpectomy with radiation (Kimmick & Muss, 1997). The presence of comorbidities in older women makes treatment choices more challenging because some conditions, such as cardiovascular disease, may militate against extensive reconstructive surgery (Munster & Hudis, 1999). The use of tamoxifen after surgery appears to increase survival from breast cancer for older women with metastases to the lymph nodes. Age alone should not be the determining factor in treatment options offered to the older woman.

SEX AND THE SENIOR CITIZEN

Chronic pain and osteoarthritis are two common problems that have deleterious effects on sexual activity and older adults. Arthritis in the hip joint presents the greatest challenge to satisfying sexual activity (Butler & Lewis, 2003), but it can be ameliorated by changes in coital position, use of heat applications, and timing during the day when joints are less painful. The "spoon" position, in which partners lie on their sides with the woman in front, allows for penile penetration of the vagina without undue strain to either partner (Monga et al., 1999). Warm baths can also help relieve pain and can be incorporated as foreplay.

Many older adults who suffer from cardiovascular disease are concerned about the safety of sex. In general, if an older adult can climb two flights of stairs or walk at a rate of 2 miles per hour without chest pain or shortness of breath, he or she should have no cardiac problems during sexual intercourse (Butler & Lewis, 2003).

Dyspareunia, painful intercourse for the older woman, may be related to decreased vaginal lubrication as well as lack of elevation of the labia during sexual arousal (Monga et al., 1999). Penetration is difficult as the vaginal opening may be partially obscured by the labia, and the lack of lubrication further inhibits entrance of the penis. Alternative expressions of sexuality, such as body caressing, manipulation of the partner's genitals with the hand, or mutual masturbation, may be suggested.

Discussing Sexuality with Older Adults

The PLISSIT model of intervention for sexual concerns was developed over 30 years ago, but is still a valid method for nurses to use with older adults (Annon, 1974; Hartford Institute for Geriatric Nursing, 2001). **P** stands for permission, in which the nurse validates the older adult's desire for sexual activity. **LI** is limited information, and the nurse offers specific, factual information pertinent to the older patient. **SS** stands for specific suggestions, such as coital positions or timing of pain medication. **IT** is intensive therapy, which requires a referral to an advanced practice nurse or other expert.

Sexuality in Long-Term Care

If one or both of the older adults involved in physical intimacy is cognitively impaired, both legal and ethical responsibilities arise. The nurse must intervene to ensure that both parties are making an informed decision to participate in sexual activity, or at least that there is no exploitation involved (Lichtenberg, 1997). Some older adults with dementias will engage in sexual activity that is inappropriate, for example, masturbation in public. One nursing intervention is to redirect the older adult to a private area or provide distraction (Monga et al., 1999). It is important to consider the motive that may be driving the sexual behavior and attempt to meet those needs (Duffy, 1998).

Erectile Dysfunction

There are no universally recommended diagnostics for ED. Treatment is dependent on etiology, so some laboratory studies and specific physical examinations may be conducted. Thyroid-stimulating hormone and serum testosterone may give important information, as may imaging studies (Stern, 1997). A review of the medications an older man takes is critical, as many drugs have ED as a side effect. A neurologic examination and assessment for depression may also be performed (Carbone & Seftel, 2002).

A variety of treatments are available for ED, including oral medication, self-administered injections into the penis, vacuum erection devices, and surgical implants (Carbone & Seftel, 2002). The nurse may act as an advocate to ensure the older man is offered all appropriate treatment options.

Sexually Transmitted Diseases

Sexually active older adults are at risk for the same sexually transmitted diseases that affect younger adults including HIV/AIDS, syphilis, and gonorrhea. They should be offered the same education about safer sex, including the use of condoms. This may be a reflection of greater acceptance of sexuality among older persons in these populations. Questions related to symptoms of sexually transmitted diseases should be included in the review of systems and nursing assessment of an older adult.

PATIENT-FAMILY TEACHING GUIDELINES

Instructing Older Persons About Urinary Tract Infections

The following are guidelines that the nurse may find useful when instructing older persons and their families about urinary tract infections.

1. What is a urinary tract infection?

   A urinary tract infection is the result of the growth of bacteria (germs) in the kidney or bladder, or in the tubes that connect them. It might also be called a bladder infection, cystitis, or UTI.

2. Who gets urinary tract infections?

   Women who have been through menopause are likely to get urinary tract infections.

   Men with prostate problems are also likely to get urinary tract infections.

   Men or women who have a urinary catheter may also get them.

3. What are the symptoms?

   Common symptoms of UTI may include:
   - Burning or itching during urination.
   - Feeling of urgency and need to urinate frequently.
   - Involuntary loss of urine or urinary incontinence.

(continued)

- Back pain, fatigue, nausea, and dull pain or ache in the lower abdomen.
- Sometimes confusion, especially in those who already have memory problems.

4. How does the healthcare provider know a patient has a urinary tract infection?

A simple urine test may show white blood cells and the bacteria causing the infection. The healthcare provider will test your urine as a result of your complaints and symptoms. One test can be done quickly in the office or clinic, and the other test (culture and sensitivity) must be sent to the laboratory and takes about 3 days to obtain the final results. If you are very uncomfortable and having severe urinary symptoms, your healthcare provider will probably treat you right away with an antibiotic while awaiting the final test results.

5. What is the treatment for urinary tract infections?

If you are found to have a UTI with troubling symptoms and bacteria, white blood cells, or blood in your urine, you will probably be given an antibiotic by your healthcare provider. It is very important to take *all* the medicine, even if you start to feel better before it is all gone. Drink at least 8 large glasses of water per day.

6. How do I prevent another infection?

Many older people are prone to frequent UTIs. You can help prevent recurrent infections by taking the following steps:
- Make sure you keep drinking at least 8 large glasses of water per day.

- Drink a few glasses of cranberry juice if you feel the symptoms of UTI starting to bother you.
- Wear all-cotton underwear, and put on a clean set every day.
- Go to the toilet as soon as you need to urinate—do not wait.
- Wipe from the front to the back after you use the toilet.
- Make sure to pass a few drops of urine after you have sexual intercourse.

CHAPTER 16

THE MUSCULOSKELETAL SYSTEM

THE NORMAL MUSCULOSKELETAL SYSTEM AND JOINTS

The musculoskeletal system consists of the body's skeleton, muscles, **ligaments,** bursae, and joints. The skeleton provides form and support for the body. Bones provide protection for delicate body parts and are an important source of minerals as well as blood cells. The skeletal muscles provide movement of various body parts. All components of the system work together to produce the normal movement and actions that allow individuals to function independently in daily life.

Normal changes of aging often bring about complaints of musculoskeletal pain and various joint limitations, and aging appears to predispose an individual to the development of diseases such as osteoporosis and arthritis, resulting in loss of mobility and function.

NORMAL CHANGES OF AGING

Skeleton

In the older person, bones become stiff, weaker, and more brittle. An average loss of height is 1 to 2 cm every two decades, from about 20 to 70 years of age. Thinning of the vertebral disks occurs more commonly in midlife; in later years, there is a decrease in the height of individual vertebrae. The result is a shortening of the trunk and the appearance of long extremities. Additional postural changes are kyphosis and a backward tilt of the head to make eye contact. The result is a forward bent, or "jutting out" posture, with the hips and knees assuming a flex position.

Muscles

By age 75, most people lose one half of the skeletal muscle mass they had at the age of 30 (Metter et al., 1999). This process is known as **sarcopenia.** Muscle tone and tension decreases steadily after the third decade. Some muscles decrease in size, resulting in weakness.

Joints, Ligaments, Tendons, and Cartilage

Ligaments, tendons, and joint capsules lose elasticity and become less flexible. There is a decrease in the range of motion of the joints due to changes in ligaments and muscles. Nonarticular cartilage, such as the ears and nose, grows throughout life, which may cause the nose to look large in relation to the face.

COMMON MUSCULOSKELETAL ILLNESSES OF OLDER PERSONS

Osteoporosis is the most common metabolic disease, affecting 50% of women during their lifetime. Major risk factors for osteoporosis are increased age, female sex, White or Asian race, positive family history of osteoporosis, and thin body habitus. Additional risk factors include low calcium intake, prolonged immobility, excessive alcohol intake, cigarette smoking, and the long-term use of corticosteroids, anticonvulsants, or thyroid hormones.

Pathophysiology

Osteoporosis is characterized by low bone mass and deterioration of bone tissue leading to compromised bone strength that increases the risk for fractures. Bone loss in the older person is considered normal when bone mineral density is within 1 standard deviation (SD) of the young adult mean. Bone density between 1 and 2.5 SD below the young adult mean is termed osteopenic. Osteoporosis is defined as bone density 2.5 SD below the young adult mean. The three factors most likely to contribute to decreased bone mass in the older person (1) failure to reach peak bone mass in early adulthood, (2) increased bone resorption, and (3) decreased bone formation.

Osteomalacia

Osteomalacia is a metabolic disease in which there is inadequate mineralization of newly formed bone matrix, usually resulting from vitamin D deficiency.

Pathophysiological Mechanisms

The most common causes of osteomalacia are vitamin D deficiency, abnormal metabolism of vitamin D, and phosphate depletion. Older persons are at risk for osteomalacia because of the inability to get outdoors, limited dietary intake of milk, as well as aging skin that is less able to produce vitamin D.

Paget's Disease

Paget's disease, or **osteitis deformans,** is a chronic, localized bone disorder of unknown etiology in which normal bone is removed and replaced with abnormal bone. Paget's disease may be asymptomatic, the diagnosis made by abnormal x-ray findings for an unrelated problem.

Clinical Manifestations

Bone pain, the most frequently reported symptom, may be described as deep and aching, and may be accompanied by muscle spasms. When Paget's disease affects the skull, it may cause enlargement and disfigurement of the cranium, resulting in complications of the central nervous system such as mental deterioration and dementia. The older person may also experience headaches, tinnitus, and vertigo.

Joint Disorders

Noninflammatory Joint Disease: Osteoarthritis

Primary or idiopathic osteoarthritis has no single, clear cause. The typical changes can occur in several joints but have various causes. Secondary arthritis has an underlying condition such as trauma, bone disease, or inflammatory joint disease.

Pathophysiology

Osteoarthritis is characterized by the progressive erosion of the joint articular cartilage with the formation of new bone in the joint. The joints most commonly involved in OA are joints of the hands, the weight-bearing joints of the knee and hip, and the central joints of the cervical and lumbar spine.

Clinical Manifestations

The most common symptoms are early morning stiffness and joint pain. Morning stiffness in the joints usually resolves in about 30 minutes. Pain usually occurs during activity and is relieved by rest. As the disease progresses, the pain may be present at rest and interrupt sleep patterns. Joints affected may have crepitus (a grating sound on movement), deficits in range of motion, and muscle weakness. Osteoarthritis of the hands may show new bone growth with the appearance of Heberden's nodes (distal interphalangeal joint) and Bouchard's nodes (proximal interphalangeal joint). Pain can be elicited on both active and passive motion. The joint damage, chronic pain, and muscle weakness of OA result in impaired balance and decreased activity.

Inflammatory Joint Disease

Rheumatoid Arthritis

Rheumatoid arthritis (RA) is the most prevalent inflammatory arthritis of any age group. Women are affected more than men by a 3 to 1 ratio and tend to have more severe articular disease symptoms. For some patients, it may be a mild remitting disease; for others, it brings severe disability, joint deformity, and even premature death (Gornisiewicz & Moreland, 2001).

Pathophysiology

Rheumatoid arthritis is a chronic syndrome, characterized by symmetrical inflammation of the peripheral joints, with pain, swelling, significant morning stiffness, as well as general symptoms of fatigue and malaise. RA is most likely due to a variety of unknown environmental factors (infectious agents, chemical exposures) that trigger an autoimmune response to an unidentified antigen. Genetic predisposition is a major factor in both the susceptibility and the severity of RA (Gornisiewicz & Moreland, 2001; Workman, 2000).

Clinical Manifestations

The course of RA may be slow and insidious, or it may present with an acute process affecting several joints (polyarticular). RA causes tenderness and limitation of movement. Clinical manifestations include disabling morning stiffness and marked pain in the joints, chiefly in the upper extremities. The morning stiffness of RA lasts more than an hour and may also occur after a period of rest. On assessment, the joints will have severe redness, swelling, and warmth of the soft tissue. These symptoms cause severe pain on movement, limitation of movement, and a disrupted sleep pattern. Although RA is characterized by joint symptoms, it is a systemic inflammatory disease. Most patients with RA experience nonspecific systemic symptoms such as fatigue, malaise, weight loss, and fever, which often occur several weeks or months before the typical joint symptoms.

Subcutaneous nodules also occur with advanced disease in more than one fourth of RA patients. They are located on pressure areas such as the elbows or sacrum, and are not attached to bone or underlying skin.

Gout

Gouty arthritis is the most common form of inflammatory joint disease in men over 25 years of age (Meiner, 2001).

Pathophysiology

The pathophysiology of gout is closely linked to purine metabolism and kidney function. Serum urate levels greater than 7 mg/dl are associated with an increased risk of gout, the risk increasing as the duration and level of urate increases (Kase & Ostrov, 2001). The main predisposing factors for gout include family history, high purine diet, and obesity. Although genetics play a major role, drugs such as alcohol and acetylsalicylic acid (ASA) also result in low urate renal clearance.

Gout results from the deposit of urate crystals in a peripheral joint where it initiates pain, inflammation, and destruction. Acute pain, warmth, and swelling in the metatarsophalangeal joint of the big toe are typically the first signs of gouty arthritis. Over time, the attacks continue and may affect other joints, including the knee, wrist, ankle, elbow, joints of the hand or feet, or bursa. General malaise, fever, and chills accompany these painful joint symptoms. Pain and tenderness are often so severe that the older person cannot tolerate the weight of a sheet or blanket, or even move the affected joint (Ettinger, 2003).

Chronic gout, also known as tophaceous gout, can begin as early as 3 years or as late as 40 years after the initial acute attack (McCance & Mourad, 2000). The person with chronic gout will have persistent complaints of aching joints, soreness, and morning stiffness, most commonly in the hands and feet. The development of tophi is directly related to the duration and severity of hyperuricemia (Ettinger 2003; Kase & Ostrov, 2001).

Pseudogout

Pseudogout, or calcium pyrophosphate deposition disease, is a form of arthritis. It is caused by the formation of calcium pyrophosphate-dihydrate crystals in large joints. Affected joints include the knee, shoulder, hip, and elbow (Kerr, 2003).

Tendinitis and Bursitis

Bursitis is an irritation of subcutaneous tissue and inflammation of the underlying bursae. Acute bursitis is characterized by a deep aching pain on movement of any structure adjacent to the bursae. Tendinitis refers to inflammation of the tendon sheath (tenosynovitis). The course of soft tissue rheumatism, such as tendinitis and bursitis, is benign and responds to therapeutic regimens. The pain, however, is significant and will often temporarily decrease mobility.

FALLS AND THE OLDER PERSON

Prevention of falls in the clinical setting is a priority. The goals are to recognize older persons at risk for falling; to identify and correct fall risk factors; to improve balance, gait, mobility, and functional independence using a structured interdisciplinary approach; to reduce or eliminate environmental factors that contribute to fall risk; and to evaluate outcomes with revision of the plan as needed. The Hartford Institute for Geriatric Nursing recommends using the Hendrich Fall Assessment Tool (page 310) when evaluating fall risk in the older adult.

Hip Fracture

Hip fractures include those in the upper third of the femur, and may be intracapsular or extracapsular. Intracapsular fractures are those located within the joint capsule and are further categorized as femoral neck and subcapital fractures. Extracapsular fractures include intertrochanteric (in the trochanter) and subtrochanteric (below the trochanter).

Selected Diagnostic Tests and Values

Some of the laboratory and radiological tests that can assist in the diagnosis and evaluation of musculoskeletal problems in the older adult include the following:

• Bone mineral density test (DEXA) of the spine and hip is recommended. The results are expressed in standard deviations, and compare the patient's results with the young adult mean. Results can also be compared with a norm group of the same age. For instance, a BMD of 1 SD below the mean (-1 SD) indicates osteopenia. A BMD of 2.5 SD below the mean (-2.5 SD) indicates severe osteoporosis, according to the World Health Organization.

- Bone and joint radiography and computerized tomography
- Magnetic resonance imaging
- Bone and joint scanning

Blood Serum Tests

Several blood tests are important in diagnosing and treating musculoskeletal disorders. They are as follows:

- Electrolytes: calcium level (increased in Paget's disease, bone fracture, and immobility; decreased in osteomalacia)
- Serum uric acid (higher levels are associated with gout attacks)
- Joint tests: rheumatoid factor (RF). A high RF (positive RF high titers $\geq$ 1:320) is a predictor of an increase in the severity of symptoms such as greater disability and extra-articular disease. RF is also elevated in patients with liver disease, lung disease, and other conditions. Rheumatoid factor is not diagnostic for RA, but it can confirm the diagnosis. RF does not change rapidly, so once the titer is high, the test is not repeated.
- Acute-phase reactants: C-reactive protein (CRP) and erythrocyte sedimentation rate (ESR) are common acute-phase reactants. ESR is the most common measurement of acute-phase proteins in rheumatic disease. Sedimentation of red cells is directly related to the acute-phase proteins. CRP is used for determining if an inflammatory process is present, such as a bacterial infection or rheumatic

disease. CRP increases and goes back to normal quicker than ESR.

- Bone and muscle enzymes: Alkaline phosphatase is an enzyme associated with bone activity. Normal values for men are 45 to 115 U/L, and for women 30 to 100 U/L. Values tend to increase after the age of 50. ALP studies identify increases in osteoblastic activity and inflammatory conditions. A person with Paget's disease will have a pronounced elevation of ALP.

Synovial Fluid Analysis

Synovial fluid analysis involves evaluation of fluids drawn from a joint with a sterile needle. Synovial fluid is normally a viscous, straw-colored substance that is found in small amounts in a normal joint to provide lubrication and prevent friction during joint movement. The fluid is initially analyzed for color and clarity. Additional routine analysis may include evaluation of white blood cells, red blood cells, neutrophils, protein, glucose crystals; tests for rheumatoid factor (RA), uric acid for gout; and bacteria to establish the presence of infection. Abnormal joint fluid may look cloudy or abnormally thick.

Pharmacology and Nursing Responsibilities for Osteoporosis

Bisphosphonates, selective estrogen receptor modulators (SERMs), and calcitonin are antiresorptive drugs prescribed for the treatment and prevention of osteoporosis in both men and women. Antiresorptive therapy preserves or increases bone density, and decreases the rate of bone resorption.

Bisphosphonates—alendronate (Fosamax) and risedronate (Actonel)—are potent drugs that inhibit osteoclastic activity and have decreased the incidence of vertebral and nonvertebral fractures by 40 to 50% in postmenopausal women (National Osteoporosis Foundation, 2002). Calcium should not be taken at the same time as bisphosphonates since this will interfere with the absorption of the drug. The older person must (1) take either drug on an empty stomach, first thing in the morning with 8 oz of water, (2) remain upright for 30 minutes, and (3) not eat or drink anything else for 30 minutes.

SERMs have been developed to provide the benefits of estrogens without the disadvantages. Raloxifene has been approved by the U.S. Food and Drug Administration (FDA) for the prevention and treatment of osteoporosis in postmenopausal women. SERMS are less effective antiresorptive drugs than bisphosphonates, but do reduce bone loss and decrease fracture risk (National Osteoporosis Foundation, 2002; Wilson, Shannon, & Stang, 2003).

Calcitonin is generally considered to be a safe but less effective treatment for osteoporosis. It has been found to decrease spinal fractures by up to 35%. It may be given intranasally or subcutaneously. It is approved for women who are at least 5 years postmenopausal (National Osteoporosis Foundation, 2002).

For many years, hormone replacement therapy (HRT) has been taken by postmenopausal women to reduce the risk of fractures and treat the symptoms of menopause. However, the FDA has withdrawn its approval of estrogen replacement for the treatment of osteoporosis.

Pharmacology and Nursing Responsibilities for Osteomalacia

The goal of the pharmacological treatment of osteomalacia is to remineralize the bone. The treatment of osteomalacia will depend on the cause. Vitamin D replacement is given in doses of 50,000 to 100,000 U/day for 1 to 2 weeks and followed by a daily dose of 400 to 800 U/day. The older person should be monitored for serum and urine calcium levels. Other forms of vitamin D such as calcidiol and calcitriol are given for the specific cause of vitamin D deficiency. All older persons with osteomalacia need to have adequate calcium intake (1,000 to 1,500 mg/day).

Pharmacology and Nursing Responsibilities for Osteoarthritis

At present, there is no therapy that will slow or halt the progression of OA (Lozada & Altman, 2001). Current therapy is directed at relief of pain and minimizing functional disability. Agents for pain relief for OA include topical agents, systemic oral agents, adjuvant agents, and intra-articular agents. Treatments include topical Capsaicin, Tylenol, NSAIDs, and intra-articular corticosteroids when inflammation is present.

Pharmacology and Nursing Responsibilities for Rheumatoid Arthritis

Pharmacological therapies for RA include prednisone, NSAIDs, and disease-modifying antirheumatic drugs (DMARDs). Corticosteroids such as prednisone are potent anti-inflammatory drugs used in the treatment of rheumatic diseases such as RA. NSAIDs are another common drug category used for RA.

Pharmacology and Nursing Responsibilities for Acute Gout and Chronic Gout

Pharmacological options for the treatment of acute gout include: NSAIDs, oral colchicine loading, intra-articular steroid injections, and systemic steroids (Kerr, 2003).

Prompt treatment in the older person is indicated to improve symptoms and ensure a better quality of life.

Treatment for chronic gout includes colchicine, allopurinol, probenecid, and sulfinpyrazone. Colchicine (0.5 mg), an NSAID, is used to decrease inflammation. Colchicine may be given long term to reduce repeated attacks of gout. The maximum dose should be lowered for elderly patients. Drugs such as probenecid, sulfinpyrazone, and allopurinol prevent long-term complications by lowering serum uric acid blood level. Probenecid and sulfinpyrazone are uricosuric agents that work by increasing the excretion of uric acid. Allopurinol is a uric acid synthesis inhibitor, which means it lowers formation of uric acid. It is more versatile than uricosurics because it may be given at all levels of renal function. The goal of therapy with these agents is to decrease serum urate levels to 6.5 mg/d or less (Ettinger, 2003; Miller, 2001).

NON-PHARMACOLOGICAL TREATMENT OF MUSCULOSKELETAL PROBLEMS

Non-pharmacological treatment of osteoporosis for the older person focuses on assessment of risk factors and education to promote positive behaviors related to healthy bones. Modifiable risk factors include low calcium intake, prolonged immobility, excessive alcohol intake, and cigarette smoking. Prevention programs should be aimed at older persons with risk factors and those with osteoporosis as determined by bone density of 2 SD below the young adult mean. However, all older people will benefit from positive lifestyle changes for osteoporosis such as diet, exercise, and other risk modifications.

The most important risk factor for OA that can be modified is obesity. Reducing weight can improve quality of life and reduce healthcare costs associated with OA. Many older persons with OA (and other joint diseases) believe that exercise will cause a flare-up of their arthritis and lead to more pain. If the muscles are not used, atrophy may result and lead to weakness, falls, and mobility limitations.

Additional non-pharmacological strategies to enhance comfort for those with musculoskeletal problems such as OA and RA include applying heat to painful joints; cold packs to reduce pain and swelling; use of canes, crutches, and walkers to protect joints; use of adaptive aids (kitchen grips, motor scooters, etc.) to increase function.

Non-pharmacological Treatment to Prevent Falls and Fall-Related Injuries

Changes in vision, balance, or judgment; cardiovascular problems; medications; urinary incontinence; and other physical conditions can all contribute to an increased risk of falling (Brown et al., 2000). Many of the so-called safety measures that have been used in the past such as restraints and side rails have not been found to be effective and may even cause injury (Capezuti, 2002). Assessment of functional mobility, such as gait, balance, and position changes, provides valuable clues regarding a person's risk for future falls.

A simple assessment of routine mobility tasks can provide clinical information to determine fall risk. The older person is observed while doing the following activities: (1) getting up from a chair, (2) turning while walking, (3) raising the foot completely off the floor, and (4) sitting down. Difficulty with any of these activities often points to an increased risk for falls. The

Fall Risk Assessment: Hendrich II Scale
By: Deanna Gray-Miceli, DNSc, APRN, FAANP

Why

Fall among older adults, unlike other ages tend to occur from multifactorial etiology such as acute[1,2,3] and chronic[4] illness, medications[5] as a prodrome to other diseases[6] or as idiopathic phenomena. Because the rate of falling increases proportionally with increased number of pre-existing conditions and risk factors,[7] fall risk assessment is a useful guideline for practitioners. Determining the "why" the fall occurred however, involves critical analysis of potential underlying etiology (i.e. a comprehensive post-fall assessment) extending beyond fall risk assessment, but inclusive of it. Fall risk assessment and post-fall assessment are two interrelated, but distinct approaches to fall evaluation, both recommended by the American Geriatrics Society Guidelines[8] (2001) for fall prevention.

Best Practice Approach

In the acute care setting, the best practice approach incorporates use of the Hendrich II Scale[9] for it is quick to administer and provides a determination of risk for falling based on mental status, emotional status, symptoms of dizziness, gender, and is inclusive of categories of known increased risk medications. It can serve as a screen for primary prevention of falls or following a fall, as an integral component of the post-fall assessment used for their secondary prevention.

Target Population

The Hendrich II Fall Risk Model is intended to be used in the acute care and the skilled nursing environment to identify adults at risk for falls. This includes rehabilitation, emergency department, and the behavioral care areas. The tool is being validated for further application of the specific risk factors in pediatrics and obstetrical populations and it is being used successfully in the home setting as well.

Validity and Reliability

The Hendrich II Fall Risk Model was validated in a large case control study in an acute care tertiary facility with skilled nursing and rehabilitation populations. The risk factors in the model had a statistically significant relationship with patient falls (Odds Ratio 10.12-1.00, .01 > p <.0001). The instrument is sensitive (74.9%) and specific (73.9%).[10] Inter-rater reliability was measured in 17 randomly selected patients and was found to be 100% agreement negating the need for further matching during the study period. Content validity was established through an exhaustive literature review, use of accepted nursing nomenclature and the extensive experience of the principal investigators in this area.

Strengths and Limitations

The major strengths of the Hendrich II Scale are its brevity, the inclusion of medications, and that the instrument focuses interventions on specific areas of risk rather than on a single, summed general risk score. Medication risk is included in the tool in two ways 1) categories of 'true' increased fall risk medications (benzodiazepines and antiepileptics) are built into the tool and 2) the risk model construction found the most common side effects of drug therapies (confusion, dizziness, altered elimination, gait and mobility disturbances) were contained within intrinsic fall risk factors. This model assures medication risk is measured while preventing the over targeting of fall risk or duplication in medication risk assessment. The tool can be inserted into existing documentation forms or a single document and it has been built into electronic health records with targeted interventions that prompt and alert the caregiver to modify and/ or reduce specific risk factors' presence.[9]

References

1. Ooi, W. L., Hossain, M., Lipsitz, I. A. (2000). The association between orthostatic hypotension and

(*continued*)

recurrent falls in nursing home residents. American Journal of Medicine 108(2): 106–11.

2. Davies, A. J., Steen, N., Kenny, R. A. (2001). Carotid sinus hypersensitivity is common in older patients presenting to an accident and emergency department with unexplained falls. Age and Ageing 30(4): 273–4.

3. Heitterachi, E., Lord, S. R., Meyerkort, P., McCloskey, I., Fitzpatrick, R. (2002). Blood pressure changes on upright tilting predict falls in older people. Age and Ageing 31(3): 181–6.

4. Stolze, H., Klebe, S., Zechlin, C., Baecker, C., Friege, L., Deuschl, G. (2004). Falls in frequent neurological diseases-prevalence, risk factors and etiology. Journal of Neurology 251(1): 79–84.

5. Leipzig, R. M., Cumming, R. G., Tinetti, M. E. (1999). Drugs and falls in older people: a systematic review and meta-analysis: Cardiac and analgesic drugs. JAGS 47(1): 40–50.

6. Gray-Miceli, D., Waxman, H., Cavalieri, T., Lage, S. Prodromal falls among older nursing home residents. Applied Nursing Research 7:1, 18–27.

7. Tinetti, M. E., Williams, T. S., Mayewski, R. (1986). Fall risk index for elderly patients based on number of chronic disabilities. American Journal of Medicine 80(3): 429–34.

8. American Geriatrics Society, et al. (2001). Guidelines for the prevention of falls in older persons. JAGS 49: 664–672.

9. Hendrich, A., Nyhuuis, A., Kippenbrock, T., Soga, M. E. (1995). Hospital falls: development of a predictive model for clinical practice. Applied Nursing Research 8: 129–139.

10. Hendrich, A. L., Bender, P. S., & Nyhuis, A. (2003). Validation of the Hendrich II Fall Risk Model: A Large Concurrent CASE/Control Study of Hospitalized Patients, Applied Nursing Research 16(1): 9–21.

Case Example: Fall Risk Assessment with prior falls history

An 80-year-old woman with new onset confusion and urinary incontinence who has fallen repeatedly at home in the past 2 months is hospitalized for further observation and possible long-term care placement. On admission she is anxious and confused, and unable to move. Medications include Haldol 0.5 mg BID started 1 week prior to admission. Admission laboratory work shows a normal CBC and SMA-12. The urinalysis has 50 WBC per high power field and $+2$ Bacteria. The Hendrich risk score was 9. A comprehensive post-fall evaluation and review of the high risk parameters led to a presumptive diagnosis of the underlying cause of the fall; acute confusion due to urinary tract infection. Haldol was stopped and Bactrim DS BID was started. Two weeks later, the urinary incontinence and confusion lessened and the falling stopped. She was discharged home to live with her daughter.

Case Discussion

This woman possesses several "red flag" areas of a dynamic nature, e.g., falls occurring on an acute, potentially reversible basis, acute urinary incontinence, urinary track infection, poly-pharmacy and delirium. Falling is related to these dynamic events and once treated the falling stopped. Note that the FRAT surfaced no past or static

(continued)

events associated with falls, such as non-reversible past medical problems like dementia or Parkinson's disease. But, use of the Hendrich scale captured significant risk factors including confusion (4 points), prescribed benzodiazepines (1 point) and inability to rise (4 points). These risks elicited from the Hendrich Scale coupled with a comprehensive post-fall assessment informed the nursing interventions.

Hendrich II Fall Risk Model©

Risk Factor		Risk Points
Confusion/Disorientation	4	☐
Depression	2	☐
Altered Elimination	1	☐
Dizziness/Vertigo	1	☐
Gender (Male)	1	☐
Any administered-prescribed antiepileptics (anticonvulsants): *(carbamazepine, divalproex sodium, ethotoin, ethosuximide, felbamate, fosphenytoin, gabapentin, lamotrigine, mephenytoin, methsuximide, phenobarbitol, phenytoin, primidone, topiramate, trimethadione, valproic acid)*	2	☐
Any administered-prescribed benzodiazepines: *(alprazolam, buspirone, chlordiazepoxide, clonazepam, clorazepate dipotassium, diazepam, flurazepam, halazepam, lorazepam, midazolam, oxazepam, temazepam, triazolam)*	1	☐
Get-up-and-go* Test: "Rising from Chair" (select one) **If unable to assess (unconscious, drug-induced coma, traction, extreme dehabilitation atrophy), monitor for change in activity level and use all other risk factor scores.*		

Able to rise in single movement	0	☐
Pushes up, successful in one attempt	1	☐
Multiple attempts but successful	3	☐
Unable to rise without assistance	4	☐

TOTAL (5 or greater = High Risk)

nurse should develop an individualized plan to increase muscle strength and prevent falls.

The older person should also be taught how to get up from a fall and how to get help. One method would be to turn over on the stomach and crawl to the phone. Another would be to scoot on the bottom or side to reach a phone, or the person may be able to crawl to a stairway and climb up until able to stand. The older person should have an emergency plan such as a bell or a phone near the floor (versus a wall phone). Daily calls to the elderly person to check on his or her safety will also give a feeling of reassurance.

Treatment of Hip Fractures

Trained emergency staff should take the older person with a hip fracture to a hospital that offers 24-hour surgical care. Fractures must be immobilized immediately to prevent further damage. Surgery is the treatment of choice and should be performed as soon as possible. Older people will benefit from the increased mobility and pain relief that is experienced after surgery. The type of injury, the overall condition of the person, and any preexisting orthopedic conditions will determine the type of surgical procedure. In general, the more invasive the surgical procedure, the more risk involved for the older person.

The goals of joint replacement surgery are to decrease pain and increase joint function. In a total hip replacement, surgeons replace the head of the femur (the ball) and the acetabulum (the socket) with new parts that allow a natural gliding motion of the joint.

Nursing care of the older person with total hip replacement or internal fixation of the hip includes assessment and prevention for common complications, including dislocation of the device, avascular necrosis, infection, and delayed healing.

PATIENT-FAMILY TEACHING GUIDELINES

Mobility Problems

1. I have osteoarthritis and chronic pain. What should I do to control my pain?

   The pain of osteoarthritis should be managed with a variety of modalities. Pain initially occurs with increased activity and may be relieved by rest. As time goes on, the pain may take longer to subside and occur at rest as well. It is important that pain be managed effectively early in the disease in order to prevent inactivity that leads to muscle weakness and joint instability. Try Tylenol, topical rubs, hot and cold packs, and regular moderate exercise.

2. Why is it important to exercise?

   In order to maintain or regain an active lifestyle you need to maintain muscle strength, coordination, balance, flexibility, and endurance. Exercise can do all of that for you plus benefit your heart and keep off excess weight that can further stress your joints.

3. What exercise can I do to keep myself moving?

   Key exercises and activities that will help you to maintain functional performance include walking, pool or water aerobics, yoga or stretching exercises, dancing, golfing, fishing, or anything that is enjoyable and gets you moving.

4. What are some precautions I should take when I exercise?

   Dress appropriately, wear proper footwear, and check with your doctor if you have chest pain, irregular heartbeat, shortness of breath, hernia, foot or ankle sores that do not heal, hot or red joints with pain, and certain eye conditions like bleeding in the retina or detached retina. If you have any of these conditions, it does not mean you cannot exercise, but modifications and precautions might be needed. See an expert who can help you get going.

5. How do I know if exercise is helping me?

   Begin by seeing how far you can walk in 5 minutes. (Use a watch and record your distance in feet or blocks.) Then time yourself as you walk up a flight of stairs (at least 10 steps). After 1 month of exercising, repeat these tests and compare your times. If you are on the right track, it should be taking less time. Keep a diary and bring it with you the next time you come to the clinic.

   If the goal has not been met, the nurse and patient need to evaluate the data and revise the care plan to reflect the abilities of the older person.

(continued)

Compassion and understanding are important so that the older person does not get discouraged. If the patient is having an episode of acute joint pain, range of motion should continue on all noninvolved joints. Stiffness, muscle weakness, and atrophy can occur quickly if the person becomes immobile. Prescribed pain medication, as well as non-pharmacological pain management techniques, should be implemented to allow the patient to remain as active as possible during the acute pain.

CHAPTER 17

THE ENDOCRINE SYSTEM

The endocrine glands control the body's metabolic processes. Two major endocrine problems are diabetes mellitus and thyroid disease. Thyroid disease and diabetes mellitus are common, often undiagnosed, and easily treated in people of all ages.

DIABETES MELLITUS

Diabetes mellitus (DM) is highly prevalent and increasing in persons over 65, particularly in racial and ethnic minorities (California Healthcare Foundation/American Geriatrics Society, 2003). DM is classified as type 1 (the result of a lack of insulin production) and type 2 (the result of insulin resistance). In general, age-specific prevalence of diagnosed DM is higher for African Americans and Hispanics than for Caucasians. Among those less than 75 years of age, Black women have the highest prevalence.

Complications of Diabetes Mellitus

Poor glycemic control may synergistically interact with normal changes of aging and other coexisting diseases to accelerate diabetes complications (Blair, 1999). Complications that can develop due to poor glycemic control include the following:

- Eye disease leading to loss of vision or even blindness
- Kidney failure

- Heart disease
- Nerve damage that may cause a loss of feeling or pain in the hands, feet, legs, or other parts of the body (peripheral neuropathies)
- Stroke
- Poor wound healing due to impaired immune response and poor tissue perfusion in peripheral vascular disease

The diagnosis of DM can shorten the average life span up to 15 years. Additionally, DM leads to higher death rates from other illness such as pneumonia, influenza, and heart disease.

Pathophysiology of Diabetes Mellitus

Type 1 DM develops due to B-cell destruction and results in a lack or underproduction of insulin in the body. Type 1 DM can be the result of (1) autoimmune disease in which cell-mediated destruction of the B cells in the pancreas occurs, or (2) idiopathic DM that occurs for no apparent reason. Regardless of cause, patients with type 1 DM are insulin dependent and at risk for ketoacidosis.

Type 2 DM, the most prevalent form of diabetes in all age groups, results from a combination of insulin resistance and an insulin secretory defect. The insulin secretion is insufficient to compensate for the insulin resistance, which occurs in response to decreased insulin effectiveness in stimulating glucose uptake by skeletal muscle and failure to inhibit hepatic glucose production. The body attempts to compensate for rising blood glucose levels by producing more insulin. In some cases, this is adequate and the person does not go on to develop DM. In others, genetic influences may play a role, and heightened insulin production results in hyperinsulinemia. This leads to further insulin resistance, characterized by visceral/abdominal obesity, hypertension, hyperlipidemia, and coronary artery disease (Barzilai, 2003). Autoimmune destruction of B cells does not occur, ketoacidosis seldom occurs spontaneously, and insulin treatment is often not needed for survival.

Risk Factors for Development of Diabetes Mellitus

Risk factors for the development of type 2 DM include:

- Age over 45 (the risk of DM increases with age).
- Being overweight (body mass index greater than 25) and having a waist-to-hip ratio approaching 1.
- Being African American, Hispanic or Latino American, Asian American or Pacific Islander, or American Indian.
- Having a parent, brother, or sister with DM.
- Having a blood pressure above 140/90.
- Having low levels of high-density lipoprotein (less than 40 for men and less than 50 for women) (good cholesterol) and high levels of triglycerides (above 250 mg/dl).
- Having had diabetes while pregnant or giving birth to a large baby (over 9 lbs).
- Having a sedentary lifestyle and exercising less than three times per week.

(National Diabetes Education Program, 2003)

Diagnostic Criteria

When an older person is identified as high risk for diabetes, appropriate testing includes a fasting plasma glucose (FPG) level or a 2-hour oral glucose tolerance test (OGTT). The FPG is performed by obtaining a blood sample and measuring the person's blood glucose after an overnight fast (8 to 12 hours). The 2-hour OGTT is performed after an overnight fast by measuring the person's blood glucose immediately before and 2 hours after drinking a 75-g glucose solution. The diagnostic criteria include FPG >126 mg/dl and OGTT >200 mg/dl.

Use of glucocorticoids or diuretics can greatly and suddenly increase blood glucose levels both in older patients with DM and in those without DM.

Older patients with DM may complain of symptoms of hyperglycemia (usually above 200 mg/dl), including polydipsia (excessive thirst), weight loss, polyuria (excessive urination), polyphagia (excessive hunger), blurred vision, fatigue, nausea, and fungal and bacterial infections (Barzilai, 2003). Older women may complain of perineal itching due to vaginal candidiasis. Additionally, older women with DM may experience frequent urinary tract infections.

The initial physical examination should include blood pressure measurement (including orthostatic changes), weight, dilated retinal examination by an ophthalmologist or eye specialist, cardiovascular examination for evidence of cardiac or peripheral vascular disease, and neurologic examination to rule out any peripheral or autonomic **neuropathy** (American Diabetes Association, 2001). Fundoscopic examination may reveal the presence of microaneurysms, hemorrhages, exudates, or increased intraocular pressure indicative of glaucoma. Peripheral pulses, capillary filling, and warmth of extremities should be assessed to indicate the presence of macrovascular pathology. Mental status, deep tendon reflexes, and ability to detect peripheral sensation are key components of the neurologic examination. Smoking status and a visual foot examination (without shoes and socks) is recommended for every older person with DM initially and at every subsequent clinical visit to the healthcare provider. Patients who smoke cigarettes should be counseled to discontinue smoking. Those ready to undertake smoking cessation should be referred to ongoing support groups and counseling centers. Patients with diabetes who are overweight should be counseled regarding weight loss.

The following laboratory tests are recommended:

- Thyroid function tests (thyroid-stimulating hormone)
- Urinalysis to test for albuminuria, serum creatinine for renal function
- Electrocardiogram if patient has not had one within 10 years
- Fasting lipid profile to assess cardiovascular risk
- **Glycosylated hemoglobin** (HbA_{1c})

(Diabetes Guidelines Work Group, 1999)

The HbA_{1c} is not specific for diagnosing diabetes; however, elevated HbA_{1c} levels confirm the degree of estimated blood glucose control over the last 3 months. The HbA_{1c} measures how much glucose attaches to the hemoglobin in the red cells. As the average life of a red cell is about 4 months, the test summarizes how high the glucose levels have been during the life of the cell. The ideal HbA_{1c} goal is less than 7.0%. Levels of 8.0% or greater indicate the need to adjust the treatment plan (Diabetes Guidelines Work Group, 1999).

An in-depth foot examination should include the presence of protective sensation, vascular status, skin integrity, and foot structure. Approximately 15% of all patients with DM will develop a foot or leg ulcer during the course of their disease (Halpin-Landry & Goldsmith, 1999). Patients with DM have sensory, motor, and autonomic neuropathies; lower extremity peripheral vascular disease; impaired host defenses against infection; and delayed wound healing. When a diabetic ulcer occurs, ischemia, neuropathy, and infection delay healing and raise the risk of complications.

A monofilament or a tuning fork can be used to assess for the presence of protective sensation that can alert the patient to the development of a blister or foot ulcer. It is recommended that a visual examination of the diabetic foot be conducted at each healthcare encounter and a more in-depth inspection be done annually. Saving the diabetic foot and preventing amputation requires the following:

- Identification of feet at risk
- Prevention of foot ulcers
- Treatment of foot ulcers
- Prevention of recurrence of foot ulcers

(NIDDK, 2004)

Foot care in the patient with DM includes hygiene and protection. It is important to lubricate dry areas with lotion, carefully dry moist areas (between toes), and care for the nails. Patients with DM should not cut their own toenails and are urged to see the podiatrist regularly and use an emery board to keep nails short and smooth between visits.

In addition to the history and physical examination, assessment of the patient with DM includes the following components:

- Nutritional assessment
- Medication review
- Functional assessment
- Psychosocial assessment
- Gait and balance evaluation

GOALS OF MANAGEMENT

The goals of management of DM in the older person include control of hyperglycemia and its symptoms;

prevention, evaluation, and treatment of macrovascular and microvascular complications; DM self-management through education; and maintenance or improvement of general health status (California Healthcare Foundation, 2003). The goals must reflect the fact that older adults with DM have varying degrees of frailty, differences in underlying chronic conditions, varying degrees of DM-related comorbidity, and highly variable life expectancies. In general, the more functional the older person and the longer the life expectancy, the more aggressively the DM will be treated by the healthcare provider to decrease the probability of DM-related complications. If an older patient is close to death, then multiple insulin injections and frequent (4 to 6 times/day) blood glucose monitoring may not be justified (Mooradian, McLaughlin, Boyer, & Winter, 1999). A less aggressive approach may be indicated because long-term complications of hyperglycemia are not relevant.

The goals of therapy for the highly functional older person include:

- A fasting blood glucose level between 100 and 120 mg/dl.
- A postprandial glucose level of less than 180 mg/dl.
- An HbA_{1c} under 8%.

The goals of therapy for the older patient with advanced microvascular complications (neuropathy or **retinopathy**), cognitive deficits, serious associated cardiovascular problems, or frailty or underlying serious illness are more conservative and include the following:

- A fasting glucose level of less than 140 mg/dl
- A postprandial glucose level of less than 200 to 220 mg/dl
- An HbA_{1c} under 10%

(Berenbeim, Parrott, Purnell, & Pennachio, 2001)

Weight Management

Maintenance of near-normal blood glucose levels, achievement of optimal serum lipid levels, provision of adequate caloric intake to attain or maintain normal weight, prevention and treatment of complications, and improvement of overall health through optimal nutrition comprise the nutrition goals for the older patient with DM (American Diabetes Association, 2001). For obese older patients with DM, weight loss is encouraged. Insulin sensitivity increases when obese patients begin to lose weight. When insulin sensitivity is improved, medication doses may be lowered and blood glucose levels are more responsive to medications. Ideally, the patient with DM should attempt to keep blood glucose levels stable throughout the day by eating smaller portions of carbohydrates and fats at mealtime and scheduling snacks during peak times of insulin or oral hypoglycemic medication action.

Patients with diabetes should be encouraged to eat at regular times and never skip meals. Snacks should be taken at the same time each day. Older patients with DM should eat a variety of foods to keep the meal plan interesting and to meet nutritional needs. Once the older patient becomes skilled at choosing healthy foods that are consistent with nutritional needs and blood glucose control, nutritional status and overall health often improve.

Additional nutritional guidelines for patients with DM include:

- Eat less fat.
- Eat less sugar.
- Eat less salt.
- Eat foods with higher fiber.
- Avoid or reduce alcohol.

Physical exercise slows the progression of DM, improves weight control, and maintains overall function. Regular physical activity is encouraged for all older people with DM. Strenuous exercise should be avoided because of the risk of injury, retinal detachment, or vitreous hemorrhage (Berenbeim et al., 2001). Additionally, patients taking insulin who engage in strenuous physical exercise may suffer from hypoglycemia, primarily because absorption from the injection site increases (Barzilai, 2003). Older patients taking insulin should check their blood glucose levels before exercising and eat additional carbohydrates if their glucose levels are below 100 mg/dl prior to exercise. Monitoring blood glucose before and after exercise helps to identify when changes in insulin or food intake are necessary to learn how the glycemic response changes as the result of exercise. The goal is to adjust the insulin and food regimen to allow safe participation in exercise that is consistent with the older person's desires. To avoid hypoglycemia, the patient should have carbohydrate foods available during and after exercise. The older person should avoid exercise if fasting glucose levels are greater than 250 mg/dl (American Diabetes Association, 2001).

Walking is one of the easiest ways to be active. It can be done almost anywhere and anytime. The older person should purchase a good pair of walking shoes and enjoy the following benefits:

- Getting more energy
- Reducing stress
- Improving sleep
- Toning muscles
- Controlling appetite

- Increasing the number of calories burned daily
- Preventing complications of diabetes

(National Diabetes Education Program, 2003)

Medications Used to Control Diabetes Mellitus

Oral hypoglycemic drugs are used for type 2 DM only. Single or combination drugs can achieve good glycemic control and have been used successfully for years. However, newer drugs have emerged during the last 10 years. Each medication addresses a different glycemic problem, and they can be used as monotherapy or in combination with other drugs.

Oral antidiabetic drugs include the antihyperglycemic drugs (biguanides, alpha-glucosidase inhibitors, and thiazolidinediones) and oral hypoglycemic drugs (sulfonylureas and meglitinide). The oldest class of oral hypoglycemic drugs is the sulfonylureas, and these drugs have been improved over the last 20 years to increase effectiveness. These second-generation sulfonylureas stimulate the **beta cells** in the pancreas to secrete insulin. They are effective drugs, but sometimes can stimulate the release of too much insulin, resulting in hypoglycemia. Hypoglycemia occurs most often with long-acting sulfonylureas (glyburide). Sulfonylurea-induced hypoglycemia can be severe and last or recur for days after treatment is stopped. All older patients treated with sulfonylureas who develop hypoglycemia should be closely monitored in the hospital for 2 to 3 days (Barzilai, 2003). An additional adverse effect is that weight gain occurs in many older patients taking these drugs. The extended-release formulations offer the advantage of simplifying dosing to once a day. Because they contain sulfa, they should not be used by patients who are sulfa-allergic.

Metformin is a biguanide introduced in 1994 that improves insulin sensitivity by enhancing glucose uptake and use by the muscles (Coyle, 2003). Additional benefits include mild weight loss and favorable changes in lipid profiles for patients with high lipid levels. Gastrointestinal side effects are common during initial dosing but are usually mild and resolve spontaneously. Metformin should not be used by patients over 80 or those with renal insufficiency (serum creatinine above 1.4 in women and above 1.5 in men) (Coyle, 2003). In contrast with oral antihyperglycemics, these drugs rarely cause hypoglycemia and may be safer for older persons (Barzilai, 2003).

Alpha-glucosidase inhibitors decrease postprandial hyperglycemia by slowing digestion and delaying intestinal absorption of carbohydrates. These drugs are helpful in older patients who exhibit baseline blood glucose levels in the normal range but become hyperglycemic immediately after eating a meal. The major side effects of these drugs are gastrointestinal and include flatulence and bloating, so many patients wish to discontinue taking these medications (Coyle, 2003). Sometimes starting at a low dose and slowly titrating up to the therapeutic dose will minimize adverse effects.

Thiazolidinediones were introduced in 1997 with the introduction of troglitazone (Rezulin). This drug was withdrawn in 2000 after it was associated with several deaths and liver transplants resulting from hepatotoxicity (Coyle, 2003). Since then, two new thiazolidinediones have been approved. These drugs enhance insulin sensitivity through activation of intracellular receptors and also suppress hepatic glucose production. Absolute contraindications include active liver disease (alanine aminotransferase (ALT) more than 2.5 times the upper limit of normal) and congestive heart failure (New York

Heart Association class III or IV) (Coyle, 2003). Regular monitoring of liver function tests is recommended at baseline and every 2 months for the first year and periodically thereafter. An additional side effect is weight gain (Coyle, 2003).

The final class of oral hypoglycemics is meglitinides. Drugs in this class are insulin secretagogues and act by stimulating insulin release in response to a meal. Although they are considered rapid-onset drugs, their duration of action is short and they must be taken with each meal for maximum effect. They should not be taken without food, in the event that a patient skips a meal or ingests a meal that is very low in carbohydrate content (Coyle, 2003).

Some patients take combination drugs such as glyburide-metformin (Glucovance), glipizide-metformin (Metaglip), and rosiglitazone-metformin (Avandamet). These drugs simplify the dosing requirements and may be less expensive in some cases. They combine drugs with different mechanisms of action to achieve better basal glucose levels and prevent postprandial peaks. However, the use of combination drugs incurs more risk in the older patient. Should an adverse effect occur, it may not be clear which drug in the combination is responsible. Extra caution and monitoring are needed to prevent hypoglycemia and ensure success with combination medications.

Insulin

Insulin is used alone in type 1 DM and may be used alone or in combination with oral hypoglycemic medications in type 2 DM (Coyle, 2003). Although most patients with type 2 DM will not need insulin, it may be used in patients whose diabetes cannot be adequately controlled with oral agents alone. Insulin is injected subcutaneously with special insulin syringes. The 0.5-ml syringes are preferred by older patients who inject doses of 50 U or less, because these syringes facilitate the accurate measurement of smaller insulin doses. A multiple-dose insulin injection device (e.g., Novolin Pen) uses a cartridge containing several days' dosage. The accuracy and ease of use of the insulin pen is ideal for some older patients. Insulin should be refrigerated but never frozen. Most insulin is stable at room temperature, but it should not be stored near a heat source or transported in an overheated car or trunk (Barzilai, 2003). For patients with visual difficulties, magnifying glasses can be helpful or the medication can be drawn up by the visiting nurse or a family member. Prefilled syringes should be used within a week.

As with oral hypoglycemics, the insulin regimen should mimic normal physiology with control of both basal and postprandial glucose levels. Long-acting insulin controls blood glucose levels and uses glucose as a fuel long after the meal has been digested (basal insulin). Short-acting insulin satisfies the need for insulin after meals or ingestion of food and is usually injected around mealtime. Newer insulins are made from recombinant DNA and do not require extraction from the pancreas of animals. NPH, Lente, Ultralente, and Regular Insulin are still available but are being used less often (Coyle, 2003). Lispro (Humalog) and Aspart (NovoLog) are the newest rapid-acting insulins with onset of action within 15 minutes. They are usually injected immediately prior to eating a meal several times daily. Longer acting insulins such as glargine (Lantus) are designed to release insulin evenly throughout the day and control basal glucose levels. Patients who take Lantus experience less overnight hypoglycemia compared to those using NPH (Coyle, 2003).

Mixtures of insulin preparations with different onsets and durations of action are often given in a single injection to simplify the dosing and better control blood glucose levels. These insulin combinations are more suitable for patients with type 2 DM because patients with type 1 DM are totally reliant on insulin and would lose the ability to make individual dose adjustments based on food consumption and metabolic demands imposed by exercise (Coyle, 2003).

Table 17–1 lists the available insulins and duration of action.

Table 17–1   Available Insulins and Duration of Action

Insulin	Duration of Action
Short-Acting	
Regular	3–6 hours
Lispro (Humalog)	1–2 hours
Aspart (NovoLog)	1–2 hours
Intermediate-Acting	
NPH	18–24 hours
Lente	18–24 hours
Long-Acting	
Ultralente	24–36 hours
Glargine (Lantus)	24 hours
Premixed Combinations	
50/50 NPH-Regular Mixture	Up to 24 hours
70/30 NPH-Regular Mixture	Up to 24 hours
75/25 Humalog Mix—NPH—Lispro	Up to 24 hours
70/30 NovoLog Mix—NPH—NovoLog	Up to 24 hours

Source: Barzilai, 2003; Coyle, 2003; epocrates.com, 2004

Hypoglycemia as a Complication of Insulin Treatment

Hypoglycemia can be caused by too high a dose of insulin, missing a meal or eating a smaller meal, unplanned exercise, or the onset of illness that alters metabolic need. Older patients should be taught to recognize the symptoms of hypoglycemia, including feeling nervous, shaky, sweaty, or excessively fatigued. Older patients should test their blood glucose levels if they experience these symptoms. If it is less than 60 to 70 mg/dl, they should treat themselves right away. If they are unable to test their glucose levels, they should treat it anyway. The usual treatment recommendation is to eat 10 to 15 g of carbohydrates right away.

After ingesting 10 to 15 g of carbohydrate, the older person should wait 15 minutes and test the blood glucose level again. Patients must be cautioned that eating the foods on this list will keep the blood glucose level up for only about 30 minutes. All patients with DM should carry an identification card that identifies them as having diabetes and wear a medical bracelet or necklace.

Morning Hyperglycemia

The dawn phenomenon refers to the normal tendency of blood glucose levels to rise in the early morning before breakfast. This normal phenomenon is exaggerated in older patients with type 1 and type 2 diabetes. The liver may produce increased glucose as a result of a midnight surge of growth hormone. In some patients, nocturnal hypoglycemia may be followed by a marked increase in fasting blood glucose with an increase in plasma ketones (Somogyi phenomenon) (Barzilai, 2003).

Injection Site Reactions

At the injection site, local fat atrophy or allergic reactions can occur. Pain and burning at the injection site may last for a few hours, followed by redness, itching, and induration. These reactions usually disappear on their own as the body becomes desensitized to the insulin. Injection sites should be routinely rotated to prevent fat atrophy.

Effect of Acute Illness

Should an older patient with DM experience an acute illness such as pneumonia or urinary tract infection, hyperglycemia can be the result. However, if the patient has lost his or her appetite or is vomiting, continuing to take the same dose of oral hypoglycemics or insulin can result in hypoglycemia. If the patient is hospitalized or in a long-term care facility, the nurses will routinely check blood glucose levels and "cover" the patient with a sliding scale of insulin until the acute illness resolves and the blood glucose levels stabilize. The physician may request that hypoglycemic drugs be withheld during an acute condition associated with decreased food intake or persistent nausea and vomiting. The effects of surgical procedure (anesthesia, surgical trauma, emotional stress) can markedly increase blood glucose levels. Every attempt should be made by the nurse and other members of the healthcare team to regulate medications and oral intake to prevent dangerous variations in blood glucose levels.

Patients and their families should be instructed to call their healthcare provider if any of the following conditions occur:

- Unable to keep food or liquids down or eat normally for over 6 hours
- Severe diarrhea

- Unintentional weight loss of 5 lb
- Oral temperature over 101°F
- Blood glucose levels lower than 60 mg/dl or over 300 mg/dl
- Presence of large amounts of ketones in the urine
- Difficulty breathing
- Feeling sleepy or unable to think clearly

(Centers for Disease Control, 1999)

Nonketotic Hyperglycemic-Hyperosmolar Coma

Nonketotic hyperglycemic-hyperosmolar coma (NKHHC) is a complication of type 2 DM that has a high mortality rate (Barzilai, 2003). It usually develops after a period of symptomatic hyperglycemia during which fluid intake is inadequate to prevent extreme dehydration from osmotic diuresis. Symptoms of hyperglycemia include dry mouth, extreme thirst, excessive urination, fatigue, blurred vision, weight loss, nausea, abdominal pain, and vomiting. NKHHC can occur in some older patients with undiagnosed or untreated type 2 DM when they receive drugs that impair glucose tolerance such as glucocorticoids or drugs that increase fluid loss such as diuretics. Older persons with severe dementia may also be at risk because the decreased thirst and hunger drive may prevent them from eating and drinking adequate amounts of fluid and nutritious foods.

NKHHC may begin as mild confusion and progress to coma or seizures. Laboratory studies reveal hyperglycemia (above 500 mg/dl), hyperosmolarity, and metabolic acidosis. Serum sodium and potassium levels are usually normal, but blood urea nitrogen (BUN) and serum creatinine levels are increased. Treatment must begin immediately and intravenous fluids are needed to expand the intravascular volume, stabilize blood pressure, and improve circulation and urine flow. Insulin treatment is not always necessary, because adequate hydration may decrease blood glucose levels.

Difficulties in Caring for Older Patients with DM

1. *Polypharmacy*—Older patients with DM may require several medications to manage their overall health problems, including elevated blood glucose levels, hypertension, hyperlipidemia, and other associated conditions.
2. *Depression*—Older adults with DM are at an increased risk for depression that may be undetected and untreated.
3. *Cognitive impairment*—Older adults with DM are at increased risk for cognitive impairment. Subtle or unrecognized cognitive impairment may interfere with the patient's ability to manage this complicated disease.
4. *Urinary incontinence*—Older women with DM are at increased risk of urinary incontinence. Urinary incontinence should be assessed initially and periodically thereafter.
5. *Injurious falls*—Falls in older people are associated with higher rates of morbidity, mortality, and functional decline. Older persons with DM are at increased risk for injurious falls because of higher rates of frailty and functional disability, visual impairment, peripheral neuropathy, hypoglycemia, and polypharmacy.
6. *Pain*—Older persons with DM are at risk for neuropathic pain, which often goes untreated. Older patients should be screened for persistent pain initially and periodically thereafter.

General Health Promotion for the Older Person with Diabetes

Older persons with DM and their families should be taught self-management skills including self-monitoring for signs of hypoglycemia, blood glucose monitoring skills and medication adjustment, nutrition management, and development and maintenance of a physical activity plan. Older persons with DM should receive the influenza vaccine every fall. The pneumococcal vaccine is recommended at age 65. Revaccination is suggested if the patient is over the age of 65 and the initial vaccine was given over 5 years ago and the patient was under 65 at that time.

At each visit, the older patient is weighed and has blood pressure recorded. The feet and skin are carefully examined. Any irritation, ulceration, deformity, or loss of sensation is carefully noted and referred for treatment.

THYROID DISORDERS

Because thyroid dysfunction often occurs gradually, the signs and symptoms may be imperceptible to the patient and family and may be attributed to normal changes of aging. Hypothyroidism is characterized by a generalized reduction in metabolic function that most often manifests as a slowing of physical and mental activity. The complaints may vary from asymptomatic, mild, moderate, or severe, and depend on a variety of factors such as the patient's age, general health status, cognitive abilities, and rate at which the disease develops (Burman, 2000). As older patients do not complain of classic symptoms of thyroid disease, their complaints may be attributed to other causes. Undiagnosed thyroid disease can have a profound effect on the body, making early and accurate diagnosis and treatment a necessity.

Normal Anatomy and Physiology

The thyroid is an endocrine gland that produces thyroxine (T_4) and triiodothyronine (T_3), two hormones that play a key role in regulating the body's energy levels and metabolic function. Normally, thyrotropin-releasing hormone (TRH) is produced by the hypothalamus, stimulating the anterior pituitary gland to produce thyroid-stimulating hormone (TSH). This in turn stimulates the thyroid to produce T_4 and T_3. Additionally, TSH increases carbohydrate, protein, and lipid metabolism and stimulates cell proliferation, thus affecting many systems of the body (Burman, 2000). High levels of T_4 and T_3 provide negative feedback to the pituitary gland and hypothalamus, decreasing the production of TSH and TRH. If free T_4 and T_3 levels are low, feedback to the pituitary gland and hypothalamus stimulates increased production of TRH and TSH, which stimulates the thyroid to produce more hormone. More than 99% of T_4 and T_3 is bound to thyroxine-binding globulin (TBG) and albumin, leaving only a small amount free to influence metabolic effect.

Normal Changes of Thyroid Function with Aging

Thyroid function is significantly altered with aging, and the thyroid gradually loses function and undergoes atrophy. The gland becomes more nodular, especially in areas with low iodine levels in the food and water. Fortunately, only about 2% of thyroid nodules are cancerous, and the presence of hypothyroidism and thyroid nodules rises dramatically with age (Solomon, 2003). Additionally, thyroid antibody levels rise with age, making it difficult to discern at what levels these antibodies indicate thyroiditis. Serum T_4 levels remain unchanged, Serum T_3 levels decrease slowly with age, while the average serum TSH levels rise with age.

Thyroid Function Testing

Thyroid function tests help to diagnose and detect the presence of thyroid disease. Table 17–2 lists common laboratory tests of thyroid function and interpretation of abnormal findings.

Hypothyroidism

Hypothyroidism is relatively common and can be caused by dysfunction of the thyroid gland (primary), pituitary (secondary), or hypothalamus (tertiary). The most common cause of primary hypothyroidism is Hashimoto's thyroiditis, an autoimmune disease with subtle onset and minimal symptoms while the thyroid gland undergoes progressive inflammatory destruction. Hypothyroidism may also be caused by factors that negatively affect the synthesis of thyroid hormones such as iodine deficiency or excess and inherited defects in thyroid hormone biosynthesis (Burman, 2001).

Table 17–2   Common Laboratory Tests of Thyroid Function

	Normal Value	Value in Hypothyroidism	Value in Hyperthyroidism
TSH	0.32–5.0 mU/ml	↑Usually > 10–20	↓Usually low (<0.30) or undetectable
Free T4	4.5–12 µg/dl	↓decreased	↑increased
Free T3	75–200 ng/dl	Normal	↑increased

Medications associated with hypothyroidism include lithium, amiodarone, sulfonylureas, salicylates, furosemide, phenytoin, rifampin, and radioactive contrast dyes (Burman, 2000).

Older patients with goiter or enlarged thyroid glands detected through physical examination are euthyroid with the goiter representing a proliferation of thyroid tissue in response to inadequate serum levels of T_3. Patients with goiter will often undergo thyroid function tests, antithyroid antibody tests, and thyroid scans to rule out Graves' disease, nodular goiter, hypothyroidism, or some other thyroid dysfunction (Kuritzky, 2001).

Effects of Hypothyroidism

Typical symptoms include the following:

- Fatigue
- Increased need for sleep
- Muscle aches
- Dry skin
- Bradycardia
- Increased cholesterol levels (elevations in LDL)
- Ataxia and balance difficulties
- Hearing loss
- Depression
- Cold intolerance
- Hair loss
- Voice changes
- Hypothermia
- Periorbital swelling
- Decreased appetite and weight loss

(Burman, 2000; Kuritzky, 2001)

Hypothyroidism can cause a variety of symptoms associated with all of the major body systems including the neurologic system (vertigo, tinnitus, depression), cardiovascular system (bradycardia, CHF), musculoskeletal system (fatigue, cramps, osteoporosis), gastrointestinal system (constipation delayed gastric emptying), and pernicious anemia. The manifestations of hypothyroidism are diverse and numerous. Thyroid hormone is important for normal metabolic functioning (Burman, 2000).

Diagnosis of Hypothyroidism

Hypothyroidism is diagnosed by precise measurement of serum TSH and T_4 levels. In primary hypothyroidism, the TSH is elevated and free serum T_4 levels are below normal. The free serum T_3 level has little value because it is normal in about one third of older patients with hypothyroidism and because low T_3 levels are associated with acute illness and inadequate caloric intake (Solomon, 2003). Thyroid nodules or sudden enlargement of the thyroid requires thyroid scans or ultrasounds (American Association of Clinical Endocrinologists, 2002).

The thyroid is examined first with a visual inspection of the neck to identify any enlargements or irregularities. The nurse observes the neck using tangential lighting and stands a foot or two away to identify any shadows. Asking the patient to swallow will accentuate any irregularities during movement. The nurse begins to palpate the thyroid by placing fingers on the trachea at either side of the larynx and moving them gently up and down.

A comprehensive health assessment and history may suggest the development of hypothyroidism. However, because the symptoms are vague and many older patients experience few symptoms, laboratory assessment of thyroid function is required to confirm the diagnosis.

Treatment and Nursing Management of Hypothyroidism

The goals of therapy are to relieve symptoms and to provide sufficient thyroid hormone to decrease raised serum TSH levels to the normal range. The treatment of choice is T_4 replacement with levothyroxine sodium. The average dose for patients over 65 years of age is 0.075 to 0.1 mg/day by mouth. If the patient has coronary artery disease, the initial dose should only be 0.0125 to 0.025 mg/day. The dose should be increased gradually (0.025 mg) over 4-week intervals and the serum TSH level monitored to assess the effectiveness of treatment. If the TSH levels are below normal, the dose of levothyroxine should be decreased. If the TSH levels are above normal, the dose should be increased slowly until the TSH is normal. Close monitoring of blood levels, overall function, cardiac status, and cognitive function is indicated during the initial period. After the TSH has stabilized in the normal range, thyroid function should be assessed every 6 to 12 months by an appropriate health assessment and laboratory testing (Burman, 2000). Overly suppressed TSH levels indicate that the patient is at increased risk for osteoporosis; however, T_4 replacement with carefully monitored TSH levels has not been associated with decreased bone density (Kuritzky, 2001).

The American Thyroid Association recommends screening every 5 years by measuring serum TSH for all men and women over age 35. For those with risk factors for thyroid disease, the serum TSH level should be checked more often and as indicated by the presence of new or unexplained symptoms of decreased metabolism. Screening of thyroid function should be performed in populations that have a high incidence of thyroid dysfunction because of disease state, drug therapy, or other predisposing factor, and when early intervention is crucial to prevent irreversible pathology once the diagnosis of hypothyroidism is made (American Association of Clinical Endocrinologists, 2002). The TSH assay is the screening method of choice for identifying hypothyroidism.

Hyperthyroidism

Hyperthyroidism, or thyrotoxicosis, is the result of excess thyroid hormone with metabolic overstimulation of body function. Hyperthyroidism in the older patient is often due to Graves' disease or toxic goiter, an autoimmune disorder associated with the production of immunoglobulins that attach to and stimulate the TSH receptor, leading to sustained thyroid overactivity (Cobin, Weisen, & Trotto, 1999). Hyperthyroidism may also result from overtreatment with levothyroxine. Less common causes include pituitary tumors, pituitary resistance to thyroid hormones, and malignancies such as thyroid cancer (Cobin et al., 1999). Regardless of the cause, hyperthyroidism is the result of high levels of thyroid hormones, especially T_3 and to a lesser extent T_4 as the peripheral tissue will convert excess T_4 to T_3 (Solomon, 2003).

Signs and Symptoms of Hyperthyroidism

Only about 25% of hyperthyroid patients over the age of 65 exhibit classic symptoms (Solomon, 2003). The severity of signs and symptoms relates to duration of the illness, magnitude of the hormone excess, and age of the patient (2002, American Association of Clinical Endocrinologists). Common clinical features of hyperthyroidism in the older person may include the following:

- Cardiac arrhythmias and tachycardia
- Tremor
- Weight loss and appetite changes

- Sleep disturbances
- Changes in vision, photophobia, diplopia, eye irritation
- Fatigue and muscle weakness

Cardiac symptoms are experienced by 27% of older persons with hyperthyroidism. New-onset atrial fibrillation, heart failure, and angina are common presentations. Because cardiac disease is common in the older person, underlying hyperthyroidism may not be suspected. Gastrointestinal symptoms may be confused with malignancy or other bowel disease. Other commonly overlooked symptoms of hyperthyroidism in the older person include depression (called apathetic thyroidism), myopathy, and osteoporosis (Solomon, 2003).

Thyroid storm is a rare, life-threatening situation that can occur when a physical illness is superimposed on an older person with hyperthyroidism. Extreme tachycardia, fever, nausea, vomiting, heart failure, and changes in mental status or level of consciousness in a patient with hyperthyroidism should be immediately reported to the physician. Emergency treatment will be required. Treatment includes large doses of propylthiouracil and intravenous propranolol to slow the heartbeat to 90 to 110 beats per minute. Intravenous glucocorticoid and oral ipodate sodium are also given to decrease inflammation and lower serum T_3 levels (Solomon, 2003).

Diagnosis of Hyperthyroidism

A comprehensive health history and physical assessment should be performed with emphasis on weight and blood pressure, pulse rate and rhythm, thyroid palpation, neuromuscular examination, eye examination, vision assessment, and cardiovascular assessment. The TSH is the best screening test for hyperthyroidism, and subnormal or undetectable values are considered to be diagnostic (Solomon, 2003). Serum T_4, T_3, and thyroglobulin levels are on average lower in older patients with hyperthyroidism than in younger patients, but are not considered diagnostic of the disease. Ultrasound and radioisotope scans are needed when nodules are detected by palpation. Fine-needle aspiration may be done to rule out malignancies. Thyroid cancer is rare over the age of 60 and should be suspected when masses are painless and rapidly growing, the gland is hard and fixed, lymph nodes are palpable, and hoarseness or vocal cord paralysis is present as indication of laryngeal nerve involvement.

Treatment and Nursing Management of Hyperthyroidism

The treatment of choice for most older persons is ingestion of radioactive sodium iodide (^{131}I). It is easy to administer and avoids the option of surgery with all the complications related to anesthesia and hospitalization. No consensus exists on the appropriate dose of ^{131}I for hyperthyroidism. One option is to administer a low dose and monitor for return to euthyroid state; another option is to administer a single large dose intended to produce hypothyroidism and treat with levothyroxine to achieve normal thyroid function. The large dose option may provide the patient with more years of well-being because the relief of hyperthyroidism is faster and more reliable (Solomon, 2003).

Drugs other than ^{131}I may be used to treat hyperthyroidism under the following circumstances: (1) ^{131}I is refused by the patient; (2) to control symptoms before the administration of ^{131}I; or (3) to deplete the thyroid gland of stored hormone in order to prevent hyperthyroidism or "dumping" of hormone into the blood after treatment with ^{131}I (Solomon, 2003). These drugs are designed to block thyroid hormone production. Propylthiouracil (PTU) is given initially at 150 to 300 mg/day in divided doses every 8 hours. Side effects of propylthiouracil are dose related and include skin rash, nausea, hepatitis, and arthritis. The most serious side effect is granulocytopenia. Patients should be warned to stop taking the medications and to seek medical attention when a sore throat or generalized infection occurs (Cobin et al., 1999).

Propranolol and other beta-blockers can help to manage symptoms of hyperthyroidism, including atrial fibrillation. Although it protects the heart from the effects of excessive thyroid hormone, it can cause adverse effects such as hypotension, heart failure, and bronchospasm. It will conceal the symptoms of thyrotoxicosis, but does not affect thyroxine levels or readings on thyroid function tests.

When hyperthyroidism is due to subacute thyroiditis, Hashimoto's disease, or radiation damage, the only effective treatment is to administer beta-blockers and closely observe the patient's function and cardiac status for complications. Antithyroid drugs are ineffective because they do not decrease the uncontrolled output of hormone from the damaged thyroid follicles (Solomon, 2003).

Another therapeutic option for hyperthyroidism is surgery to remove a significant portion of the thyroid gland. This procedure is usually a last option for older patients and reserved for those with suspicious nodules, those allergic or intolerant of antithyroid drugs, and those with symptoms so severe that they cannot wait for ^{131}I to become effective (Cobin et al., 1999).

2. What are some things I need to know right away?

Some basic information that you need to begin to manage your thyroid problem includes:

- The importance of taking thyroid medication daily and avoiding other drugs that are known to interact with thyroid medications.
- Awareness of the signs and symptoms of thyroid disease such as appetite changes, fatigue, cardiovascular symptoms, change in bowel movement, weight changes, and mood changes.
- Need for careful ongoing monitoring of TSH by the healthcare provider and importance of keeping appointments.
- Need to tell all healthcare providers about the diagnosis and treatment of hypo- or hyperthyroidism.
- Importance of not changing brand of levothyroxine without careful monitoring of thyroid function.

PATIENT-FAMILY TEACHING GUIDELINES–DIABETES MELLITUS

1. I have diabetes. What can I do to stay healthy?

   General goals of health maintenance for older persons with diabetes include:

   - Achieving and maintaining near normal blood glucose levels by balancing food intake and medication with physical activity.
   - Achieving optimal serum lipid levels.
   - Providing adequate calories for attaining and maintaining reasonable weight.
   - Preventing and treating the acute and long-term complications of diabetes (damage to the eyes, kidneys, nerves, and heart).
   - Improving overall health through optimum nutrition.

2. I have just been diagnosed with diabetes. What are the most important things for me to know?

   Important things to know include:

   a. The relationship of food and meals to blood glucose levels, medication, and activity including action, side effects, timing, and interactions of all medications.

      - Recognition, causes, treatment, and prevention of hypo- and hyperglycemia.
      - Benefits of control.
      - Importance of lifestyle modification.
      - Use of glucagon if appropriate.
      - Use of blood glucose meter and establishment of blood glucose target with guidelines for reporting high or low levels.
      - Disposal of lancets and other contaminated materials.

(continued)

b. Basic food and meal plan guidelines—referral to the dietitian if necessary.

c. Consistent times each day for meals and snacks.

d. Recognition, prevention, and treatment of hypoglycemia.

e. Sick day management.

f. Self-monitoring of blood glucose.

g. Complication prevention and recognition.

- Self foot care and podiatry consultation.
- Need for yearly eye examination.
- Impact of lipids and need for yearly lipid evaluation.
- Need for blood pressure control and establishment of regular monitoring schedule.
- Identification of symptoms; treatment and methods for preventing kidney disease, peripheral vascular disease, cardiovascular disease, periodontal disease, and peripheral neuropathy.
- Need for pneumococcal vaccine and annual flu immunization.

3. What are some things I will need to know over time?

As you and your family become more familiar with the management of DM and blood glucose levels, additional content beyond basic meal planning is needed. As you make changes in your weight, exercise regimen, medications, and functional status, we will schedule follow-up sessions and focus on increasing your knowledge, skills, and flexibility to improve the quality of your life. Additional content may include:

- Sources of essential nutrients and their effect on blood glucose and lipid levels.

- Label reading and grocery shopping guidelines.
- Dining out and restaurant guidelines.
- Modifying fat intake.
- Use of sugar-containing foods, and dietetic foods and sweeteners.
- Alcohol guidelines.
- When to modify blood glucose testing schedules for glucose patterning and increased control.
- Adjusting mealtimes.
- Adjusting food for exercise.
- Special occasions and holidays.
- Travel and schedule changes.
- Vitamin and mineral supplementation.

PATIENT-FAMILY TEACHING GUIDELINES–THYROID PROBLEMS

1. I have just been diagnosed with a thyroid problem. What should I know about my thyroid?

People live long and healthy lives with thyroid problems. The essential knowledge for you to understand about your thyroid disorder include

- Understanding the relationship between thyroid hormones and the body's metabolic rate.
- Correctly identifying the body's reaction to excess or deficient thyroid hormone levels (signs and symptoms of hypo- or hypermetabolic state).
- Preventing or delaying complications resulting from hypo- or hyperthyroidism.
- Participating in the plan of care and improving your disease management skills.

(continued)

CHAPTER 18

THE GASTROINTESTINAL SYSTEM

NORMAL CHANGES OF AGING

Biological changes in GI function that occur in older persons result from the physical, mental, and psychological changes of aging and other factors associated with aging, such as immobility, impaired fluid balance, neuromuscular disorders, endocrine and metabolic problems, and the effects of medications. Age-related changes in the gastrointestinal system begin before age 50 and continue gradually throughout life (McCance & Huether, 2001). These changes include:

- Changes in the mouth, including loss of teeth, periodontal disease, decline in sense of taste and smell, and decreases in salivary secretion.
- Decreased esophageal motility.
- Diminished gastric motility with increased stomach-emptying time.
- Diminished capacity of the gastric mucosa to resist damage from factors such as nonsteroidal anti-inflammatory drugs (NSAIDs) and *Helicobacter pylori.*
- Achlorhydria or insufficient hydrochloric acid in the stomach.
- Decreased production of intrinsic factor leading to pernicious anemia.

- Decreased intestinal absorption, motility, and blood flow.
- Decreased pancreas size with duct hyperplasia and lobular fibrosis.
- Increased incidence of cholelithiasis (gallstones) and decreased production of bile acid synthesis.
- Decreased liver size and blood flow.
- Decreased thirst and hunger drive due to cognitive changes or psychological conditions such as depression.
- Increased medication use and possible adverse drug reactions.

(Horowitz, 2004; McCance & Huether, 2001)

Medications with great potential to affect the GI tract include the anticholinergics (antidepressants, neuroleptics, antihistamines, antiparkinsonian agents), antihypertensives (calcium channel blockers, ACE inhibitors, diuretics), iron and calcium supplements, aluminum-containing antacids, opiates, and laxatives (Camilleri, Lee, Viramontes, Bharucha, & Tangalos, 2000).

COMMON DISORDERS IN AGING
Esophageal Disorders

In healthy older persons, aging has only minor effects on esophageal motor and sensory function. Older patients with significant esophageal disorders usually have vascular or neurologic problems.

Dysphagia

Dysphagia is the most common esophageal disorder in older people (Borum, 2004). Dysphagia is defined as difficulty in any part of the process involved with swallowing solid foods or liquids. Whether acute or chronic, the condition affects oral intake and is usually indicative of some other disease process.

Patients at Risk for Dysphagia

Signs and symptoms observable in older patients at risk for dysphagia include the following:

- Reports from the older person or his or her family that swallowing food or medications is difficult
- Difficulty in controlling food or saliva in the mouth (drooling, dribbling)
- Facial droop, open mouth
- Dementia, frailty, confusion, extreme lethargy, decreased level of consciousness
- Inability to sit in an upright position and maintain trunk position for a reasonable length of time
- Choking or coughing while eating or drinking
- Increased nasal or oral congestion or secretion after a meal
- Weak voice, cough, and tongue movements
- Slurred speech
- Change in voice during meal (wet, gurgling, or hoarse voice)
- Recurrent upper respiratory infections or pneumonia
- Retention or pocketing of food in mouth
- Oral thrush
- Refusal to open mouth or accept a large bite of food
- Unexplained weight loss

(Dahlin, 2004; Kayser-Jones & Pengilly, 1999)

Early detection of dysphagia is vital because its complications can be life-threatening. Aspiration of food or fluid into the respiratory tract can cause choking, airway obstruction, hypoxia, and aspiration pneumonia. Risk factors associated with nursing home residents and dysphagia include the following:

- Residents not positioned properly.
- Residents fed inappropriate food and liquid.

- Residents fed quickly with large bites of food.
- Residents labeled as "difficult" or "uncooperative."

(Kayser-Jones & Pengilly, 1999)

Because dysphagia is associated with underlying illness or disorders, the older person with multiple co-morbidities is considered to be at risk for aspiration. Causes of dysphagia include:

1. Neurological disorders
2. Muscular disorders
3. Anatomical abnormalities

Nursing Assessment of Dysphagia

Often, the gerontological nurse is aware that the patient has a swallowing disorder based on the signs and symptoms presented above. In other cases, the nurse must carefully observe the older patient at rest and during the process of eating and drinking. Speech and occupational therapists can assist the nurse and provide valuable professional opinions during the assessment process. The following questions should be included in a dysphagia assessment:

- Have you ever choked while eating or drinking? If so, how recently? Does choking occur frequently?
- Does your mouth feel dry? Do you have enough saliva to chew your food easily?
- Do you have problems with drooling or controlling saliva?
- Does food ever fall out or get stuck in your mouth?
- Do you ever spit up food after a meal?
- Do you feel the need to clear your throat frequently?
- Do you have problems sitting upright during mealtime?

If the answer to any of these questions is positive, notify the primary care provider and request a formal swallowing evaluation by the speech pathologist. A bedside evaluation may be carried out with the older person drinking a variety of liquids (thin to thickened) and observed for swallowing functionality. In some cases, videofluoroscopic radiographic evaluation of the swallowing process is conducted.

Residents at risk for aspiration should have a notation made on the nursing care plan to inform all involved with the patient's care regarding this risk and appropriate interventions to facilitate safe eating and drinking. Nurses and others caring for the patient should follow these guidelines:

- Try to minimize distractions during eating. Provide a pleasant and calm environment during mealtime.
- Try to use consistent feeding techniques with notations as to the older person's likes, dislikes, eating and drinking habits, and consumption patterns.
- Make sure the older patient is properly positioned and supported during mealtime.
- Try to maintain the upright position for at least 1 hour after eating.
- Ensure the patient has swallowed one bite before giving another. Do not try to rush. The patient may become resistive.
- Monitor the patient's respirations. A change in breathing pattern or rate can signal the onset of aspiration.
- Provide oral hygiene before and after the meal. A clean, fresh, odor-free mouth will stimulate the patient's appetite. Ensure dentures are in place and in good repair.
- Plan meals at times when the patient is rested. Present meals to persons with dementia according to routine.

- Offer food and liquid consistencies according to the speech pathologist's and dietitcian's recommendations. Do not overly thicken liquids. The older person will resist "chewing" juice or liquids (rightly so).
- Keep conversation to a minimum and focus attention on the task at hand. For instance, "Now here's a bite of vegetables. Chew them slowly and let me know when you are ready to swallow." Assess mental status to ensure the patient can understand instructions and follow commands.
- Instruct all persons who assist the patient with feeding in the appropriate techniques. Nurses' assistants should feed no more than two or three patients at mealtime and they should sit comfortably at the same level as the patient.
- Never engage in forceful feeding techniques. Everyone has times when they are not hungry and do not feel like eating. Forcing an older patient to eat may set the stage for a power struggle at the next meal.

(Kayser-Jones & Pengilly, 1999;
http://www.geronurseonline.org, 2004)

Nursing Outcomes Related to Caring for Older Patients with Dysphagia

Nurse sensitive outcomes that would indicate an appropriate nursing intervention include no new aspiration events; adequate food and fluid intake to maintain weight and body functions; maintenance of good skin turgor; normal or improving hemoglobin, hematocrit, and serum albumin levels; patient and family satisfaction with oral intake and meals; maintenance of good oral hygiene; and patient's report or observation that the patient possesses appropriate levels of energy.

Gastroesophageal Reflux Disease

Gastroesophageal reflux disease (GERD) involves reflux of gastric contents into the esophagus. Older adults are more at risk for GERD complications because of prolonged esophageal acid exposure over a period of years. Additionally, the higher frequency of hiatal hernia, decreased saliva volume, and use of drugs that reduce lower esophageal sphincter tone may contribute to the development and progression of GERD in older adults (Ray, Secrest, Ch'ien, & Corey, 2002). Hiatal hernias, or diaphragmatic hernias that allow a small portion of the stomach to slide into the chest, are common in older people and are usually asymptomatic.

The symptoms of GERD include heartburn (sensation of burning in the substernal or sternal area), indigestion, belching, hiccups, and regurgitation of gastric contents into the mouth (sour mouth). The heartburn will typically worsen with lying flat or bending over. Chest pain can be so severe and persistent that it is sometimes confused with cardiac pain or angina. The older person may seek emergency evaluation because he or she fears the onset of a heart attack. Erosive esophagitis occurs when the caustic gastric contents remain in contact with the esophageal mucosa and begin to cause damage to the esophageal lining. Chronic laryngeal irritation can cause voice hoarseness, wheezing, bronchitis, asthma, and aspiration pneumonia. Symptoms may be worsened by eating large meals, using certain medications, eating foods and drinking beverages high in fat or caffeine, using tobacco and alcohol, reclining after eating, and obesity (Borum, 2004).

Complications from untreated GERD include esophagitis, bleeding, scarring, and stricture formation. Hemorrhage can occur from deep erosions and ulcerations resulting in anemia, black tarry stools, or vomiting of bright red blood.

Nursing Assessment of Gastroesophageal Reflux Disease

The patient's report of symptoms, past medical history, medications, and dietary and sleep habits are the most useful sources of information to diagnose GERD. Patients with atypical pain, weight loss, or anemia should be referred to a gastroenterologist for diagnostic testing. The most frequently used diagnostic test is the barium swallow. Upper **endoscopy** is the best method to assess mucosal injury.

Treatment Goals for Gastroesophageal Reflux Disease

The goal of treatment is to control symptoms and heal esophageal mucosal injury. Lifestyle modifications include elevation of the head of the bed, reducing meal size, weight loss, stopping drugs that may worsen the condition, staying upright for 1 to 3 hours after a meal, and drinking 8 ounces of water when taking medications.

Medications Used to Manage Gastroesophageal Reflux Disease

Over-the-counter antacids buffer the gastric pH and are widely available. The cost is reasonable, but side effects may include diarrhea, constipation, altered mineral metabolism, and acid-base disturbances. Magnesium-containing antacids can cause diarrhea and should be used with caution in older patients with renal dysfunction, including chronic or acute renal failure, because of the potential for hypermagnesemia and related toxicity. Aluminum-containing antacids can cause constipation, osteomalacia, hypophosphatemia, and related toxicity (Borum, 2004).

Histamine$_2$ receptor agonists decrease acid production by inhibiting histamine stimulation of the parietal cells. These medications are potent inhibitors of gastric acid secretion and are generally well tolerated in older people with a low incidence of side effects. Risk factors for side effects include advanced age, hepatic or renal impairment, and diagnoses of additional medical conditions. Cimetidine, a drug available without prescription, has the greatest chance for adverse effects, including erectile dysfunction, gynecomastia, confusion, agitation, anxiety, and depression, and should be used with caution. Further, cimetidine inhibits the cytochrome P-450 oxidase system, increasing the probability of interactions with other medications.

Proton pump inhibitors suppress acid secretion by inhibiting the hydrogen/potassium adenosinetriphosphatase pump at the parietal cell. Common side effects of proton pump inhibitors include atrophic **gastritis,** headache, diarrhea and constipation, dizziness, rash, cough, backache, and abdominal pain (Borum, 2004; epocrates.com, 2004; Reuben et al., 2002).

Other medications besides acid-suppression agents can help control the symptoms of GERD, including promotility agents that enhance esophageal clearance and gastric emptying. However, these drugs are considered second-line treatments because of the prevalence of adverse effects, including abdominal cramping, diarrhea, gynecomastia, galactorrhea, fatigue, drowsiness, and movement disorders (tremor, rigidity, and tardive dyskinesia).

The mucosal protectant agent sucralfate aids in mucosal healing by reducing direct tissue exposure to acid. It is minimally absorbed, but bowel function should be carefully monitored as it may cause constipation. Sucralfate should be used with caution in older patients with renal impairment because of the potential for aluminum absorption and associated toxicity. Further, sucralfate can reduce the absorption of other drugs, including quinolone antibiotics, phenytoin, and warfarin (Borum, 2004). Older patients taking these drugs should have drug levels carefully monitored if sucralfate is added to the medication regimen.

Misoprostol, a combination drug that has an antisecretory and mucosal protective effect, is a synthetic prostaglandin E analogue. It is indicated only for prophylactic treatment in older patients taking NSAIDs (Borum, 2004). The major side effects are diarrhea (13 to 40% of patients) and abdominal pain (7 to 20%).

Older patients with GERD and with Barrett's esophagus require aggressive treatment with proton pump inhibitors and regular endoscopic examination. Surgery may be required if esophageal erosion does not reverse with treatment.

Gastritis

Gastritis, or inflammation of the gastric mucosa, is classified by the severity of the mucosal inflammation, the site of involvement, and the inflammatory cell type. Erosive (hemorrhagic) gastritis may be caused by ingestion of substances that irritate the gastric mucosa such as NSAIDs, alcohol, radiation therapy, gastric trauma, or ischemia as a result of arterial insufficiency or circulatory problems. Diagnosis is based upon endoscopic appearance of the stomach lining, and biopsy is usually not necessary to confirm the diagnosis. Older patients with severe gastritis may be diagnosed with anemia and require transfusion, careful ongoing monitoring of hemoglobin and hematocrit levels, and periodic evaluation of stool for occult blood testing.

Peptic and Duodenal Ulcer Disease

Peptic ulcer disease is defined as an excoriated area of the gastric mucosa (peptic ulcer) or first few centimeters of the duodenum (duodenal ulcer) that penetrates through to the muscularis mucosae. Duodenal ulcers are more common than gastric ulcers. Bleeding from duodenal ulcers occurs more frequently in older patients (Borum, 2004). Chronic or slow upper gastrointestinal bleeding may present with anemia, melena (black, tarry stools), or a positive fecal occult blood test. Upper gastrointestinal endoscopy is required for evaluation of the cause of upper gastrointestinal bleeding (Ali & Lacy, 2004).

H. pylori is an important factor in the development of ulcers, and the prevalence of *H. pylori* infections increases with age. Eradication of *H. pylori* is associated with more rapid ulcer healing and decrease in recurrence rates (Borum, 2004).

NSAID use increases the incidence of peptic ulcer disease, especially early in treatment (during the first 3 months). Higher doses of NSAIDs, history of peptic ulcer disease, and concurrent use of anticoagulants (warfarin, aspirin) predispose older patients to larger ulcers. These patients often do not experience abdominal pain. The first signs of peptic ulcer disease may be serious gastrointestinal bleeding episodes requiring emergency evaluation, treatment, and transfusion.

Zollinger-Ellison syndrome is characterized by gastric hypersecretion and peptic ulceration caused by a gastrin-producing tumor (gastrinoma) of the pancreas or duodenal wall. The continuous high gastrin output stimulates the parietal cells to produce acid. Peptic ulcer occurs in 95% of patients with Zollinger-Ellison syndrome with persistent symptoms that progress and do not respond to drug treatment. For these patients, referral to a gastroenterologist for additional testing and assessment of gastrin levels is indicated. Treatment may include tumor removal and surgical resection for older patients without surgical risk or treatment with omeprazole.

Signs and Symptoms of Peptic and Duodenal Ulcer Disease

In older people, the classic signs and symptoms of peptic ulcer disease are rare. Often the presenting sign is blood loss and iron deficiency anemia. **Dyspepsia** (indigestion with bloating, early satiety, abdominal distention, or nausea) is a common symptom but often is not vigorously investigated and is attributed to normal changes of aging.

Diagnosis of Peptic and Duodenal Ulcer Disease

The patient's report of symptoms, past medical history, use of medications, and dietary habits are the most useful sources of information to diagnose peptic ulcer disease. A history of anemia or occurrence of new-onset anemia should be aggressively investigated by the healthcare provider. Generally, pain resulting from peptic ulcer disease is described as dyspepsia localized in the epigastric area, occurring hours after a meal (on an empty stomach), and relieved by food or antacids. Abdominal pain that awakens the patient at night can be a symptom of peptic ulcer disease. Upper endoscopy is the most sensitive and specific test for assessing abnormalities in the upper GI tract. Biopsies can be taken, if needed, during the procedure. Gastric ulcers are often difficult to distinguish from stomach cancer, and biopsy is required to eliminate the possibility of malignancy.

Treatment Goals for Peptic and Duodenal Ulcer Disease

In older patients with documented *H. pylori* infection, the use of antisecretory drugs combined with antibiotic results in more rapid duodenal ulcer healing. Although no standard therapy exists, triple or quadruple therapy regimens are advocated based on efficacy, tolerability, compliance, and cost (Borum, 2004). Usually two or three antibiotics are combined with a proton pump inhibitor. The most effective combination for eradicating *H. pylori* includes oral lansoprazole 30 mg bid, clarithromycin 500 mg bid, and amoxicillin 1,000 mg bid for 2 weeks. Ranitidine bismuth citrate 400 mg po bid for 4 weeks and clarithromycin 500 mg po tid for 2 weeks may also be effective.

Nurse Sensitive Outcomes Related to Care of Older Patients with Peptic Ulcer Disease

Nurse sensitive outcomes that would indicate an appropriate nursing intervention include positive relief of signs and symptoms, no significant side effects of medications, sustained progress on lifestyle modification plan, adequate nutrition as measured by weight and nutritional markers, and resolution of ulcer disease as evidenced by tissue healing and stable hemoglobin and hematocrit levels.

Lower Gastrointestinal Tract Disorders

Normal Changes of Aging

Aging is associated with diminished anal sphincter tone and strength (Wald, 2004). The structural weakening of colonic muscle may contribute to the development of **diverticula,** or saclike mucosal projections through the muscle wall. Older persons with the presence of diverticula are diagnosed with **diverticulosis.** Several factors can alter colonic function and lead to alterations in the lower bowel function, including diagnosis with a metabolic or endocrine disorder, lifestyle and environmental factors such as insufficient fiber or fluid in the diet, neurologic disorders or injury, mobility problems, cognitive impairment or mood disorders, and many medications. These factors may make the older person more susceptible to fecal incontinence, constipation, or diarrhea.

Common Lower Gastrointestinal Disorders

Diverticula are acquired saclike mucosal projections that protrude through the muscular layer of the GI tract. They can potentially trap feces, become inflamed and infected, and rupture. Usually diverticula are found in the sigmoid and descending colon where blood vessels penetrate to the submucosa (Wald, 2004). Lifestyle-related factors include inadequate intake of dietary fiber. A low-fiber diet increases the density of the stool with increases in intraluminal pressure, forcing the saclike projections of the colon wall through the muscular layers of the colon.

Diverticulitis is an infection from colonic diverticula. Diverticulitis is caused when normal bowel flora (aerobic and anaerobic gram-negative bacilli) overgrow and flourish in the diverticular pouch when stool becomes entrapped, causing inflammation. With inflammation, the diverticular opening becomes obstructed and a pouch forms, trapping the infection. Fever, leukocytosis, pain, or abdominal tenderness may be indicators of diverticulitis, but the very old or frail older person may exhibit none of these classic symptoms (Wald, 2004).

Nursing Assessment for Diverticular Disease

Examination of the abdomen for abnormal peristaltic waves and auscultation of bowel sounds should always precede palpation because palpation may stimulate or alter peristaltic movement. Hyperactive bowel sounds, rebound tenderness, or the presence of an abdominal mass may indicate a bowel obstruction or perforation and require immediate referral and medical attention. Note the time and nature of the last bowel movement. Diarrhea and fecal oozing may accompany bowel obstruction and complicate recognition of the problem.

Most often, a gastroenterologist will obtain an abdominal computerized tomography (CT) scan or ultrasound to assess colonic wall thickness and extraluminal structures for suspected diverticulitis. Surgery may be recommended for some older patients who fail to respond to medical therapy within 72 hours, for those with repeated attacks of diverticulitis, and for the immunocompromised older patient (including those on chemotherapy, chronic steroid users, and those with diabetes mellitus). Emergency surgery is required for generalized peritonitis, persistent bowel obstruction, and uncontrollable GI bleeding (Wald, 2004).

Goals of Treatment

Mild infections may be treated with oral antibiotics on an outpatient basis, whereas severe infections may require hospitalization with intravenous antibiotics. Sometimes a liquid diet progressing to a low-fiber diet may be suggested to allow the colon to rest and heal (Wald, 2004).

To prevent recurrence of diverticulitis and manage diverticular disease, the nurse may suggest the following interventions:

- Eat more fiber and drink plenty of fluids (try to drink 8 full glasses of water per day). This will decrease intraluminal pressure and soften the consistency of the stool.

- Do not ignore the urge to have a bowel movement.
- Exercise regularly (walking, swimming, etc.) to aid digestion and increase colonic peristalsis.
- Avoid foods that precipitate painful attacks.

Inflammatory Bowel Disease

Ulcerative Colitis

Ulcerative colitis is a chronic inflammatory process that affects the superficial layers of the wall of the colon in a continuous distribution. Pathological changes to the epithelial lining of the colon include inflammatory changes such as widespread ulceration, epithelial necrosis, depletion of goblet cells, and leukocyte infiltration (Wald, 2004).

The major signs and symptoms of ulcerative colitis include bloody diarrhea, left lower quadrant abdominal pain, and weight loss. Systemic manifestations may also occur and include uveitis and arthralgia. Diagnosis is made by referral to a gastroenterologist for sigmoidoscopy, colonoscopy, and rectal mucosa biopsy. Stool samples may be obtained and cultured or examined for toxins indicating the presence of pathogens such as *Salmonella, Shigella*, and ***Clostridium difficile*** in older patients with recent history of antibiotic use.

Toxic megacolon may occur in the older patient as a result of chronic ulcerative colitis. Symptoms of toxic megacolon include abdominal distention, fever, colonic dilatation, and rapid deterioration. The risk of developing colorectal cancer increases substantially in older patients with ulcerative colitis. Annual colonoscopy with biopsy to detect mucosal dysplasia (premalignant lesions in ulcerative colitis) is recommended in older patients diagnosed with toxic megacolon (Wald, 2004).

Goals of Treatment for Inflammatory Bowel Disease

For older patients with severe ulcerative colitis or toxic megacolon, hospitalization for administration of intravenous corticosteroids may be necessary. For older patients with moderate disease, oral corticosteroids are used to decrease inflammation. Prednisone 40 to 60 mg per day may be given initially and then tapered to 20 mg every morning as symptoms resolve. To avoid adverse effects from long-term corticosteroid use, the dose of prednisone should be tapered by 5 mg per week as long as symptoms do not recur. Long-term corticosteroid use may cause or induce hyperglycemia in patients with diabetes, induce steroid psychosis or acute delirium, accelerate osteoporosis, and worsen heart failure and hypertension. Corticosteroid retention enemas may be used for patients with left-sided disease; however, approximately 60% of rectal corticosteroid may be absorbed and systemic effects may occur (Wald, 2004).

Sulfasalazine, olsalazine, or mesalamine (5-ASA drugs) are often given with oral corticosteroids; however, adverse effects occur in up to 30% of patients. Adverse effects are dose related and include nausea, anorexia, diarrhea, headache, and rash. Treatment should be maintained indefinitely for older patients who can tolerate these drugs. The usual maintenance dose of sulfasalazine is 1 g po bid (Wald, 2004).

Surgery may be necessary for functional older patients with acute disease, when drug therapy fails, and when multiple precancerous lesions are detected. The most common surgical procedure is subtotal colectomy and ileostomy.

Crohn's Disease

Crohn's disease is a chronic inflammatory process that usually affects the terminal ileum or colon and is characterized by inflammation, linear ulcerations, and granulomas. The inflammatory process affects all layers of the bowel and can often result in scarring and fibrosis. Unlike ulcerative colitis, Crohn's disease exhibits "skip areas" or areas where normal bowel exists between areas of inflammation (Wald, 2004).

Signs and symptoms of Crohn's disease in the older person include diarrhea, fever, abdominal pain, and weight loss. The diagnosis is confirmed by barium enema or colonoscopy when visualization of the colon reveals discontinuous or skip areas of ulceration and inflammation followed by areas of healthy bowel. Abdominal CT scans are being used more to diagnose Crohn's disease as they are noninvasive and identify abnormalities of the colon wall more easily. A complete blood count may confirm leukocytosis or elevated white cell count and elevated sedimentation rate as a result of the inflammatory process. If the disease is long-standing or severe, the older patient may exhibit signs of systemic illness such as hypoalbuminemia or anemia due to chronic blood loss and malabsorption syndromes. Drug therapy includes all the drugs used for ulcerative colitis. In some older patients, antibiotics are used to supplement treatment (Wald, 2004). Unlike ulcerative colitis, Crohn's disease is not cured by surgery.

Benign and Malignant Tumors

Most benign tumors are polyps. Predisposing factors include age, diet, family history, and prior diagnosis of polyps. Most polyps are asymptomatic, but occasionally rectal bleeding can occur. Diagnosis is usually confirmed by sigmoidoscopy, colonoscopy, or barium enema. During colonoscopy, polyps can be removed for biopsy.

In early stages, colorectal cancer is asymptomatic and diagnosis is most often made by barium enema or endoscopy. Later stage tumors may be accompanied by change in bowel habits, abdominal pain, abdominal mass, onset of anemia, rectal bleeding, and weight loss. Carcinoembryonic antigen levels may be elevated in patients with cancer of the colon as well as those with benign conditions. Therefore, it cannot be considered a diagnostic tool but it may be used to follow the effectiveness of treatment and management of those diagnosed with colon cancer (Tompkins, 2004).

Surgical resection of the primary tumor is needed to prevent perforation, bleeding, and obstruction of the bowel. Segmental resection, subtotal colectomy, or colostomy may be performed, depending on the stage and extent of the disease and the older patient's underlying health status. About 25% of patients with colorectal cancer develop hepatic metastases, and adjuvant chemotherapy is frequently used as a treatment in these patients. Radiation therapy can ease the pain of recurrent rectal cancer, and laser therapy has been used to reduce inoperable rectal tumors and prevent obstruction (Tompkins, 2004). For end-stage patients with bowel obstruction, nasogastric tubes can be used to relieve distention and prevent the vomiting of fecal material.

Annual fecal occult blood testing increases detection of colorectal tumors in the early and curable stage and improves long-term survival. Sigmoidoscopy and colonoscopy have been established as cost-effective screening tools. Initial screening should begin at age 50 and be repeated every 10 years until the age of 85. If polyps are identified, the procedures should be repeated every 3 to 5 years (Ali & Lacy, 2004).

Antibiotic-Associated Colitis and Diarrhea

Diarrhea that occurs during or shortly after the administration of antibiotics is caused by a cytotoxin produced by *C. difficile,* an organism that is part of the normal bowel flora but overgrows as a result of elimination of other bowel organisms during antibiotic treatment. *C. difficile*–induced diarrhea and colitis are more common in older people receiving treatment in hospitals or residing in nursing homes and may indicate underlying frailty and the presence of acute and chronic illnesses. Risk factors for the acquisition of *C. difficile* include recent surgery, spending time in the intensive care unit, nasogastric or gastric intubation, and extended hospital stays. Although most antibiotics are associated with the development of *C. difficile* infection, cephalosporins, extended-spectrum pencillins (ampicillin), and clindamycin are implicated most often (Wald, 2004).

Careful hand washing done on a regular basis is the best way to stop the spread of nosocomial infections like *C. difficile.* It is easier and safer to prevent an infection than to cure one.

The signs and symptoms of *C. difficile* infection range from mild diarrhea to severe colitis often associated with pseudomembranes that adhere to necrotic colonic tissue. Typically, the patient passes watery nonbloody diarrhea, complains of lower abdominal pain and cramping, and exhibits a low-grade fever. In severe cases and in those who are not treated, dehydration, hypotension, and colonic perforation may occur. The stools have a characteristic odor that many nurses over time recognize as associated with this infection.

Diagnosis is confirmed by stool analysis and examination by enzyme-linked immunoassay or stool culture. Often several stool samples are necessary to diagnose the condition.

Treatment includes metronidazole 250 mg by mouth qid for 7 to 10 days. Refractory cases are treated with vancomycin 125 mg by mouth QID for 7 to 14 days. Metronidazole is about as effective as vancomycin in mild to moderate cases and much less expensive, making it the drug of choice under these circumstances. Fever usually resolves within 24 hours, and diarrhea decreases over 4 to 5 days. Antidiarrhea drugs should not be used because they expose the colonic tissue to the toxin for longer periods of time and place the patient at risk for the development of necrotic tissue and pseudomembranes. Aggressive nursing interventions to prevent dehydration should be implemented, including frequently assessing pulse and blood pressure, assessing postural blood pressure if the patient is ambulatory, establishing a schedule to offer the patient oral fluids (water, juice, and the beverage of choice) every 15 to 30 minutes, monitoring urinary output and skin turgor, and notifying the primary care provider of imminent dehydration so that intravenous fluids may be initiated if necessary. If the older person is receiving diuretics, these drugs should be held until the diarrhea subsides as they may exacerbate dehydration.

Constipation

Constipation is defined as two or fewer stools per week, straining at stool, or difficult passage of hard feces, often with fecal impaction and feeling of incomplete evacuation (Howard, West, & Ossip-Klein, 2000; Prather, 2004). Factors contributing to constipation include dehydration, side effects of medication, insufficient fiber intake, cognitive impairment, and immobility. Presence of physical illness can also predispose an older person to constipation, including metabolic and endocrine disorders (diabetes, hypothyroidism, chronic renal failure), muscular dystrophy, neurologic disorders (spinal cord injury, multiple sclerosis, Parkinson's disease, cerebrovascular accident, Alzheimer's disease), and recent abdominal surgery (McCrea, 2003). Constipation can lead to abdominal discomfort, loss of appetite, and nausea and vomiting.

Drugs known to cause constipation include all of those with anticholinergic side effects (antidepressants, neuroleptics, antihistamines, antiparkinsonian agents), some antihypertensive agents (calcium channel blockers, ACE inhibitors, diuretics), iron supplements, calcium supplements, aluminum-containing antacids, benzodiazepines, antiarrhythmics, and opiates. The nurse should carefully monitor bowel function in patients taking these medications.

The major complication of constipation is fecal impaction, which can result in intestinal obstruction, colonic ulceration, overflow incontinence with leakage of stool around the obstructing feces, and paradoxical diarrhea (Prather, 2004). Urinary incontinence, urinary tract infection, and urinary retention are also associated with fecal impaction. Excessive straining to pass stool is associated with syncope, transient ischemic attacks, **hemorrhoids,** anal **fissures,** and rectal prolapse. Over time, older patients with chronic constipation and straining at stool will dread having a bowel movement and may ignore the need to defecate, further compounding the problem.

Nursing Assessment of Constipation

The older person should be questioned as to frequency of bowel movement (fewer than three per week), consistency of stool (hard or difficult to pass), presence of excessive straining, or feeling of fullness in the rectum after completing a bowel movement. The presence of bright red blood on the stool or toilet tissue may indicate bleeding from internal or external hemorrhoids or perhaps a more serious underlying condition such as a rectal fissure or tumor.

A careful review of the older person's medications, medical conditions, level of exercise, fluid and fiber, and psychological status (somatization, anxiety, and depression) is indicated. The nursing assessment should also include an abdominal examination with auscultation of bowel sounds and palpation to detect the presence of large amounts of stool in the colon. The rectum may be examined digitally for the presence of hard impacted stool in the rectal vault. The primary healthcare provider may, when appropriate, seek further diagnostic testing such as barium enema, colonoscopy, or x-ray of the abdomen.

Constipation is often relieved by adequate hydration, increased mobility, fiber supplementation (20 to 35 g/day), and use of laxatives. One nursing study reported that laxatives can sometimes be discontinued for an older person with bran intake that reached 25 g daily (Howard et al., 2000). A bran mixture that significantly reduces laxative use for older patients includes 3 cups unsweetened applesauce, 2 cups coarse wheat bran, and 1 1/2 cups unsweetened prune juice. Administering 4 tablespoons per day (2 before breakfast and 2 before supper) will stimulate natural bowel movements and decrease dependence on laxatives (Smith & Newman, 1989). Fiber should be consumed as wheat or oat bran, fruits, vegetables, or nuts. When fiber intake is increased, excessive gas may be initially present but this annoying problem usually resolves as the body becomes accustomed to the change. It is recommended to increase fiber intake slowly with 5 g daily, adding small increments until the desired results are achieved with good tolerance and minimal gas and bloating. Contraindications to use of the fiber mixture include bowel obstruction, severe dysphagia, dietary restriction to low-fiber diet, and limited fluid intake. Lack of sufficient fluid intake with increased fiber diets or use of fiber supplements is associated with impaction, bowel obstruction, and large amounts of dry stool accumulating in the colon. The older person should be instructed in techniques of bowel training and urged not to delay the urge to have a bowel movement and to take advantage of the natural defecation reflex that usually occurs about 30 minutes after a meal.

Laxatives

Bulk laxatives contain soluble and insoluble fibers that absorb water (in states of adequate hydration) into the intestinal tract and increase stool mass. The increased mass will stimulate colonic peristalsis. Bulk laxatives are contraindicated in the presence of intestinal obstruction or when peristaltic activity is compromised (paralytic ileus). Stool softeners should be limited to patients who complain of straining at stool, painful defecation with the presence of hemorrhoids, or anal fissures. Stool softeners are sometimes used to facilitate bowel movements and prevent constipation in high-risk patients (postoperative abdominal surgery). Osmotic laxatives draw water into the colon by osmotic pressure. If the osmotic laxative is metabolized by bacteria in the colon, production of gases may lead to flatulence, abdominal bloating, or cramping. Magnesium-containing products should not be used in older persons with chronic renal failure, and sodium agents should be avoided in the presence of congestive heart failure and hypernatremia (Thomas, Goode, & LaMaster, 2003). Laxatives containing senna increase peristalsis and secretion of water into the bowel. These agents tend to be more harsh than other agents and can sometimes cause unpleasant cramping. Suppositories and enemas are usually reserved for those patients who have not responded to the other laxatives, and are invasive and sometimes uncomfortable for the older patient; therefore, they should be used as a last resort. Enemas are the treatment of choice if colonic fecal impaction is suspected. Plain tap water or sodium phosphate enemas are recommended. Soapsuds enemas produce mucosal damage and cramping and should be avoided. Because rectal volumes increase with age, the enema should be administered slowly to prevent cramping and should generally contain about 150−300 milliliters or 5−10 fluid ounces of solution. After the initial blockage has been passed or removed manually, a second enema may be needed to remove additional stool that has moved into the proximal colon (Prather, 2004). As this procedure is uncomfortable and unpleasant, fecal impaction should be avoided by paying close attention to the older person's bowel function.

For drug-induced constipation, the best action is to seek advice from the primary care provider as to whether the offending medication may be discontinued. Some drugs (verapamil) cause more constipation than others, and these drugs should be discontinued if possible. However, when the medication cannot be discontinued (for example, opioids for pain), a careful bowel management plan is needed to prevent constipation and fecal impaction. Correction of constipation associated with opioid use requires a senna or osmotic laxative to overcome the strong opioid effect. Stool softeners and bulking agents alone are inadequate because of the opioid-related constipation resulting from slowed gut motility. A prophylactic bowel regimen should be initiated whenever an older person is started on an opioid pain medication to prevent fecal impaction (Thomas et al., 2003). Fecal impactions high in the rectum or in the sigmoid can lead to nausea and vomiting, anorexia, pain, obstruction, perforation, and fecal peritonitis.

Diarrhea

Diarrhea is defined as abnormally loose stool accompanied by a change in frequency or volume (Prather, 2004). A history of gastric tube feeding or recent antibiotic use may suggest the presence of *C. difficile.*

Diarrhea of less than 2 weeks duration is considered acute; diarrhea occurring longer than 4 weeks is defined as chronic. Most diarrhea in the older person is acute and self-limited. Causes include infection (viral, bacterial, or parasitic), medications and drug changes, and food intolerances. Acute bloody diarrhea needs immediate medical evaluation. Causes include ischemia, diverticulitis, or inflammatory bowel disease. Viruses responsible for infectious diarrhea include the Norwalk virus and rotavirus. Both viruses are spread by the fecal-oral route and have caused epidemic diarrhea in nursing homes. Toxic diarrhea can result from food poisoning *(Salmonella, Staphylococcus aureus, E. colt)* or ingestion of contaminated food. Careful hand washing and food preparation in sanitary conditions are required to prevent infectious diarrhea in the older person.

Chronic diarrhea may occur as a result of tumors, surgery, and medications. Almost all drugs can cause diarrhea. Commonly associated drugs include NSAIDs, magnesium-containing antacids, antiarrhythmics, beta-blockers, quinidine, colchicine, and digoxin (Prather, 2004). If the pattern of diarrhea suggests lactose intolerance (diarrhea after ingestion of dairy products), a trial lactose-free diet or treatment with lactase can be tried and bowel function carefully monitored. Older patients who are immunosuppressed, such as those receiving chemotherapy or those diagnosed with HIV/AIDS, may experience chronic diarrhea secondary to bowel infections caused by giardiasis, microsporidiosis, and *Mycobacterium avium-intracellulare* (Prather, 2004).

Nursing Assessment of Diarrhea

Nursing assessment should include a careful examination of the abdomen, including visual examination for bloating or excessive peristaltic movements, auscultation of bowel sounds, palpation to identify masses or rebound tenderness, and digital rectal examination to determine presence of impacted stool. Older patients with recent antibiotic use, those who have experienced recent foreign travel, and those who may have been exposed to food poisoning should have stool collected for culture and analysis. A plain abdominal x-ray (kidneys, ureter, bladder) may indicate the presence of an intestinal obstruction or fecal impaction.

If toxin-producing and infectious diarrhea are not suspected, antidiarrheal agents can be administered. However, administration of these drugs in the presence of toxins and infectious agents can lead to colon damage and systemic adverse effects by allowing the toxic substance to remain in the bowel for longer periods of time and thus to be absorbed into the general circulation. Soluble fiber (Metamucil) adds bulk to the stool and is sometimes helpful to slow bowel movements in persons requiring bulk. Kaopectate, Pepto-Bismol, and Imodium A-D can be administered after each loose stool in divided doses. Lomotil should be avoided because of significant atropine-like side effects (Prather, 2004).

Fecal Incontinence

Fecal incontinence is embarrassing and can cause an older person to severely limit social activity. Immobilized and functionally impaired older persons may be unable to suppress the urge to defecate and suffer fecal incontinence while waiting for assistance to use the bedpan or toilet. A regular toileting program, administration of a high-fiber diet, elimination of medications associated with diarrhea, and treatment of infections are appropriate interventions for older persons with fecal incontinence.

Hemorrhoids and Rectal Bleeding

Hemorrhoids and colorectal cancer are the most common causes of rectal bleeding (Tompkins, 2004). Hemorrhoids are varicose veins of the anorectal junction and are separated as internal or external if they protrude through the anus (Schulz, 2004). A thrombosed external hemorrhoid is a localized clot that forms in the vein of an external hemorrhoid or arises from a ruptured blood vessel (Schulz, 2004). Thrombosed hemorrhoids appear bluish in color and may be painful.

Hemorrhoids tend to be asymptomatic in the early stages but may bleed over time. Bleeding is usually scant and involves bright red blood on toilet tissue. External hemorrhoids may be easily seen, but internal hemorrhoids require visualization by sigmoidoscopy or colonoscopy because they cannot be reliably felt with a digital examination. Any rectal bleeding should be referred to a gastroenterologist for an accurate diagnosis and followed up with endoscopic examination to rule out malignancy.

Treatment of hemorrhoids depends on size. Heavy lifting and straining at stool should be avoided as they can worsen prolapse. Sitz baths and suppositories with benzocaine can relieve symptoms. Sclerotherapy, cryosurgery, and laser therapy may also be effective options for some older patients. Hemorrhoidectomy should be reserved for those patients with persistent symptoms who have not been helped by nonsurgical techniques (Ali & Lacy, 2004).

Rectal prolapse or passage of the rectum through the anus is common in older persons, affecting women more than men (Schulz, 2004). The main symptom is protrusion of the rectum with the passage of stool or upon standing. Continued rectal prolapse can lead to fecal incontinence, and surgical repair may be necessary. Conservative therapy includes instruction on avoiding heavy lifting and prolonged standing and prevention of constipation and straining at stool.

Liver and Biliary Disorders

With aging, the liver is more susceptible to the effects of drugs and other toxins. An older person with liver disease may present with vague and ambiguous symptoms, including fatigue, weight loss, anorexia, and malaise. The older patient with viral **hepatitis** may complain of nausea, fatigue, and loose stools.

Hepatic cysts are common in the older person and are usually benign. If a cyst enlarges and causes discomfort, excision or draining may be necessary. Hemangioma, a common benign liver tumor, is found in about 5% of older persons. Benign tumors and cysts are usually asymptomatic and are often found when a CT scan or ultrasound is done for another reason. Liver function tests are usually normal. Typically no treatment is required; however, for patients with complaints of abdominal discomfort, the cysts may be aspirated under local anesthesia as needed for comfort.

Metastatic carcinoma is the most common form of liver cancer, and many cancers metastasize to the liver. Primary liver cancer or hepatocellular cancer rates are higher in parts of the world where the incidence of viral hepatitis is higher. In most cases, the tumor develops in cirrhosis resulting from hepatitis B or C infection. Other predisposing factors include excessive alcohol and tobacco use.

Only 20% of older patients with hepatocellular cancer will have symptoms at the time of diagnosis. These symptoms usually include jaundice, variceal bleeding, ascites, right upper quadrant abdominal pain, weight loss, or an enlarged liver. Liver function tests are usually abnormal with increased serum bilirubin levels, elevated serum alkaline phosphatase, and decreased serum albumin concentrations. Definitive diagnosis follows after abdominal ultrasound, CT scan, and liver biopsy (Castells, 2004).

Treatment is determined by the tumor stage and the older person's functional status. Options include tumor embolization, chemotherapy, and immunotherapy (Castells, 2004). Liver transplantation may be curative for nonmetastasized tumors, but most centers will not perform liver transplantation in patients over 65, especially if they have coexisting medical conditions (Castells, 2004).

In the United States, gallbladder cancer is the fourth most common GI cancer. Bile duct cancer, usually adenocarcinoma, is more common in men. Adenocarcinoma also accounts for 80% of all gallbladder cancers (more common in women), and gallstones are present in 85% of cases. Symptoms include intermittent vague pain in the upper right quadrant. Later in the progression of the disease, jaundice and weight loss are common. Abdominal ultrasound and CT provide definitive diagnosis.

The prognosis for cure is poor with only 5% of older patients experiencing 5-year survival. Radical cholecystectomy is the treatment of choice for nonmetastasized tumors of the gallbladder. Radiation therapy and chemotherapy are ineffective (Castells, 2004). Whipple operation (radical resection of the bile duct and pancreatoduodenectomy) provides some promising benefit for bile duct cancer with 5-year survival rates about 20 to 30%, but patients over the age of 70 have a high surgical risk (Castells, 2004).

Gallstones

The incidence of gallstones rises with age. Typical symptoms include right upper quadrant pain, gas, distention, and nausea and vomiting. Acute cholecystitis, a complication of gallstones, is characterized by increased local tenderness, fever, and increased white blood count. If a gallstone migrates into the common bile duct, blockage and pancreatitis can result with increases in serum amylase levels (Tompkins, 2004). Surgery should be performed within 2 or 3 days from the onset of symptoms of acute cholecystitis, especially after several acute attacks.

Ultrasound visualizes gallstones in 95% of cases, and abdominal CT scans will diagnose biliary problems. Treatment includes laparoscopic cholecystectomy, stone dissolution by chenodeoxycholic acid, and extracorporeal shock wave lithotripsy (Ali & Lacy, 2004). Many older persons decide to avoid aggressive treatment for gallstones and instead manage their symptoms by avoiding high-fat and other foods that cause them pain or distress.

Pancreatitis

Acute pancreatitis occurs more frequently and is more severe in older persons than in younger persons. Factors that increase risk include gallstone, medications, alcohol abuse, and cancer. Drugs increasing the risk of pancreatitis include estrogen, furosemide, ACE inhibitors, and mesalamine. Diagnosed hyperlipidemia and hypercalcemia also increase the risk. Typical presenting symptoms are epigastric pain, nausea, and vomiting. Serum amylase, lipase, bilirubin, and alkaline phosphatase levels may be elevated. Abdominal ultrasonography or CT scanning should be done to confirm the diagnosis (Ali & Lacy, 2004).

Treatment for acute pancreatitis includes nasogastric suction, pain management, hyperalimentation, and fluid replacement. In 90% of older persons, acute pancreatitis is self-limiting and conservative measures are sufficient.

Chronic pancreatitis results in weight loss, diarrhea, diabetes, and presence of persistent pain. Diagnosis is based on symptoms and specialized testing. All older patients with chronic pancreatitis must refrain from alcohol (Tompkins, 2004). Surgical treatment may be necessary when conservative measures fail.

Pancreatic cancer accounts for 5% of all cancer deaths in the United States (Ali & Lacy, 2004). Painless jaundice, pruritus, and weight loss are common presenting symptoms. The prognosis of pancreatic cancer is poor (Ali & Lacy, 2004).

ENDOSCOPIC GASTROINTESTINAL PROCEDURES

Upper or lower gastrointestinal endoscopic procedures can be done to view body cavities with fiberoptic tubing. Conventional x-rays cannot identify color changes, bleeding, or vascular malformations. Endoscopy allows biopsy of abnormalities, allows stent placement, and helps surgeons determine if surgery is needed (Waye, 2004).

Esophagogastroduodenoscopy visualizes the upper gastrointestinal tract. Inspection of the esophagus to the duodenum is indicated for evaluation of the esophageal and gastric areas and provides information on upper gastrointestinal bleeding. Therapeutic indications include dilating esophageal strictures, vaporizing gastric and esophageal neoplasms, endoscopic injection therapy or thermal coagulation of upper gastrointestinal bleeding, sclerotherapy for esophageal varices, and removal of polyps.

Most endoscopies are performed while the patient is consciously sedated. Usually benzodiazepines are given for relaxation. Midazolam is given for conscious sedation. Aggressive cleansing protocols are difficult for some older patients to tolerate. Harsh cathartics can result in dehydration in an older person, and adequate fluid intake must be maintained during preparation for the procedure.

A sigmoidoscopy permits inspection of the rectum and distal sigmoid colon, and most of the descending colon. The flexible sigmoidoscope (about 60 cm in length) may be used to evaluate the left side of the colon where two thirds of neoplasms appear (Waye, 2004). Polyps are usually not removed during examination with the flexible sigmoidoscope. Sedation is not required, and one or two phosphate enemas cleanse the bowel adequately. The patient usually lies on the left side during the procedure.

Colonoscopy allows visual examination of the entire colon. Colonoscopy is indicated for routine testing or when anemia is present, positive fecal occult blood testing is noted, or polyps are suspected. Screening in asymptomatic older people should begin at age 50 and continue every 10 years until the age of 85 (Waye, 2004). Colonoscopy allows the removal of colonic polyps and evaluation of bleeding sites with electrocautery treatment. Strictures may be dilated and stents may be placed in strictures resulting from malignant growths to prevent bowel obstruction. Contraindications to colonoscopy include fulminant colitis, acute diverticulitis, perforated bowel, and recent myocardial infarctions (Waye, 2004).

The colon must be cleansed to allow complete visualization. One or 2 days of a liquid diet and administration of a cathartic the night before the procedure are the typical preparation. Even the smallest amount of feces in the colon can hide important details and compromise the examination. Two doses of sodium phosphate should be administered.

Complications from colonoscopy when performed by a skilled clinician are minimal. Colonoscopy is a relatively safe procedure and reliable results are valuable for accurate diagnosis. Risk of colonic perforation and excessive bleeding is low. Complications from sedative use include arrhythmias, aspiration, and rarely cardiac arrest (Waye, 2004). Patients should be instructed to bring a friend or relative to the procedure because they will be unable to drive for at least 24 hours after the administration of the sedation. The older person will usually receive a smaller dose of the sedating drug but still may be lethargic and sleepy for 24 hours.

PATIENT-FAMILY TEACHING GUIDELINES

The following are guidelines that the nurse may find useful when instructing older persons and their families about gastrointestinal problems.

1. How can I prevent gastrointestinal disease?

    Many people experience heartburn, constipation, diarrhea, and other problems with the gastrointestinal tract as they get older. Some problems are common and will go away on their own such as occasional constipation or diarrhea. Other problems are more serious and require further investigation such as blood in the stool and change in normal elimination patterns. Some suggestions for general health of the gastrointestinal tract include the following:

- Know your family history. Do you have a blood relative with polyps in the colon, colon cancer, Crohn's disease, or diverticulitis? If so, you may be more at risk than others without a family history.
- Eat a balanced diet that is high in fiber and low in fat.
- Maintain a normal weight.
- Stop smoking or using tobacco products.
- Decrease the size of portions at mealtime and avoid lying down for 2 to 3 hours after eating.
- Ask your healthcare provider to provide you with occult blood stool testing cards every year, and begin having colonoscopies at age 50 and periodically thereafter.
- Take medications with 8 oz of water and sit upright for 20 minutes after taking them.
- Limit the use of nonsteroidal anti-inflammatory agents such as ibuprofen because they can interfere with the protective covering in the stomach and cause ulcers.

2. If I already have gastrointestinal disease, is there anything I can do to stop it?

Yes. Take medications prescribed by your healthcare provider and begin lifestyle changes immediately. Also carry out all suggestions previously discussed. If your doctor prescribes medication

(continued)

for you, take it exactly as directed. Report any worsening of your condition or new symptoms to your doctor or nurse. Avoid straining at stool and heavy lifting if you have hemorrhoids. Drink plenty of fluids and try to get daily exercise. With treatment and lifestyle changes, most gastrointestinal problems can be successfully treated.

3. Is there anything else I should do to make the most of living with gastrointestinal disease?

   Yes. Exercise to keep your muscles fit and strong, eat a healthy diet, control your weight, and see your healthcare provider on a regular basis. Screening tests, no matter how unpleasant, save lives. Your healthcare provider can give you specific instructions that will help you to lead a long and healthy life.

CHAPTER 19

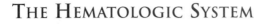

THE HEMATOLOGIC SYSTEM

Erythrocytes, or red blood cells (RBCs), have a life span of about 120 days. They are flexible concave disks that arise from stem cells in the **bone marrow.** Erythrocytes are composed of **hemoglobin,** a protein that binds with oxygen to form oxyhemoglobin. Old RBCs are destroyed in the spleen, liver, bone marrow, and lymph nodes by **phagocytes** that save and reuse key materials from the destroyed RBCs, including proteins and iron. The number of circulating RBCs remains fairly stable under normal conditions, but illness, blood loss, toxic substances, and nutritional deficiencies can decrease the number of circulating cells and result in **anemia.** Anemia occurs whenever the hemoglobin content of the blood is insufficient to satisfy body demands (LeMone & Burke, 2004). Erythropoiesis, or the production of RBCs, is regulated by erythropoietin, a hormone secreted by the kidneys that stimulates the cells in the bone marrow. Erythropoietin is released by the kidneys in response to hypoxia and stimulates the bone marrow to produce RBCs. This process usually takes about 5 days to reach a maximum and will result in the release of a higher percentage of reticulocytes or immature RBCs in the circulation (LeMone & Burke, 2004).

Anemia is a sign and symptom of disease—not a disease itself. When an older person is diagnosed with

383

anemia, the underlying condition should be diagnosed before the anemia is corrected.

NORMAL CHANGES OF AGING

Most of the changes of aging in the hematologic system are the result of reduced capacity of the bone marrow to produce RBCs quickly when disease or blood loss has occurred. However, without major blood loss or the diagnosis of a serious illness, the bone marrow changes are not clinically significant.

At about age 70, the amount of bone marrow in the long bones begins to decline steadily. Additional changes of aging in the hematologic system include the following:

- The number of stem cells in the marrow is decreased.
- The administration of erythropoietin to stimulate use of iron to form RBCs is less effective in older persons than in younger persons.
- Lymphocyte function, especially cellular immunity, appears to decrease with age.
- Platelet adhesiveness increases with age.
- Average hemoglobin and **hematocrit** values decrease slightly with age but remain within normal limits.

Many functions of the hematologic system remain constant in healthy older persons, including RBC life span, total blood volume, RBC volume, total lymphocyte and granulocyte counts, and platelet structure and function (Berne & Levy, 2000; Friedman, 2004; McCance & Huether, 2001).

COMMON DISORDERS IN AGING
Anemia

Anemia, or insufficient hemoglobin content to meet the body's needs, is defined as decreases in the number of circulating RBCs or hemoglobin resulting from blood loss, impaired production of RBCs, or increased RBC destruction. Anemia is common in older persons. Although old age alone does not increase the chances of developing anemia, many chronic illnesses that occur with aging can be responsible.

All anemias result in a loss of oxygen-carrying capacity of the blood and produce generalized tissue hypoxia. The body tries to compensate by raising the heart and respiratory rates, shunting blood to vital organs away from the skin, and increasing blood viscosity to supply oxygen to hypoxic tissues. The physiological results may include skin pallor, chronic fatigue, dyspnea on exertion, and bone and joint pain (LeMone & Burke, 2004).

Anemias are usually classified by measuring the size of the RBCs and computing the **mean corpuscular volume** (MCV). The resulting groups include **microcytic** (smaller RBCs), **macrocytic** (larger RBCs), and **normocytic** (RBCs of normal size). However, some anemias fall into more than one category, and sometimes an older person may be diagnosed with more than one type or a mixed anemia.

Symptoms include fatigue, shortness of breath, worsening of angina, and developing or worsening of peripheral edema. Dizziness and mental status changes such as confusion, depression, agitation, and apathy may also occur as symptoms of anemia, especially in the frail older adult who is less likely to be physically active and to exhibit the more common musculoskeletal and cardiac symptoms. Pallor, usually less noticeable in the older person and persons of color, may be noticed in the oral mucosa and conjunctiva (Friedman, 2004). Severe anemia may result in tachycardia, palpitations, systolic murmurs, and angina with ischemic changes evident on electrocardiogram.

Judicious blood testing in hospitalized patients would minimize anemia resulting from blood loss for laboratory testing, especially in intensive care patients and others subjected to frequent blood drawing (Toy, 2004).

Evaluation of the older person with suspected anemia should begin with laboratory tests including measurement of hemoglobin, hematocrit, red blood cell count and indices, reticulocyte count, white blood cell count and differential, and platelet count. A man is considered anemic with a hemoglobin concentration below 13 g/dl, and the cutoff for a woman is below 12 g/dl. Hemoglobin concentrations will be artificially higher in a dehydrated older person and in those who smoke cigarettes or live at high altitudes. Hemoglobin concentrations are 0.5 to 1.0 g/dl lower in African Americans of both sexes (Toy, 2004).

Microcytic Anemias

Anemias are classified as microcytic if the MCV is less than 80 fl. In older people, microcytic anemias can result from iron deficiency and thalassemia minor (a result of inadequate globin synthesis). Anemia of chronic disease can be microcytic but is more commonly normocytic, especially early in the disease process (Friedman, 2004). Iron deficiency anemia is characterized by small, pale RBCs and eventual depletion of iron stores. Serum ferritin levels usually accurately reflect bone marrow iron stores; however, these may remain normal early in the process before iron stores are depleted. The reticulocyte count is usually decreased. Serum ferritin levels of less than 10 µg/L are highly diagnostic of iron deficiency (Friedman, 2004).

Serum ferritin concentrations can be falsely elevated in patients with liver damage or certain cancers (Blackwell & Hendrix, 2001).

Iron deficiency can occur as the result of acute blood loss (from surgery or trauma) or chronic blood loss (from gastrointestinal bleeding, hemorrhoids, or cancer). It may also result from inadequate dietary intake of iron or malabsorption of iron. In men or postmenopausal women, the first site to consider for possible blood loss is the gastrointestinal tract. Excessive blood donation and frequent phlebotomies (patients who are on warfarin or hospitalized) are causes that are often overlooked (Blackwell & Hendrix, 2001).

Once the cause of the iron deficiency has been identified, oral iron therapy is the preferred treatment. Stool should be tested for occult blood, and additional gastrointestinal testing (colonoscopy or barium studies) may be necessary. Iron therapy should never be recommended for an older person with iron deficiency anemia without identifying the reason for occult blood loss. Correcting the symptom without knowing the underlying cause of the problem can mask the symptoms of serious disease like cancer.

The usual treatment is ferrous sulfate 325 mg daily. Enteric-coated and sustained-release formulations should be avoided, because they are poorly absorbed. A single daily dose of ferrous sulfate reduces the risk of constipation and gastric irritation. Increasing the dose only minimally increases iron absorption; however, the nurse should carefully monitor the older person taking iron supplements and report new-onset constipation and symptoms of gastrointestinal distress. Therapeutic response is monitored by measuring the serum hemoglobin, hematocrit, and ferritin levels in about 2 months, and it may take up to a year to fully replenish iron stores in the marrow (Friedman, 2004).

Thalassemia is an inherited disorder of hemoglobin synthesis in which parts of the hemoglobin molecular chain are missing or defective. As a result the RBC is fragile, hypochromic, and microcytic. Thalassemia occurs mostly in persons of Mediterranean (Greek or Italian) descent, but may be found in persons of Asian or African descent (LeMone & Burke, 2004). The diagnosis is made by a hematologist using serum electrophoresis. Iron replacement is not indicated and may result in iron overload (Friedman, 2004).

Normocytic Anemia

The most common types of normocytic anemia in the older person are anemia of chronic disease, hemolytic anemia, and aplastic anemia. Anemia in which the MCV is 30 to 100 fl is considered normocytic as the RBCs are of normal size. Normocytic anemia is usually caused by concurrent chronic illness (heart, respiratory, or renal disease, or malignancy), and anemia of chronic disease is the most common type of normocytic anemia.

Anemia of chronic disease is usually associated with malnutrition or conditions such as chronic infection or inflammation, cancer, renal insufficiency, chronic liver disease, endocrine disorders, and malnutrition. These diseases influence RBC production:

- Chronic infection and inflammation.
- Renal insufficiency.
- Chronic liver disease.
- Malnutrition.
- Malignancies.

Diseases associated with anemia of chronic disease include:

- Acute infections—bacterial, fungal, or viral.
- Chronic infections—osteomyelitis, infective endocarditis, chronic urinary tract infection, tuberculosis, or chronic fungal disease.

- Inflammatory disorders—rheumatoid disease, systemic lupus erythematosus, burns, severe trauma, and acute and chronic hepatitis.
- Malignancy—carcinoma, myeloma, lymphoma, leukemia.
- Chronic renal failure.

(Rasul & Kandel, 2001)

Hemolytic anemia is also a normocytic anemia that can occur at any age, but it becomes more common with aging. When the **hemolysis** or premature destruction of RBCs increases, the body compensates by increasing production of immature RBCs in the bone marrow, resulting in increased numbers of circulating reticulocytes in the blood. The causes of increased RBC destruction may be associated with increased autoimmune antibodies, inherited enzyme deficits (G6PD deficiency), infections such as syphilis, leukemia, Hodgkin's disease and non-Hodgkin's lymphoma, trauma, mechanical factors (prosthetic heart valves), burns, exposure to toxic chemicals and venoms, and drugs (Friedman, 2004; LeMone & Burke, 2004).

Drugs capable of causing hemolytic anemia include ibuprofen, l-dopa, penicillin, drugs classified as cephalosporins, tetracycline, acetaminophen, aspirin, erythromycin, hydralazine, hydrochlorothiazide, insulin isoniazid, methadone, phenacetin, procainamide, quinidine, rifampin, streptomycin, sulfonamides, and triamterene (Epocrates.com, 2004; Friedman, 2004). Increased destruction results in increased levels of unconjugated bilirubin. The indirect Coombs' test is used to detect antibody of complement on the RBC. Hemolysis usually stops quickly when the drug is withdrawn (Friedman, 2004).

All hemolytic anemias require folic acid treatment because this vitamin is used up with increased bone marrow production of RBCs. Folic acid is absorbed from the intestine and is found in green leafy vegetables, fruits, cereals, and meats. Deficiencies are often found in chronically undernourished persons. When the cause of the hemolytic anemia cannot be found, prednisone is sometimes used to treat this idiopathic autoimmune hemolysis. More commonly, the identifying drug can be identified. Drug-induced hemolysis is usually treated by simply discontinuing the responsible drug.

Aplastic anemia is not very common and is usually a disease of adolescents and young adults, but it can occur in old age. The cause of aplastic anemia is unknown in the majority of cases, but this anemia may sometimes develop as a result of damage to the cells in the bone marrow by radiation or chemical substances (benzene, arsenic, chloramphenicol, and chemotherapeutic agents). Treatment involves discontinuation of all medications and administration of ongoing blood transfusions. Bone marrow transplantation is usually not effective in patients over the age of 65 (Friedman, 2004).

Macrocytic Anemias

Anemias are classified as macrocytic if the MCV is greater than 100 fl. The most common cause of macrocytic anemia in the older person is B_{12} or folate deficiency. Vitamin B_{12} deficiencies can occur when the amount of the vitamin in the diet is inadequate or, more commonly, when sufficient amounts are not absorbed from the gastrointestinal tract. Failure to absorb vitamin B_{12} from the gastrointestinal tract is called pernicious anemia and results from a lack of intrinsic factor. Neurologic damage, such as neuropathies, paresthesias, and cognitive impairment, may occur before the anemia is discovered. Additional causes of macrocytic anemia include hypothyroidism, chronic liver disease, and drugs such as chemotherapeutic agents and anticonvulsants (Friedman, 2004).

Pernicious anemia results when an older person lacks the needed intrinsic factor to absorb vitamin B_{12}. As only about 1% of older persons lack intrinsic factor, a more common cause of low serum vitamin B_{12} results from the inability to split vitamin B_{12} from proteins in food. This inability may be the result of a deficiency of hydrochloric acid or pancreatic enzymes. Other causes of B_{12} deficiency include gastrectomy, small bowel disease, *Helicobacter pylori* infection, prolonged use of antacids, intestinal bacterial overgrowth, cachexia, and adherence to a strict vegetarian diet (Friedman, 2004).

The signs and symptoms of B_{12} deficiency may take years to develop and are often subtle. Mental status may be affected, and cognitive impairment, depression, mania, and other psychiatric syndromes may develop. Neurologic findings will include peripheral neuropathies, numbness and tingling in the extremities, and ataxia and difficulty walking and maintaining balance. Unfortunately, correcting the B_{12} deficiency does not usually reverse or improve mental status but may halt the progression of the symptoms. Laboratory tests used to detect low levels of B_{12} may not be abnormal until the older person becomes overtly anemic. In addition to a large MCV, leukopenia and thrombocytopenia may occur.

The diagnosis of vitamin B_{12} deficiency has traditionally been based on low serum vitamin B_{12} levels, usually less than 200 pg/ml, along with clinical evidence of disease. Furthermore, measurements of metabolites such as methylmalonic acid and homocysteine have been shown to be more sensitive in the diagnosis of vitamin B_{12} deficiency than measurement of serum B_{12} levels alone (Oh & Brown, 2003).

The widespread use of gastric acid–blocking agents may contribute to the eventual development of vitamin B_{12} deficiency because these medications neutralize the acidic environment that is needed to break down and release vitamin B_{12} bound to the ingested food. When caring for an older patient on long-term acid suppression therapy, methylmalonic acid and homocysteine levels should be monitored periodically.

For those with pernicious anemia, treatment usually consists of lifelong B_{12} replacement. Because most clinicians are generally unaware that oral vitamin B_{12} therapy is effective, the traditional treatment for B_{12} deficiency has been intramuscular injections. The usual intramuscular dose is 1,000 µg/day for the first week, then 1,000 µg/week for 4 weeks, and then 1,000 µg/month for life. Although the daily requirement of vitamin B_{12} is approximately 2 µg, the initial oral replacement dosage consists of a single daily dose of 1,000 to 2,000 µg. This high dose is required because of the variable absorption of oral vitamin B_{12} in smaller doses. The oral replacement should be taken on an empty stomach. It has been shown to be safe, cost-effective, and well tolerated by patients (Oh & Brown, 2003). Approximately 1 month of treatment is needed to correct the anemia. Treatment with folic acid alone may improve the anemia, but it will not prevent further decline or improve existing neurologic changes associated with the B_{12} deficiency (Friedman, 2004). Folic acid supplementation may mask an occult vitamin B_{12} deficiency and further exacerbate or initiate neurologic disease (Oh & Brown, 2003).

Folic acid deficiency produces laboratory results similar to those found with B_{12} deficiency. Serum folate levels will measure below 4 ng/ml, and B_{12} levels are normal in early folate deficiencies. Folate deficiency is not common in the healthy older person but may be found in older people with malabsorption syndromes, poor nutrition, alcoholism, and underlying malignancies. Foods high in folate include liver, orange juice, cereals, whole grains, beans, nuts, and dark green leafy vegetables like spinach. Chronic use of certain drugs such as triamterene, trimethoprim, anticonvulsants, and nitrofurantoin can also cause folic acid deficiency by blocking folic acid metabolism. It usually takes about 6 months to deplete the folic acid from body storage (Kado et al., 2004).

Laboratory testing usually reveals a macrocytic RBC and low serum folate levels (<2 ng/ml) or low RBC folate levels (<100 ng/ml). However, RBC folate levels are a more stable marker and more clinically reliable. Treatment consists of folic acid 1 mg/day by mouth (Friedman, 2004).

In older patients with macrocytic anemia due to a B_{12} deficiency, treatment with folic acid alone may correct the anemia but will not prevent or reverse neurologic damage as a result of the B_{12} deficiency.

Sickle Cell Anemia

Sickle cell anemia is an inherited disease in which the RBCs are crescent shaped. As a result, they tend to form small clots and clump together. These clots give rise to recurrent painful episodes called sickle cell crises. Symptoms of sickle cell disease begin at about 4 months of age. Complications of the disease include lung disease, kidney and liver failure, gallstones, joint destruction, blindness, neurologic symptoms, and stroke. Approximately 1 out of every 500 African Americans has sickle cell disease, and about 1 in 12 has the trait or carries the gene that can cause the disease if he or she has a child with another carrier. Persons with sickle cell disease should avoid infection, consume a balanced diet, avoid dehydration, and avoid stress as these factors can precipitate a sickle cell crisis (Medline Plus, 2004).

Transfusions

When the older patient's hematocrit is below 30% and he or she is experiencing symptoms such as shortness of breath or chest pain, a blood transfusion may be needed (Toy, 2004).

Older patients are subject to fluid overload and are at risk for acute heart failure. Therefore, the physician may request transfusion with packed red blood cells (most of the plasma removed) to reduce the volume to be transfused. Signs of fluid overload include elevated systolic blood pressure, jugular vein distention, crackles, dyspnea, tachycardia, peripheral edema, cyanosis, and headache.

Most transfusions for older people are given slowly over a 4-hour period. If several units of packed cells are to be infused, often a diuretic (20 mg furosemide) is given orally between units to prevent fluid overload and congestive heart failure. Older people may have more fragile veins, and venous access may be more difficult. Therefore, older people are at increased risk for infiltration. The IV site should be carefully secured and frequently observed for signs of infiltration including bruising, swelling, and accumulation of fluid into the soft tissue surrounding the site. The gerontological nurse should carefully monitor the older patient's vital signs and urinary output during the transfusion process.

As with all transfusions, the patient's blood type must match the donor's. To prevent transfusion errors and potentially fatal hemolytic reactions, the blood will be tested by type and crossmatch each time the patient requires a transfusion. The hemolytic reaction that can occur when a patient receives an incompatible blood transfusion is life threatening, and every precaution must be taken both in the laboratory and at the bedside to ensure that the patient and the blood type are correctly identified and matched. Hemolytic reactions can progress to oliguria, renal failure, and disseminated intravascular clotting with uncontrolled hemorrhage.

Chronic Myeloproliferative Disorders

Thrombocythemia is characterized by an increased number of circulating platelets in the blood. Older patients with thrombocythemia are more likely to exhibit uncontrolled bleeding with hemorrhage or develop clot formation. Symptoms are absent or vague and may include headache, visual disturbances, and burning pain and erythema of the hands and feet. Accurate diagnosis requires bone marrow aspiration. Usually, the treatment includes administration of hydroxyurea to suppress platelet formation, and the goal is to keep the platelet count below 400,000/µL. Older persons with thrombocythemia are at significantly increased risk of thrombosis, and careful monitoring of platelet levels and symptoms is indicated (Tefferi, 2004).

Polycythemia vera is a chronic stem cell disorder characterized by an increase in hemoglobin concentration and uncontrolled production of mature RBCs. Approximately 90% of persons with this disease are diagnosed after age 60. Symptoms of the disease are absent initially but later progress to findings common in hypervolemia, including headache, dizziness, hypertension, visual disturbances, weight loss, and night sweats. Itching after bathing is a common complaint. Phlebotomy significantly decreases the risk of thrombosis. About 500 ml of blood may be removed daily until the hematocrit is below 45% in men and 42% in women. Hydroxyurea can decrease the risk of thrombosis and can supplement phlebotomy in older persons. Gentle bathing, use of soft towels, and starch baths may decrease postbathing pruritus (Tefferi, 2004).

Myelofibrosis is a chronic disease characterized by bone marrow fibrosis (scarring of the bone marrow), splenomegaly, and teardrop-shaped RBCs. Symptoms include weight loss, pallor, abdominal distention, fatigue, low-grade fever, and night sweats. The diagnosis is made by examination of a peripheral blood smear and bone marrow biopsy. Survival time after diagnosis is about 3 to 5 years. There is no specific treatment, but blood transfusions can eliminate symptoms of anemia, and administration of erythropoietin may stimulate RBC production. Splenectomy can improve symptoms and may be indicated in some patients (Tefferi, 2004).

Hematologic Malignancies

Hematologic malignancies arise when immature lymphoid and myeloid cells are overproduced with associated bone marrow failure. Large numbers of immature WBCs accumulate in the bone marrow, liver, spleen, lymph nodes, and central nervous system, and eventually cause failure. Acute leukemia is primarily a disease of children and elderly adults (Friedman, 2004). Predisposing factors include exposure to chemical agents such as benzene, genetic factors, viruses, immune disorders, certain antineoplastic drugs, and radiation exposure (LeMone & Burke, 2004).

Often the liver, spleen, and lymph nodes are enlarged. The WBC count may or may not be elevated. Diagnosis is confirmed by bone marrow aspiration. The prognosis is poor without treatment. Advanced age, bleeding, and concurrent diagnosed chronic illness are indicators of poor prognosis. Treatment consists of a combination of drugs designed to inhibit WBC production, including vincristine, prednisone, anthracycline, and asparaginase. Most older patients experience relapse within one year. Bone marrow transplantation is rarely used for patients over 65 (Friedman, 2004).

Infections are the major cause of morbidity and mortality. Acute leukemia in older patients is most often fatal within 1 to 2 years. The risks and benefits of aggressive chemotherapy must be discussed with the older person and the family so they can make an informed decision about treatment choices. Palliative care with emphasis on pain and symptom control and hospice care (when and if appropriate) will enhance the quality of life of the older person.

Chronic lymphoid leukemia (CLL) usually progresses more slowly than acute leukemia. CLL is characterized by a proliferation and accumulation of small, abnormal mature lymphocytes in the bone marrow, peripheral blood, and body tissues. These cells are usually unable to produce adequate antibodies to maintain normal immune function (LeMone & Burke, 2004). Common symptoms include fatigue, malaise, rapid worsening of coronary artery disease, and decreased exercise tolerance. Enlarged lymph nodes occur in the cervical, axillary, and supraclavicular areas. The spleen may also be enlarged as the disease progresses.

As with acute leukemia, infections and fever are frequent complications of CLL. The diagnosis of CLL requires repeated measurement of sustained lymphocytosis and examination of the bone marrow. Oral alkylating agents combined with prednisone provide effective treatment (Mortimer & McElhaney, 2004). As the disease progresses, older patients will increasingly require nutritional support, pain control, skin care, and emotional support from the gerontological nurse.

Multiple myeloma is a malignancy that results from the overproduction and accumulation of immature plasma cells in the bone marrow, lymph nodes, spleen, and kidneys. Bone pain in the lower back or ribs is the most common early symptom of multiple myeloma. Additional symptoms include bone fractures, pallor, weakness, fatigue, dyspnea, and palpitations. Bruising and excessive bleeding from trauma are common. Renal disease occurs in about 50% of patients, including urinary tract infections, calcium or uric acid calculi, and dehydration. Most patients have a normocytic anemia and osteolytic bone lesions or osteoporosis, monoclonal proteins *(Bence Jones protein)* in blood serum, and increased plasma cells in the bone marrow. Treatment involves administration of steroids, chemotherapy, and radiation therapy for localized tumors and to relieve back pain from osteolytic lesions.

Autologous transplantation with peripheral blood stem cells is being used for people up to age 70 and older, depending on functional status. Fluid intake should be 2 to 3 L/day to increase urinary output and increase the excretion of calcium, uric acid, and other metabolites. There is no cure for multiple myeloma. The disease is progressive, with death occurring 2 to 5 years from diagnosis (LeMone & Burke, 2004). Palliative care with the emphasis on pain management and symptom control, referral to hospice (if and when appropriate), and emotional support will be needed by the patient and family.

Lymphomas

Hodgkin's Disease

Hodgkin's disease is more common in men than women and usually presents as one or more painlessly enlarged lymph nodes. Other symptoms include persistent fever, night sweats, fatigue, weight loss, malaise, pruritus, and anemia (LeMone & Burke, 2004). The diagnosis is made by lymph node biopsy. Additional testing includes computerized tomography (CT) scans, magnetic resonance imaging (MRI), splenectomy, and liver biopsy (Friedman, 2004). Treatment of the disease depends on the stage, but older people usually receive chemotherapeutic drugs for 6 to 8 months.

Non-Hodgkin's Lymphoma

Malignant disorders that originate from lymphoid tissue but are not diagnosed as Hodgkin's disease are classified as non-Hodgkin's lymphoma. Non-Hodgkin's lymphoma can begin with one node and spread throughout the lymphatic system and then metastasize to bones, the central nervous system, and the gastrointestinal tract. Because of the more systemic nature of non-Hodgkin's lymphoma, the prognosis is generally poorer than the prognosis of an older patient with Hodgkin's lymphoma. The risk of acquiring the disease increases with age. The cause is unknown, but those with impaired immune systems abnormalities or taking phenytoin are more at risk.

Symptoms include cervical or inguinal lymph node enlargement. Diagnosis is made by lymph node biopsy, bone marrow aspiration, blood testing, and chest x-ray. Chemotherapy is used to treat intermediate and high-grade lymphomas but does not prolong survival time in early disease. Aggressive chemotherapy in older persons with comorbidities can be extremely difficult, resulting in disability and inability to engage in self-care.

Older patients with early disease are closely monitored for progressive problems, and radiation can be used to treat enlarged lymph nodes. The gerontological nurse should provide ongoing pain control, symptom management, nutritional guidance, and counseling during the treatment and recuperative phases of the illness.

Both lymphomas are curable with radiation and intensive chemotherapy; however, aggressive treatment in the older person with comorbidities is often difficult and may not be tolerated. Older people living alone may need assistance with activities of daily living, nutrition, and pain and symptom control during the required 6 months of aggressive treatment (Friedman, 2004).

NURSING ASSESSMENT OF OLDER PATIENTS WITH HEMATOLOGIC ABNORMALITIES

A complete review of the older person's past medical history and current health status is needed to assess the situation of a person with anemia or other blood disorders. The complaints of an older person with anemia or a blood disorder may be vague and often confused with normal changes of aging or symptoms of chronic disease. Any complaints of fatigue, shortness of breath, loss of appetite, weight loss, mental status changes, bruising, and activity intolerance should be carefully investigated. Anemia and other blood disorders can be caused by nutritional problems, blood loss, chronic illness, medications, or a variety of other factors that may respond to treatment.

The nurse can begin by gathering the following information:

- Diagnosis of any concurrent chronic or progressive illness such as cancer or heart or kidney disease

- Medication listing, including over-the-counter and herbal remedies
- History of surgery or trauma
- Baseline level of function and activity level and documentation of change of status
- Lifestyle factors that can be related to the older person's status, including smoking, alcohol use, depression, obesity, poor nutrition, and sedentary lifestyle
- Family history and diagnosed blood disorders in first-degree relatives
- Occupational exposures during the patient's work career to chemicals or pollutants

Because anemia is a sign of disease and not an actual disease itself, further investigation and careful assessment of the person with vague symptoms of fatigue, activity intolerance, and weakness should always be carried out. The skin should be examined for pallor, bruising, and poor turgor. The axillary, cervical, and inguinal areas should be checked for lymphadenopathy. The liver and spleen should be palpated for enlargement. The presence of rashes, urticaria, and itching should be noted. Balance and endurance should be observed and documented. Although there is no single recommended test of endurance, the nurse can observe the older person walking in a protected environment for several minutes and then assess for the presence of increased heart and respiratory rate, irregular respiratory or cardiac rate, weakness, and decreasing pulse oximetry after exercise. As depression can contribute to and be a result of chronic illness, the older person should be carefully screened for depression.

Referral to a health provider for a complete health assessment is indicated for older patients who might be experiencing anemia. A complete physical examination, electrocardiogram, test of thyroid function, and complete blood count with differential are indicated. Older patients with a decreased WBC count should be protected from infection and placed in reverse isolation if necessary until their WBC count returns to normal.

Some nursing interventions that may be appropriate for the older person with hematologic problems include:

- Providing support and teaching for the patient and family.
- Protecting the skin from dryness, cracking, and injury.
- Providing teaching and administration of medications to relieve nausea and vomiting.
- Encouraging recreational and diversional activities consistent with the patient's general functional ability.
- Advising and referral regarding nutritional intake.
- Assessing and treating pain with appropriate pharmacological and non-pharmacological techniques.
- Treating associated symptoms, including constipation, diarrhea, and dry mouth.
- Involving the multidisciplinary team to address physical, social, psychological, and spiritual needs.

Nurse sensitive outcomes include lessening of symptom severity, increased effectiveness of cardiac pump, improvement of vital signs, improvement of ambulation and endurance, improvement of nutritional status, discontinuation of toxic medication, improvement in quality of life and overall functional ability, and improvement of depressive symptoms. If serious underlying disease is found during the investigation of the older person with anemia or other hematologic problems, the nurse can provide support during aggressive therapy and palliative care, with hospice referral if appropriate.

Hypercoagulability and Anticoagulation

Deep-vein thrombosis (DVT) and pulmonary embolism can lead to myocardial infarction and stroke, and the incidence increases with age. Hospitalized older patients are more at risk due to impaired mobility, surgical interventions, and orthopedic procedures. The older person is more at risk because of three components:

1. Abnormalities in the vessel walls caused by trauma, atherosclerosis, or intravenous medication administration
2. Abnormalities within the circulating blood and hypercoagulability seen with coagulation disorders, some cancers, and hormone (estrogen) use
3. Stasis of blood flow secondary to immobility, age, or heart failure

(Becker, 2004; McCance & Huether, 2001)

The major danger associated with DVT is that a portion of the thrombus will embolize to the lungs, causing pulmonary embolism (McCance & Huether, 2001). Aggressive therapy is needed to treat DVT because it is a potentially life-threatening situation. Anticoagulation and bed rest are critical to prevent movement of the clot to the lungs, heart, or brain where it can block vital circulation.

The clinical manifestations of DVT include edema, skin discoloration, and pain. The hallmark of DVT is the rapid onset of unilateral leg swelling with pitting edema. The diagnosis is made with Doppler ultrasonography, plethysmography, or venogram.

Preventive approaches are individualized to minimize the risk factors that can predispose to DVT. Specific conditions warranting prevention include:

• Orthopedic procedures.
• Atrial fibrillation.

- Acute myocardial infarction.
- Ischemic stroke.

Nursing interventions designed to prevent DVT formation include:

- Identifying patients at risk, including those with history of DVT, clotting disorders, heart failure, orthopedic surgery, and other risk factors.
- Getting patients up and walking as soon as possible after surgery or injury.
- Changing the position of bed-bound patients every 2 hours to prevent circulatory compromise.
- Urging patients at risk for DVT to wear fitted support stockings, avoid stasis, maintain adequate hydration, elevate legs during periods of rest, and perform meticulous skin care to keep skin clean and intact.
- Urging the use of intermittent pneumatic compression boots postoperatively until patients are ambulatory.
- Administering anticoagulants as prescribed.

There are many anticoagulants and each has distinct uses. In general, drugs given intravenously, such as heparin or the fibrinolytic agents, are used short term for hospitalized patients. Oral drugs, such as warfarin and antiplatelet drugs, are used long term for outpatients. Low-molecular-weight heparins, administered subcutaneously, are used in both settings (Becker, 2004). Drugs are given for prevention and treatment of thrombotic conditions.

Laboratory tests to monitor efficacy and to determine the dosage of medications are usually done every 3 to 4 days of therapy. They include the prothrombin time (PT) and the partial thromboplastin time (PTT). The PT, a measure of the time required for a firm fibrin clot to form after reagents are added to the blood sample, is the standard measure of efficacy. It is commonly reported in an international normalized ratio (INR). The higher the INR, the longer it takes the blood to clot. Guidelines suggest various target INR measurements and duration of therapy. The PTT is used to evaluate the time required for a firm fibrin clot to form after phospholipid reagents are added to the specimen. Heparin will prolong the PTT.

Anticoagulant Medications

Heparin is the most widely used anticoagulant. It accelerates the inhibitory interaction between hemostatic proteins and clotting factors. Unfractionated heparin is used in older patients to prevent and to treat venous or arterial thromboembolism.

Low-dose heparin therapy (500 U subcutaneously every 8 to 12 hours) is prophylactic therapy for DVT in patients who have the following:

- Orthopedic surgery
- Acute myocardial infarction
- Ischemic stroke with lower extremity paralysis
- Congestive heart failure

High-dose heparin therapy (intravenous administration) to maintain a PTT (1.5 to 2.5 times control) is indicated in the following patients:

- Those with DVT, pulmonary embolism, or unstable angina
- Those receiving thrombolytic therapy
- Those receiving perioperative care who are on warfarin therapy

(Becker, 2004; Reuben et al., 2003)

The most common adverse effect of heparin is hemorrhage. Other adverse effects include thrombocytopenia, alopecia, and skin necrosis. The risk of bleeding increases with increased dosage. Other risk factors include older age, low body weight, recent trauma or surgery, and performance of invasive procedures with concurrent use of aspirin. Mild bleeding can be handled by reducing the dose, and severe bleeding requires discontinuation of the heparin (Becker, 2004).

Low-molecular-weight heparins are used for DVT prophylaxis and in the treatment of DVT with acute coronary syndromes such as unstable angina and myocardial infarction. Low-molecular-weight heparins can be given intravenously or subcutaneously. Because of the predictable bioavailability, dose-independent clearance rates, and a more stable anticoagulant response, these drugs have been increasingly used in the clinical setting (Nadeau & Varrone, 2003). They do not prolong the PTT, and the predictable antithrombotic response eliminates the need for laboratory monitoring and dose adjustment. However, as a precaution, the older patient receiving low-molecular-weight heparins should be carefully monitored for signs of excessive bleeding.

Warfarin is frequently used for anticoagulation in the prevention or treatment of DVT. It is rapidly absorbed from the gastrointestinal tract, reaches maximal serum concentration in about 90 minutes, and takes up to 7 days to reach stable serum levels on fixed doses (Reuben et al., 2003). Warfarin interacts with many substances, and older patients taking the medication should be instructed to report any changes in their medication regimen to their healthcare providers so that INRs can be monitored and warfarin dosage adjusted in response.

Hepatic clearance of warfarin declines with age. The older person is more likely to experience bleeding complications, so the drug is usually started at lower doses. Frequent monitoring is required to safely titrate dosage during the induction period. In general, target INR's range from 2.0 to 3.0 in older persons following orthopedic surgery, DVT prophylaxis, atrial fibrillation, and treatment of pulmonary embolism. Higher INRs are recommended for those with mechanical heart valves and 1 to 3 months post myocardial infarction.

Contraindications to warfarin therapy include patients with bleeding disorders, frequent fallers at risk for intracranial bleeding, and those who are not compliant with dosage adjustments and laboratory testing. Some surgeons will request that warfarin be held for four doses prior to surgery to decrease the risk of intraoperative bleeding.

Excessively high INRs (3.5 and over) should be reported immediately to the healthcare provider or anticoagulation clinic so that dosage adjustment and possible action to reduce the INR reading can be accomplished. For INRs between 3.5 and 5, the usual recommendation is to omit the next dose and lower the maintenance dose. For INRs between 5 and 9, the recommendation may be to omit the next several doses and restart at a lower dose. Some healthcare providers recommend administration of vitamin K 1.0 to 2.5 mg by mouth. For INRs over 9 with or without bleeding, the warfarin would probably be discontinued and vitamin K given orally or intravenously until the INR returns to normal levels.

Protamine sulfate is indicated in the treatment of heparin overdosage. Protamine sulfate should be administered by very slow intravenous injection over a 10-minute period in doses not to exceed 50 mg. All serious or significant bleeding requires emergency treatment and evaluation for an older patient taking any anticoagulant. Signs of bleeding may occur as blood in the urine or stool, vomiting of blood, nosebleeds, blood in the sputum, bleeding gums, bruising out of proportion to or in the absence of injury, fatigue, severe headache, and loss of vision or weakness on one side of the body. All patients taking warfarin should be instructed to take the medication as ordered, regularly monitor INR levels, check for interactions before starting any new medications, recognize dietary sources of vitamin K and ingest stable amounts, and recognize the signs of bleeding and the need to seek treatment (Nadeau & Varrone, 2003).

Platelet Antagonists

Platelets participate in the thrombotic process by adhering to abnormal surfaces, aggregating to form a plug, and triggering the coagulation cascade. Aspirin irreversibly inhibits platelet aggregation by blocking enzymes in the clotting process and impairing prostaglandin metabolism. Aspirin is used for primary and secondary prevention of myocardial infarction and stroke and is used with other antiplatelet agents (clopidogrel or ticlopidine) after the placement of intracoronary stents (Becker, 2004).

Ticlopidine is a potent inhibitor of platelet aggregation by impairing platelet adhesion and inhibiting platelet release action. Ticlopidine has been used in the treatment of transient ischemic attacks, strokes where aspirin was already being taken, unstable angina, and cardiac stent placement. Side effects include two serious conditions: neutropenia and thrombocytopenic purpura. Clopidogrel reduces the risk of myocardial infarction and recurrent myocardial infarction among older patients with atherosclerotic vascular disease. It has a more favorable side-effect profile than ticlopidine, and the longer half-life requires only once-a-day dosing (Becker, 2004).

NURSING ASSESSMENT OF THE OLDER PATIENT WITH HYPERCOAGULABILITY

Older persons at risk for hypercoagulability and DVT formation include those with atherosclerosis, circulating blood abnormalities, and slowing of blood flow. Immobility and orthopedic surgery greatly increase the risk of DVT formation, and the older person should be assisted to ambulate as soon as possible after surgery. Postoperative nursing care involves use of compression stockings, intermittent pneumatic compression boots, early and consistent ambulation of older patients, maintenance of adequate hydration, and careful administration of anticoagulants. Postoperative and chronic pain should be carefully assessed and treated to prevent the hazards of immobility.

Nurse sensitive outcomes may include the following:

- Lessening of symptom severity
- Increased effectiveness of cardiac pump
- Improvement of vital signs
- Improvement of ambulation and endurance
- Improvement of mobility
- Discontinuation of toxic medication
- Adherence to monitoring and laboratory requirements

PATIENT-FAMILY TEACHING GUIDELINES

The Older Patient with Anemia

1. How do I know if I have anemia?

   There is no one main symptom of anemia. Often the symptoms are vague and may be noticed as fatigue, lack of energy, shortness of breath

   (continued)

on physical exertion, pale skin color, memory problems, and worsening of other problems like heart or lung conditions.

2. What are the most common causes of anemia?

Anemia is caused by either an underproduction of red blood cells or excessive loss or destruction of red blood cells. Iron deficiency is common in older people who have had blood loss due to injury or surgery. Unexplained blood loss should be investigated to make sure there is not hidden bleeding in the stomach or intestinal tract. Some medications can cause red blood cells to be broken down and destroyed, causing anemia. Sometimes red blood cells are not formed quickly enough to replace the ones that live a natural life span. The bone marrow slows production because of chronic illness in the heart, lungs, or kidneys. Sometimes a nutritional deficiency is responsible. Whatever the cause, it is important to pinpoint the kind of anemia and treat the cause.

3. What kinds of tests is my healthcare provider likely to order to diagnose anemia?

The most basic test is a complete blood count with differential. This test gives a measure of the number of circulating red blood cells and the types and numbers of other cells, including white blood cells and platelets. Sometimes iron studies are performed and vitamin B_{12} and folate levels examined, depending on the kind of anemia suspected. If the physician suspects bleeding in the stomach or intestine, an endoscopy or examination of the stomach or colon with a small tube and camera may be performed. Because anemia is not a disease itself but a symptom of some other condition, a careful search for the cause is indicated.

4. How often should I ask my healthcare provider to check my blood for the presence of anemia?

    Healthy older people should be checked for anemia every year. A complete blood count may be ordered and stool checked for occult bleeding. Those with chronic conditions, recent injury or trauma, or symptoms should be checked more frequently.

5. What can I do to prevent anemia?

    Eat a balanced diet, keep active, avoid taking unnecessary medications, and report any fatigue or loss of energy to your healthcare provider. Taking a once-a-day multivitamin can help. There is no need to take iron pills unless you are instructed to do so by your healthcare provider. Be sure to report any gastrointestinal distress, black stools, or red blood in the stool to your healthcare provider immediately.

CHAPTER 20

NEUROLOGIC DISORDERS

DEMENTIA

Dementia is a symptom of several acquired, progressive, life-limiting disorders that erase memory and the person's usual way of being in the world. The person with dementia has both a chronic illness and a terminal illness, first losing the ability to independently perform activities of daily living and finally becoming completely dependent in all aspects of self-care. Since the disease can affect different areas of the brain and different levels of the cortex, there is no uniform course and no predictability.

AD requires a variety of nursing interventions and an interdisciplinary approach. The following characterizations about AD should be considered when planning and providing care.

- There is currently no medicine or technology that prevents or cures AD. Symptomatic nursing care is the primary intervention for this relentlessly progressive neurologic disorder.
- AD is both a life-limiting and a chronic illness. Caregivers require expertise in long-term care and end-of-life care. Due to the nature of AD, family caregivers also require supportive care.
- AD predisposes persons to develop challenging behavioral and psychiatric symptoms. Care targeted at

alleviating symptoms and teaching patients and caregivers about the effects of AD is necessary to promote comfort and reduce feelings of distress.

- Persons with AD are cared for in a variety of settings, including their own homes, hospitals and nursing homes, congregate living facilities, and hospice settings to provide palliative care.
- AD is a family disease. All generations are affected, (e.g., grandchildren who cannot understand why a grandparent has forgotten their name, and adult children or relatives who must provide caregiving services).
- AD is a public health problem. The effects of growing numbers of persons with AD raise many caregiving concerns, including costs of care.
- Persons with AD and their families depend on nursing for promoting independence and autonomy, preventing avoidable complications, providing comfort, and promoting quality of life.

Progressive Dementias

Dementia is an acquired syndrome that causes progressive loss of intellectual abilities, such as memory, as well as **aphasia, apraxia,** and loss of **executive function.** Dementing disorders are characterized by gradual onset plus continuing cognitive decline that is not due to other brain disease. Screening tests can identify persons who should be referred for a complete diagnostic workup (Boustani et al., 2003). Early diagnosis of dementia is the goal of a diagnostic workup, which is done to exclude potentially reversible causes and initiate therapy as early as possible. Short-term memory impairment is usually the first symptom of dementia. Clinical diagnosis of dementia requires (1) loss of an intellectual ability with impairment severe enough to interfere with social or occupational functioning and (2) ruling out delirium. **Delirium** must be ruled out because cognitive impairment caused by delirium may be reversible. The development of delirium may indicate decreased reserve capacity of the brain and may signal an increased risk for dementia (Expert Consensus Panel, 2004).

Mild cognitive impairment is another risk factor for dementia. Persons with mild cognitive impairment have complaints and objective evidence of memory problems, but do not have deficits in activities of daily living or in other cognitive functions and do not meet the diagnostic criteria for dementia.

Dementia may be caused by more than one mechanism, even in the same individual. An autopsy examination is necessary to confirm the diagnosis. The most common combinations are AD with **vascular dementia** and AD with Lewy bodies. Clinically, progressive dementia symptoms are similar, especially in the later stages of the disease. Persons may differ in the onset and severity of a particular symptom.

Alzheimer's Disease

Neuropathological criteria for AD include presence of two abnormal structures: neuritic plaques and neurofibrillary tangles. The plaques and tangles each contain a specific protein that may play a role in pathogenesis of AD. Beta-amyloid protein is present in the plaques, and the tau protein is found in the tangles. AD disrupts the three processes that keep neurons healthy: (1) communication, (2) metabolism, and (3) repair. As a result, nerve cells are destroyed or die, causing memory failure, personality changes, problems carrying out activities of daily living, and other deficits. Although the definitive diagnosis is provided only after histopathological confirmation at autopsy, the clinical diagnosis can be made from history, physical examination, and neuropsychological testing (Ala, Mattson, & Frey, 2003).

Vascular Dementia

Diagnostic criteria for vascular dementia are an abrupt onset of dementia, focal neurologic findings (abnormal reflexes or nerve functions), low-density areas (indicating vascular changes in the white matter), or presence of multiple strokes in computerized tomography (CT) or magnetic resonance imaging (MRI) scans. Other criteria include fluctuation of impairment, unchanged personality, emotional lability, and a temporal relation between a stroke and development of dementia.

Lewy Body Disease

Dementia with Lewy bodies, also called diffuse Lewy body disease, may be confused with delirium and differs from AD (Marui, Iseki, Kato, Akatsu, & Kosaka, 2004). Clinical features of dementia with Lewy bodies persist over a long period and progress to severe dementia. Autopsy confirmation reveals round structures, called Lewy bodies, and Lewy neuritis in specific systems throughout the brain stem, diencephalon, basal ganglia, and neocortex (Duda, 2004). These Lewy bodies are also present in **Parkinson's disease,** but in that condition they are limited to subcortical areas of the brain.

Frontotemporal Dementia

Frontotemporal dementia, which includes **Pick's disease,** is diagnosed on the basis of personality changes and the presence of frontal brain area atrophy in neuroimaging studies (CT scan or MRI). Personality changes observed in frontotemporal dementia are similar to changes induced by damage of frontal lobes by other causes (injury, stroke) and include behavioral disinhibition, loss of social or personal awareness, or disengagement with apathy. Atrophy of the brain frontal and temporal lobes, and proliferation of nonneuronal glial cells in these areas characterize pathological findings in frontotemporal dementia. Pick's disease is characterized by two specific neuropathological findings on autopsy: (1) Pick's bodies inside nerve cells; and (2) ballooned nerve cells.

ALZHEIMER'S DISEASE

No treatments currently available reverse or stop the advancement of the pathological processes of progressive dementia, but some drugs may temporarily reverse or slow the progression of clinical symptoms. However, there is higher prevalence of AD in women, suggesting a link between gonadal hormone levels and AD. Currently, the use of HRT to prevent or delay the onset of dementia is not recommended (Shumaker et al., 2003).

Other medications, vitamins, and herbal remedies have been examined for use to prevent or slow the progression of AD including nonsteroidal anti-inflammatory drugs, vitamin E, the statins (to reduce cholesterol), and ginkgo biloba. Further research is needed.

There is a group of drugs, cholinesterase inhibitors (ChEI therapy), that slow the progression of AD symptoms. The ChEI hypothesis is that preventing the destruction of acetylcholine (a neurotransmitter) by inhibiting the acetylcholinesterase enzyme that destroys acetylcholine should result in decreasing symptoms of cognitive improvement. ChEI has been found to have a cognitive and functional benefit in the early stage of AD, lesser clinical benefit as the disease progresses, but a beneficial effect by delaying admission to nursing homes (Lopez et al., 2002). In general, ChEI therapy by cholinesterase enhancers such as donepezil (Aricept), rivastigmine (Exelon), and galantamine (Reminyl) may keep the patient in the early stage of AD for an additional 6 to 12 months. Donepezil has been found to be beneficial with good drug tolerability for use in patients with moderate to severe AD (Feldman et al., 2001).

Donepezil has been found to stabilize or retard the decline of cognitive and functional impairment and to improve problematic behaviors of dementia (Smith, 2003). Rivastigmine has been found effective in treating cognitive and behavioral symptoms in AD and in Lewy body dementia (Farlow, 2003). In general, for this class of medication, doses should be titrated to the highest therapeutic dose tolerated, but as slowly as necessary to decrease the development of gastrointestinal or other side effects. Nausea may be reduced by administering the ChEI on a full stomach, and intermittent antiemetics may be required.

The newest class of medication used for AD is based on the hypothesis that overstimulation of the N-methyl-d-aspartate (NMDA) receptor by glutamate causes neuronal degeneration induced by beta-amyloid. The drug, memantine, is an antiglutamatergic treatment that protects against beta-amyloid–induced neurotoxicity. In a clinical trial, memantine was found to reduce clinical deterioration in patients with moderate to severe AD (Reisberg et al., 2003).

Stages of Alzheimer's Disease and Implications for Nursing Care

The hallmark of AD is the cognitive symptom of memory loss. As AD worsens, other deficits appear and symptoms develop. Several classification systems have been proposed to describe stages commonly observed in the dementing diseases. In general, symptoms are clustered into four stages: mild, moderate, severe, and terminal (Volicer & Hurley, 1998). These symptoms and their consequences make planning and providing care complex during all the progressive stages and in all settings.

At the Time of Diagnosis

Both the patient and primary family caregivers must understand the clinical diagnosis of AD and receive advice regarding early-stage issues (Drickamer & Lachs, 1992). While the patient still has decision-making capacity, the clinician should initiate discussions about desired treatment modalities, selecting a healthcare proxy (power of attorney for healthcare), and informing the proxy about desired care to be provided when unable to make those decisions later in the disease (Rempusheski & Hurley, 2000). The patient may benefit from cognitive-enhancing medications (discussed earlier), which should be initiated as soon after the diagnosis as possible and may keep the patient in the early stage of AD for an additional 6 to 12 months. Referrals should be made to the local Alzheimer's Association for support groups, services, and assistance locating other community services such as the Program of All Inclusive Care for the Elderly (PACE). The patient may benefit from being in a support group with other persons who have early-stage AD. There are also specific family support groups, such as for working spouses and adult children.

Advance Directives and Establishing a Proxy (Power of Attorney for Healthcare)

Families will struggle to make decisions about care in the later stages if these issues were not discussed when persons with AD still could make their own decisions and plan for the future. Persons with AD should be given an opportunity to establish advance directives. As early as practicable, they should select a healthcare proxy to carry out their wishes (Rempusheski & Hurley, 2000).

Effect of the Disease on the Person

The AD process directly causes cognitive impairment. Progressive dementia in combination with the person's underlying personality may lead to **delusions** and hallucinations as well as mood disorders and functional impairment. Similarly, spatial disorientation may lead to **elopement,** combativeness, interference with other residents, and **agitation.** Inability to initiate meaningful activities may lead to apathy, repetitive vocalization, agitation, and insomnia.

The overall approach is first on prevention. If known triggers result in problematic behaviors, the caregiver should remove those stimuli. Second, nurses should provide and suggest behavioral strategies. When non-pharmacological strategies have been instituted and the patient still suffers from symptoms, pharmacological interventions should be added to the care plan (Table 20–1). Medications are given for the benefit of the patient and for no other reason.

Functional Impairment

Functional impairment is a primary consequence of dementia and has both cognitive and physical components. The physical component may result from the underlying dementia, other comorbid conditions, or disuse. Improving or supporting functional ability will have a positive effect on multiple behavioral consequences of dementia. The pathological processes of dementing illnesses cause receptive and expressive aphasia and similar problems with reading and writing.

Table 20–1 Useful Medications For Patients with Alzheimer's Disease

Drug Class	Name	Dose Range (mg)/Frequency	Comments
Selected Antidepressant Medications			
Selective serotonin reuptake inhibitors	Fluoxetine (Prozac)	10–40/qam	Desired dose for a person with AD may vary from traditional range, e.g., Block (2001) recommends 25–100 mg/day for sertraline dose.
	Fluvoxamine (Luvox, Faverin)	50–300/qhs	
	Paroxetine (Paxil)	20–50/qam/hs	
	Sertraline (Zoloft)	50–200/qam/hs	
	Citalopram (Celexa)	20–40/qam	
Other	Mirtazapine (Remeron)	15–45/qhs	Trazodone and mirtazapine may be useful in patients who suffer from insomnia.
	Nefazodone (Serzone)	50–300/bid	
	Trazodone (Desyrel)	50–600/tid, hs	
	Venlafaxine (Effexor)	25–75/bid–tid (up to 300 mg)	
Selected Drugs Used in Treatment of Delusions and Hallucinations			
Typical neuroleptics	Haloperidol (Haldol)	0.5–1/qd–tid	Half-lives range from 4 (thioridazine) to 30 (olanzapine) hours. Do not give a drug with a long half-life for an intermittent symptom of short duration
	Thioridazine (Mellaril)	10–40/qd–tid	
	Loxapine (Loxitane)	5–10/bid–tid	

		Selected Medications to Treat Anxiety	
Atypical neuroleptics	Risperidone (Risperdal)	0.25–1/qd–bid	
	Olanzapine (Zyprexa)	2.5–10/qd	
	Quetiapine (Seroquel)	25–100/bid–tid	
Benzodiazepines	Lorazepam (Ativan)	0.5–1/bid–tid	Side effects are sedation, impaired motor coordination, akathisia, risk of falls, memory loss, respiratory or central nervous system depression, and paradoxical reaction. Must be tapered slowly.
	Alprazolam (Xanax)	0.25–0.5/tid	
	Oxazepam (Serax)	10–20/tid–qid	
	Clonazepam (Klonopin)	0.25–0.5/bid	
Azaspirone	Buspirone (BuSpar)	5–20/tid	Side effects are headache, nausea, drowsiness, and lightheadedness.

qd = once a day, bid = twice a day, tid = three times a day, qid = four times a day, qam = every morning, qhs = every evening.

It is important to continue to talk with persons who have AD and to use other interventions of cueing, reminiscence, favorite familiar music, environmental modification, and stimulus control to facilitate communication.

Provide verbal prompts one at a time to decrease the chances of the patient becoming confused. Even when verbal language is lost, nonverbal communication by way of tone of voice, smiling, and body language may be comforting. It is important to avoid any pressure to perform and to allow persons with dementia to continue with patterns that give a sense of security. Fatigue, nonroutine activities, alcohol, and a high-stimulus environment should be avoided because they increase functional impairment.

Apraxia interferes with the ability to follow a command such as "wash your face." However, patients with AD may be able to wash their face if handed a washcloth, or to continue an activity such as eating if someone helps them get started. **Agnosia** causes functional impairment and predisposes to safety hazards.

Interventions for physical impairment should be targeted to maintain the highest level of functional capacity for as long as possible and to restore capacity that may be remediable. Often patients are restrained for no reason other than a belief that the person may fall (Hamers, Gulpers, & Strik, 2004). Some general guidelines to retard physical impairment include the following:

1. Prevent excess disability. To prevent immobility, provide assisted ambulation versus allowing the person to remain on bed rest.
2. Treat other conditions that lead to physical decline. If pain interferes with walking, be sure prn pain relief is ordered and provided.
3. Identify and respond rapidly to acute changes in function. Be alert to symptoms suggesting an infection in order to make an early diagnosis.

4. Adapt care to accommodate neuromotor changes secondary to the progression of dementia. Compensate for changes in muscle tone and reflexes that affect posture, balance, range of motion, and ability to cooperate with care. Establish a preventive program to assess mobility, prevent falls, promote proper positioning, and implement environmental adaptations, such as redesigning furniture or introducing appropriate assistive devices (Trudeau, 1999b).

An individualized assessment should be conducted to develop specific interventions to prevent excess disability, create a therapeutic environment, actualize functional potential, and promote dignity.

Mood Disorders

Depression may be a core consequence of AD and cause secondary and peripheral symptoms such as agitation and inability to initiate meaningful activities. Depression is difficult to diagnose since many of its clinical signs also result from other complications of dementia (e.g., insomnia and agitation), and many patients cannot respond to most standardized assessment instruments or express sadness. Caregivers should be alert for changes in appetite, disinterest and **anhedonia,** sleep abnormality, and fatigue. The treatment of depression in AD requires long-term administration of antidepressants.

Delusions and Hallucinations

Paranoid delusions are common psychotic symptoms in AD. Delusions and hallucinations may also be caused by delirium induced by drugs, electrolyte imbalance, hyperglycemia, urinary tract infection, seizure disorder, hypothyroidism, and Parkinson's disease. Delusions in AD may be due to (1) an intercurrent confusional state (delirium), (2) an interaction of dementia and personality, (3) a separate mental disorder that co-exists with the dementia, or (4) a disinhibition of cortical functions resulting in "released" symptomatology.

Non-pharmacological approaches targeted to presumed causes should be initiated and evaluated (Volicer, Mahoney, & Brown, 1998). If delusions and hallucinations are causing other behavioral problems, pharmacological treatment may be necessary. Very potent and effective neuroleptic medications for treatment of delusions and hallucinations are available, but they should be avoided unless absolutely necessary.

Anxiety

Anxiety may be a primary disorder or a symptom of depression. It may result from delusions, hallucinations, or functional impairment. Environmentally focused and behavioral interventions should be used before prescribing anxiolytics. The nurse should plan specific interventions to minimize stress level, enhance feelings of trust and safety, and promote stability by providing a daily routine with few variations. Diversional activities should be provided.

Spatial Disorientation

Spatial disorientation may cause misunderstanding of the environment and lead to the development of fear, anxiety, suspicions, illusions, delusions, and safety problems such as getting lost. In the early stage of dementia, the person may become confused when in an unfamiliar place. In the later stages, the person can become confused when in previously familiar places.

Elopement

Caregivers are justifiably fearful that their care recipient will wander away and become lost, get injured, or die. Elopement is a potential problem in all settings. Community-dwelling AD patients are more likely to wander if they have severe cognitive impairment, exhibit more than one challenging behavior, and spend long periods alone (Logsdon et al., 1998). Other risk factors include a darkened or unfamiliar environment, boredom, stress, tension, lack of control, lack of exercise, and nocturnal delirium.

In designing prevention strategies, the primary care provider should ask caregivers two questions: (1) Is the patient ever left alone? (2) Is the patient registered with the Alzheimer's Association Safe Return Program? Safe Return is a national program that helps to find and return registered AD patients and helps guide the family through elopement (Silverstein & Flaherty, 1996). Or call 888-572-8566 to register a patient in the national database for a reasonable fee.

It is important to remove the precipitants of elopement such as unmet physical needs, boredom, easy exit, or reminders stimulating leaving. Safe walking activities provide exercise, offer social interaction, fill time, and use energy. Exits should be locked. The caregiver must not leave cues to leaving, such as car keys or coats, by the door.

Resistiveness to Care

Resistiveness to care is common during the middle to late stages of dementia and stresses both patients and caregivers (Mahoney et al., 1999). If unmanaged, it is also a major reason for institutionalization and the use of psychotropic medications and restraints (Potts, Richie, & Kaas, 1996). Resistiveness to care occurs during interactions among care recipient, caregiver, and their environment. At times, simply responding with a relaxed and smiling manner may achieve calm and functional behavior. A time-out with a pleasant distraction should divert the patient's attention from the disturbing stimulus. There are no medications to directly prevent or treat resistiveness to care. Core consequences and secondary symptoms of AD that may lead to resistiveness can be managed by behavioral or pharmacological interventions. Because resistiveness occurs intermittently for short periods, a medication with a long duration and poor side-effect profile should not be used.

Food Refusal

Specific issues related to food refusal occur during each of the progressive stages of AD as a consequence of primary or secondary symptoms. Mealtimes should be a focal point of the day, and other activities can be built around structured eating times. The primary caregiver should know the individual's current likes and dislikes, his or her level of physical activity and degree of independence, and how to make eating pleasant and nutritious to provide adequate calories, nutrition, and hydration. A nourishment plan should specify which foods will be provided and how they will be prepared, identify the best eating areas, and establish routines for the eating process.

The person with AD may have age-related changes in the sense of taste, which can lead to decreased appetite and decreased food intake. Often persons with AD develop a fondness for sweet food.

The amount and type of food and beverages should be limited to prevent too much visual stimulation or too many choices, which can be overwhelming. It is best to use foods that are easily handled, chewed, and swallowed. Since persons with AD tend to lose weight later in the disease, caloric density should be maximized, unless they are above ideal weight. Use of finger foods (sandwiches) is one way to address misperception or inability to use a knife, fork, or spoon. In the terminal stage, when patients are bedfast, mute, dysphagic, and subject to infections, eating difficulties can become very problematic (Volicer et al., 1989). Choking may appear in the severe to terminal stage and may be prevented or at least minimized by avoiding thin liquids, feeding the person in a sitting position or keeping the head of the bed at a 90-degree angle, and using foods in which the bolus has sufficient moisture content to help passage through the pharynx and facilitate swallowing (Frisoni, Franzoni, Bellelli, Morris, & Warden, 1998).

Insomnia

Insomnia in elderly adults has been discussed, but AD may present more difficulties with insomnia since it causes death of nerve cells in many areas of the brain, including the suprachiasmatic nucleus. Circadian rhythm disruption leads to changes of sleep, body temperature, melatonin secretion, and possibly other physiological functions.

It is important to avoid using products that interfere with sleep (caffeine, nicotine, and alcohol), scheduling exercise close to bedtime, engaging in exciting or emotionally upsetting activities close to bedtime, and having a poor sleep environment, such as an uncomfortable bed or a bedroom that is too bright, stuffy, hot, cold, or noisy (Bootzin, Epstein, & Wood, 1991).

All persons with AD are choline deficient, and anticholinergic drugs have the potential to worsen the symptoms of AD. It is essential to be wary of over-the-counter sleeping medications that may contain an anticholinergic component or other drugs that may have anticholinergic properties.

Apathy and Agitation

Apathy and agitation are likely to occur as AD worsens and persons experience more functional and cognitive decline. Persons with AD are unable to make sense of their environment, to filter the stimulation that comes their way, and to handle the stress of what is happening to them. **Engagement,** the opposite of apathy, involves attention to and participation in the external environment such as involvement in a conversation or other meaningful activities. Persons with AD need help to become active and interested in what is going on around them. It is common for persons with AD to have bouts of apathy followed by agitation. By uncovering the causes, it is easier to treat agitation before it escalates into assaultive or even violent behavior.

Treatment for agitation and apathy is central to promoting psychological well-being specific for persons with dementia (Volicer et al., 1998). Worsening of AD over time restricts the capacity to express emotions. As persons with AD lose their ability to express their emotions verbally, they resort to other, primarily nonverbal, means of communication. Caregivers control the environment and can communicate emotionally with persons who have AD (Raia, 1999).

Pharmacological Interventions

Pharmacotherapy is indicated only when non-pharmacological interventions do not prevent or alleviate challenging behaviors. Prevention or treatment of challenging behaviors is critical to patients' overall well-being since behavioral dysregulation can be associated with functional impairment (Schultz, Ellingrod, Turvey, Moser, & Arndt, 2003). In all cases, medications are prescribed to promote the patient's comfort and for no other reason. Two traditional principles of geriatric nursing—start low and go slow, and monitor treatment continuously—must be followed. Exactly which medication to select is dependent on the patient's clinical condition and the balance between the desired action and side-effect profile. For example, capitalizing on the hypnotic side effect of trazodone for a depressed patient who also has insomnia uses one medication to treat two problems.

Do Not Resuscitate

For persons with late-stage Alzheimer's disease, CPR should not be offered. If the person does not have an advance plan stipulating either CPR or do not resuscitate (DNR), the DNR decision should be discussed with the surrogate decision maker. DNR does not present an ethical dilemma as clinicians recognize both the futility (Awoke, Mouton, & Parrott, 1992) and adverse effects (Applebaum, King, & Finucane, 1990) of CPR on long-term care patients in general, and its use is low (Duthie et al., 1993). Resuscitation for an unwitnessed cardiac arrest in this population has a very low probability of restoring life (Duthie et al., 1993).

Transfer to an Acute Care Site

There are many reasons why older adults in general and persons with AD in particular are transferred from a long-term care facility to a hospital, and often these reasons are not patient care centered. Once in the hospital, elderly adults with dementia are at risk for complications such as delirium, being tube-fed, relocation stress, and dying.

Feeding Tube

The "need" for feeding tubes may be avoided by promoting eating and preventing food refusal. Caregivers should sit and make eye contact, chat, and make eating an important and pleasurable component of long-term institutional care (Burger, Kayser-Jones, & Bell,

2001; Kayser-Jones & Schell, 1997). More than one third of severely cognitively impaired nursing home residents in the United States have feeding tubes (Mitchell, Teno, Roy, Kabumoto, & Mor, 2003). Even though patients with AD may refuse food, turn away when food is offered, push the spoon or hand away, or spit out food, they can be successfully fed by hand (Volicer et al., 1989).

Permanent tube feeding is not recommended for persons with advanced AD, even those who choke on food and liquids. Tube feeding does not prevent aspiration, improve functioning or quality of life, increase comfort, or promote weight gain (Finucane, Christmas, & Travis, 1999). Body functions are shutting down during the dying process, and food and liquids are no longer necessary (Smith, 1998). In fact, dehydration is beneficial during the dying process because it decreases the sensation of pain and prevents edema and excessive respiratory secretions. Dehydration also decreases the incidence of vomiting and diarrhea. The only consequence of dehydration that may lead to discomfort is dryness of the mouth, lips, or eyes, which can be prevented or alleviated by moisturizing spray, swabs or salve, or ice chips.

Treatment of Infections

Infections are an inevitable consequence of advanced AD because of several risk factors that cannot be avoided, such as changes in immune function, incontinence, decreased mobility, and aspiration (Volicer, Brandeis, & Hurley, 1998). Infections may be treated by the administration of oral antibiotics that are as effective as parenteral antibiotics and do not require restraints to prevent removal of an intravenous catheter. However, the effectiveness of antibiotic treatment is diminished in the terminal stage of AD when infections become recurrent. Pneumonia is the most common cause of death in individuals with dementia, reflecting the limited effectiveness of antibiotic therapy in this patient population. Antibiotics are not necessary to maintain comfort of the patient during an infectious episode because comfort can be maintained by administration of analgesics and antipyretics.

PARKINSON'S DISEASE

Parkinsonism is a group of symptoms and signs in which there are variable combinations of tremor, rigidity, bradykinesia, and a disturbance in gait and posture. Parkinson's disease (PD) is a chronic, progressive neurologic disorder in which idiopathic Parkinsonism appears without other widespread neurologic symptoms, such as cognitive impairment.

PD may progress to PD with dementia, and the nurse will be caring for a patient with two characteristic groups of neurologic symptoms, including movement and memory disorders.

The pathology of PD is related to the loss of the dopaminergic cells situated deep in the midbrain in the substantia nigra (the black substance so named because of the melanin seen in those neurons). Pharmacological intervention by administration of levodopa, the metabolic precursor of dopamine, provides symptomatic relief of symptoms, particularly bradykinesia.

The anticholinergics are another class of medications used for symptomatic treatment of PD. These drugs are prescribed to relieve tremors. The nurse needs to be vigilant in managing the side effects of dry mouth, constipation, blurred vision, and urinary retention. Because PD is a movement disorder, a vision problem can further increase the risk of falling. In elderly men, urinary retention could complicate symptoms of an enlarged prostate. Another drug, amantadine, alone or in combination with an anticholinergic drug, may help by potentiating the release of endogenous dopamine. However, this benefit may be transitory. Another class of medications are dopamine agonists, which directly stimulate the dopamine receptors, such as Permax (Parkinson Study Group, 2000). Dopamine agonists are often initiated in early PD before starting levodopa and are also used in combination with levodopa through the progressive course of PD. Thus, because of the on-off effects of levodopa, some patients are tried on other medications at the onset of symptoms.

Nursing care should be directed to helping the patient manage Parkinsonism—that is, to design individualized interventions to promote mobility, prevent falls, and preserve independence for as long as possible. In the very late stage, the patient cannot stand or walk, becomes cachectic, and requires constant nursing care.

Nurses should assess fall risk (Gray & Hildebrand, 2000) using an agreed upon assessment measure such as the functional reach test (Behrman, Light, Flynn, & Thigpen, 2002). Exercise is another way to preserve independence (Baatile, Langbein, Weaver, Maloney, & Jost, 2000).

STROKE

A stroke is a sudden loss of consciousness followed by paralysis. The pathology typically is caused by hemorrhage into the brain, an embolus or thrombus that occludes an artery, or rupture of an extracerebral artery causing subarachnoid hemorrhage. Immediate treatment is targeted to lifesaving techniques, prevention of extension of the stroke, and early treatment using a plasminogen activator. Stroke is an emergency, and the benefits of reducing further morbidity have to be balanced with risks of increasing the possibility of intracerebral hemorrhage. An adequate airway needs to be established and maintained with ventilation and oxygenation provided as needed. An experienced team needs to make the decision about movement of the patient and transport.

After an acute stroke, the patient is typically transferred to an emergency department. If thrombolytic therapy is not contraindicated, then often recombinant tissue plasminogen activator (rt-PA) will be administered within 3 hours to treat the acute ischemic stroke (Tanne et al., 2002). However, not all patients treated with rt-PA therapy have positive outcomes. The occurrence of symptomatic intracerebral hemorrhage after rt-PA therapy is a catastrophic event, and most of those who survive are discharged to a long-term care facility versus home (Schlegel et al., 2004).

For those stroke survivors who are able to return home, the physical, cognitive, and emotional sequelae place great burdens on the patient and family. Many of their postdischarge needs are ameliorable to nursing interventions. Structured nursing interventions during the rehabilitative period have resulted in better functional status, less depression, and higher self-perceived health, self-esteem, and dietary adherence (Nir, Zolotogorsky, & Sugarman, 2004).

Although the onset of stroke is precipitous, the risk factors have often developed over the years. Stroke prevention is best accomplished by prudent heart living. Prevention activities include maintaining normal blood pressure, not smoking, exercising, and maintaining normal weight. The nurse has an important role in prevention and health education. These interventions should begin in the formative years in elementary school.

SEIZURES

Seizure is an abnormal, abrupt release of electrical activity in the brain. A seizure can cause a variety of symptoms (e.g., spasticity, flaccidity) based on the area of the brain affected. **Epilepsy** is two or more unprovoked seizures. Seizures are either generalized, partial (focal), or unclassified seizures. Classification is based on the area of the brain that the electrical activity originated from, regardless if it then spreads to other areas. In generalized seizures, both hemispheres of the brain are involved.

Partial (focal) seizures occur in only one hemisphere of the brain and are either complex or simple. Complex partial seizures are 1 to 3 minutes in duration and involve loss of consciousness and automatisms. The patient can have autonomic changes or unilateral movement of a limb. Determining the type of seizure is important to choose the appropriate medication. In general phenytoin and caramazepine are drugs of choice for simple, complex and tonic-clonic seizures; ethosuximide for absence seizures; and valproic acid for myoclonic seizures.

There are several nursing interventions when caring for a patient with a history of seizures. It is the nurse's responsibility to obtain an accurate patient history, including age of seizure onset and frequency of attacks. In addition, the nurse should inquire about the dates and duration of the seizures as well as medication name, dosage, and frequency. It is important for the nurse to be aware of the medication dose, as many patients are not initially given a high enough dose.

If a patient has a seizure, the most important responsibility of the nurse is to prevent injury of the patient. Suction equipment should be kept by the patient's bedside so that an oral airway may be obtained and aspiration prevented. In addition, patients should be placed on their side during a seizure to prevent aspiration. If necessary, the head-tilt-chin method can be used to obtain an airway. Although it is rare for patients to die during a seizure, the chief causes of death are asphyxiation and suffocation due to turning of the face during the postictal unconscious phase. Oxygen and intravenous access should always be made available. Oxygen is used if the patient experiences signs of hypoxia (change of skin color), and intravenous access is needed in case emergency medication must be administered. Side-rail pads are used to prevent injury to the patient.

A seizure that lasts more than 10 minutes or groups of seizures that occur in rapid succession and last a combined time of 30 minutes are **status epilepticus,** a neurologic emergency. In the event of status epilepticus the physician should be notified, an airway should be established, and oxygen should be given. If an intravenous access is not already available, one should be started and the patient should receive 0.9% sodium chloride. The physician may prescribe medications to cease the motor movement (intravenous diazepam, lorazepam, or valproate) followed by a medication to prevent recurrence (Dilantin or Cerebyx). Vital signs should be closely monitored during the entire event. If the patient needs to be transported, only padded carts should be used because there is a great risk of a fall with the use of a wheelchair.

Patient-family education is an important intervention of the nurse. Patients and families should be provided with audiovisual aids they may review at their own pace (e.g., handouts and videotapes). Identifying and avoiding precipitating factors associated with seizures should be taught, such as alcohol withdrawal, stress, and lack of sleep. It is important to emphasize taking medication correctly and the dangers of not adhering to the prescribed self-care regimen. The family should be taught what to do in the event of a seizure (lay the patient on his or her side, surround with soft objects, and do not place anything in the mouth) and how long to wait before taking the patient to the emergency department as a possible status epilepticus.

PATIENT-FAMILY TEACHING GUIDELINES

Forgetfulness or Memory Problems

1. Sometimes I forget things. Should I be worried that I'm developing Alzheimer's disease?

   A lot of people forget things and experience memory lapses. Sometimes this is serious and sometimes it is not. Serious changes in memory accompanied by changes in personality, behavior, or the ability to care for oneself often accompany the diagnosis of dementia. Symptoms of dementia include asking the same question repeatedly; getting lost or disoriented in a familiar environment; being unable to follow directions; becoming disoriented to time and place; neglecting personal safety, hygiene, and nutrition; and being unable to manage personal affairs and finances. Alzheimer's disease is one of the many types of dementia.

2. What causes dementia or serious memory problems?

   Dementia has many causes, some of which are reversible by treatment and some of which are permanent and progressive. Some reversible conditions that may cause dementia include high fever, dehydration, vitamin deficiencies, poor nutrition, side effects of medications, thyroid conditions, head injuries, and undiagnosed serious illness like urinary tract infection or pneumonia. Sometimes older people who are depressed, bored, or worried can have memory problems. Seeing a doctor as soon as possible after the detection of memory problems can assist in the diagnosis and treatment of these reversible conditions.

3. How is the diagnosis of Alzheimer's disease confirmed?

Your doctor will carry out a complete medical, neurologic, psychiatric, and social evaluation of your health status. Information will be gathered about your medical history, use of medications, diet, past medical problems, and general health and function. A family member should accompany you if you have problems relating specific information regarding your symptoms or past medical history. Tests of blood and urine will also be done. A CT scan may be done to examine the brain. It usually takes one or two visits to gather all of the information needed for an accurate diagnosis.

4. How is Alzheimer's disease treated?

In the early and middle stages of Alzheimer's disease, drugs like donepezil (Aricept) and galantamine (Reminyl) are used to delay the worsening of the disease and the progression of symptoms. Medications are also used for behavioral problems like agitation, anxiety, depression, and sleep disorders. Careful use of drugs is important, and nurses will keep track of symptoms to make sure that they are improving as a result of medication administration. General healthcare like diet, exercise, social activities, and memory aids such as

(continued)

calendars, lists of important phone numbers, and other notes about day-to-day activities can help improve the quality of life of older persons with dementia.

5. What can I do to prevent dementia?

The research shows that people who remain active and engaged in life stimulate their bodies and brains to continue to function effectively. Develop hobbies and interests, enjoy your life, exercise to remain or become fit, eat a balanced diet, avoid smoking and heavy drinking, do not take unnecessary drugs, avoid stress and anxiety, and stay connected with at least one other person on a daily basis. Some physical and mental changes occur with age in healthy people; however, dementia is a disease and not a normal part of aging. Report any memory problems to your physician or nurse and seek an accurate diagnosis as soon as possible to identify reversible causes.

CHAPTER 21

THE IMMUNE SYSTEM

Three major biological defense mechanisms protect the human body from injurious chemicals, foreign bodies, microorganisms, and parasites. The first line of defense is the **anatomical and biochemical barrier** provided by the skin and mucous membranes. The second line of defense is **mechanical clearance** that prevents substances from entering the body or assists in expelling them, such as sloughing of the skin, actions of the respiratory cilia and mucous secretions, vomiting, defecation, and urination. The third line of defense is the **immune response,** a highly complicated, integrated system that is controlled by a complex communication mechanism.

The immune system identifies anything that is not a normal part of the body, and attacks and destroys the invader. However, the normal tissues of the body are left undisturbed. In this process, invaders can be blocked from entering the body, chemically neutralized, or destroyed.

Types of Immunity

Natural immunity, or innate resistance, is not produced by the immune response. One type of natural immunity that is present at birth is specific to the human species.

Acquired active immunity results from stimulation of the body's immune system to destroy or neutralize foreign substances, usually microorganisms. It occurs after an agent is introduced into the body, either from the environment or through immunization, producing either an illness or an inapparent illness.

Acquired passive immunity is obtained by introducing a serum that contains specific antibodies into a person who is susceptible to the disease. Because the person receives antibodies that have been formed elsewhere, there is no direct stimulation of the person's own immune system.

Components of the Immune Response

White blood cells are primarily associated with both inflammation and the immune response. The three primary types of white blood cells are granulocytes, monocytes, and **lymphocytes.**

Primary and Secondary Immune Responses

The characteristic of memory is involved in both primary and secondary immune responses. The first exposure to the foreign antigen results from active infection or immunization, and a **primary immune response** is begun. A latent period occurs initially, during which no antibodies can be detected. After approximately 5 days, 1 gM antibodies can be detected in the blood.

With a second exposure, however, the **secondary immune response** is evoked. Due to presence of memory cells, there is a more rapid production of large amounts of antibodies than occurred in the primary immune response. The characteristics of the primary and secondary response allow clinicians to determine the individual's stage of an infectious disease by evaluating a series of antibody titers for a specific antigen.

Cell-Mediated Immune Response

During the process of maturation in the thymus gland, T cells begin producing several types of new proteins that become attached to the surface of the T cell. Most of these become specialized receptors called T cell antigen receptors (TCRs).

The two major types of mature T cells are helper T (Th) cells and cytotoxic (Tc) cells. They produce substances that stimulate inflammation and minimum response. These functions can be affected by aging and disease.

IMMUNE CHANGES WITH AGING

Often in older people, there is a decrease in the speed, strength, and duration of both the immune response and the regulation of immune activities (Digiovanna, 2000). A decreased ability to respond to antigenic stimulation by B lymphocytes is a common characteristic of the aging immune system. Although the secondary immune response of the humoral (B cell) immune system may be normal due to the presence of memory cells, the response to new antigens is decreased. More antigenic material may be needed to prompt antibody production, and the production is slower. A lower peak antibody concentration may occur, and antibody levels decline faster as the person ages. As a result, risk of an insufficient humoral immune system response increases with the age at which antigens are first encountered.

Over time, the secondary immune response may also show changes. The number of B cells in the circulation decreases in some individuals. Therefore, vaccinations should be given by the age of 60 to have the greatest effectiveness.

Factors Affecting Aging of the Immune System

- Stress
- Diagnosis of comorbidities
- Lack of exercise
- Lack of essential nutrients
- Excessive immune responses

Hypersensitivity

Hypersensitivity is either an excessive response to antigen stimulation or a normal response that is inappropriate. It usually does not occur on the first exposure to the antigen when the primary immune response occurs (sensitization). Reexposure to the antigen and initiation of the secondary immune response can stimulate hypersensitive reactions in predisposed individuals.

Type I Hypersensitivity

Type I hypersensitivities are immediate and may be life threatening. Reactions normally occur within 15 to 30 minutes after exposure to an antigen (allergen). Manifestations vary in severity, but often include hives, localized swelling, tightening of the throat, shortness of breath, wheezing, tachycardia, and hypotension. Anaphylactic allergic reactions leading to shock can occur.

Type II Hypersensitivity

Type II hypersensitivities also occur within 15 to 30 minutes of exposure. Examples of this type of reaction include transfusion reactions, drug reactions, myasthenia gravis, thyroiditis, and autoimmune hemolytic anemia (Copstead & Banasik, 2000).

Type III Hypersensitivity

Type III hypersensitivity is characterized by a failure to remove antigen-antibody complexes from the circulation and tissues. The subsequent inflammatory reaction can lead to cell and tissue injury. The underlying cause may be a persistent low-grade infection by a viral or bacterial agent; chronic exposure to an environmental antigen from molds, plants, or animals; or an autoimmune process. This may lead to acute or chronic renal failure.

Rheumatoid arthritis is believed to be another example of type III hypersensitivity that affects the older person. About 1% of all adults have rheumatoid arthritis, and it is more frequent in women. Peak incidence is between the fourth and sixth decade of life.

Type IV Hypersensitivity

Type IV hypersensitivity is also called delayed hypersensitivity. Tissue is damaged as a result of a delayed T-cell reaction to an antigen. The reaction normally occurs within 1 to 14 days after exposure, although it is often slower in older persons. Contact hypersensitivity such as dermatitis from a latex allergy, tuberculin reactions, and transplant rejections are examples. In people with multiple sclerosis, a variety of studies have documented abnormalities in both B cells and T cells.

Deficient Immune Responses

Deficient immune responses occur when there is a functional decrease in one or more components of the immune system. These are either primary or secondary immunodeficiency disorders.

Primary Immunodeficiency Disorders

Primary immunodeficiency disorders are either congenital or acquired, and are not attributed to other causes.

HIV/AIDS

Infection with the human immunodeficiency virus (HIV) and the resulting acquired immunodeficiency syndrome (AIDS) is the best example of a primary immunodeficiency disorder. The hallmark of this infection is a decrease in cellular (T cell) immunity. Helper T (CD4) cells are primarily affected by the virus. These T cells mediate between the antigen presenting cells (macrophages) and other B and T cells. It is a chronic disease spread primarily through sexual contact with an infected person. The widespread organ involvement associated with the infection has caused much human suffering and death.

HIV infection in the older person is most likely underdiagnosed and underreported. Healthcare workers often do not take sexual histories of older patients, nor do they recommend HIV testing. Symptoms of HIV infection, such as memory loss and weight loss, are often treated as symptoms of other common age-related health problems, such as Alzheimer's disease (Szirony, 1999).

Older people have lower CD4 cell counts, are more ill at the initial diagnosis, have more comorbidity, are characterized by a more aggressive course of the disease, and have a higher risk of death from the disease (Chen, Ryan, & Ferguson, 1998; Wellons et al., 2002). It is believed that these characteristics are due to delayed diagnosis, chronic coexisting health problems, and the age-related impairments in T-cell immunity.

Antiretroviral therapy, which typically contains at least three antiretroviral medications, holds promise for treatment of older people with HIV infection. When compared to younger people, older patients in one study had somewhat better virological responses and similar immunological responses to antiretroviral therapy. Older patients had fewer interruptions in the therapy and were able to tolerate and adhere to the therapy regimen relatively well. Failure of an older patient to respond to antiretroviral therapy should not be attributed to age alone (Wellons et al., 2002). The prognosis for seniors diagnosed with HIV today is good. Although they live fewer years after diagnosis, they can still live long productive lives (Marcus, 2002).

Secondary Immunodeficiency Disorders

Secondary immunodeficiency disorders are a consequence of other disorders or treatment regimens. Many factors can lead to the development of secondary immunodeficiency disorders, including physical, nutritional, environmental, psychosocial, and pharmacological factors.

The stress of surgery, including the effects of anesthesia, can decrease the number of both B and T cells, and the deficiency can last for up to one month. This is particularly true for removal of the spleen, a structure of the immune system. Diabetes mellitus, cirrhosis, severe trauma and burns, malignancies, and severe infections are associated with secondary immune deficiencies. Medications, such as the cancer pharmacotherapeutic drugs, also cause a state of general immunosuppression. Others, such as antibiotics, anticonvulsants, antihistamines, and steroids, affect various mechanisms of the immune system. X-rays can destroy the rapidly proliferating cells of the immune system. Malnutrition can lead to protein and other deficiencies that impair immune function. Many of these factors affect older persons, many of whom already have a decreased ability to reproduce new cells of the immune system (Copstead & Banasik, 2000).

SUSCEPTIBILITY TO INFECTIONS

Infections are one of the most frequently encountered problems in the older population. Although specific relationships between an aging or compromised immune system and infection are not clear, the decline in responsiveness of the immune system to harmful foreign invaders leads to an increase in the incidence and severity of infections. Sometimes they are difficult to diagnose. The febrile response that signals infections may be blunted in the older person. Medications commonly taken may also decrease the normal fever response. The baseline body temperature in older people is approximately 1°F lower than the normal temperature in younger people. Therefore, a rise in body temperature may not be immediately evident. Any temperature of 37.8°C or 100°F when other symptoms are present may indicate an infection. Other classic signs and symptoms of infection, such as redness, swelling, and pain, may also be altered.

Pneumonia

Pneumonia is a leading cause of death in people over 65 years of age. It is the most common hospital-associated infection, and it has the highest mortality rate of all **nosocomial infections.** The combination of pneumonia and influenza causes the greatest number of deaths. *Streptococcus pneumoniae* (pneumococcus) remains the single most common cause of pneumonia in the older person, and it increases with age. It accounts for approximately 40 to 60% of the cases. Pneumococcal pneumonia may occur as a primary illness or as a complication of a chronic disease. *S. pneumoniae* is a common resident of the human upper respiratory tract, and has been isolated in up to 70% of healthy adults.

Urinary Tract Infection

Urinary tract infection is one of the most common problems in older adults, especially in women. It is important to differentiate between asymptomatic bacteriuria and symptomatic infection. The prevalence of urinary bacteriuria increases with age. Asymptomatic bacteriuria generally is not treated. Adverse reactions, reinfection, and the development of resistant organisms can occur.

Bacteremia

Microorganisms can be introduced into the bloodstream as a complication of pneumonia, urinary tract infections, infection of skin and soft tissues, and other infectious processes. The urinary tract is the most common source of bacteremia, followed by the respiratory tract. Perirectal abscesses are frequently missed and can be a source of infection. Once in the bloodstream, microorganisms are disseminated to other organs throughout the body. Increased age and associated illness contribute to a poorer prognosis, and mortality rates are between 15% and 40%. Gram-negative rods, such as *Escherichia coli, Proteus* species, and *Klebsiella* species, are the most common microorganisms. *Staphylococcus aureus* is the most common gram-positive organism and is associated with 50% mortality.

Tuberculosis

Tuberculosis still remains a worldwide problem. It is a chronic pulmonary and extrapulmonary infectious disease that is acquired through exposure to *Mycobacterium tuberculosis.* It spreads from person to person by airborne transmission. The number of cases of tuberculosis is highest in people over 65 years of age, with the exception of those who are infected with HIV. The majority of active cases occur through reactivation of a dormant infection in an older person who has not been effectively treated in the past. Older persons are also at increased risk of initial infection, particularly those who are chronically ill or debilitated and residing in nursing homes.

Skin Infections

As the skin becomes thinner and less elastic with age, the older person becomes more susceptible to injury and breakdown of tissue. Peripheral neuropathy with decreased sensation and circulation may lead to abrasions, burns, and stasis ulcers. Reduced physical activity, malnutrition, dehydration, and other systemic illnesses are also predisposing factors. Immobilized people who are convalescing at home are at high risk for the development of pressure ulcers. Any interruption of skin integrity leads to infection, especially with organisms that are a part of the normal skin flora.

The reactivation of the herpes zoster (varicella) virus that has lingered in nerve tissue for years following chickenpox infection can lead to shingles. Approximately 9 per 1,000 people over 60 years of age acquire the illness each year (Fune et al., 1998). Vesicular lesions occur along spinal nerves, most frequently affecting T3 to L2 nerves and the fifth cranial nerve. Extreme discomfort may occur. Early treatment with acyclovir or other antiviral medications should begin within 72 hours after appearance of the rash. This treatment reduces acute pain and shortens the period of infectivity. Otherwise, treatment is largely supportive with administration of analgesics and topical cleansing. Occasionally, chronic pain develops that will require longer term analgesics and possibly antidepressants.

Nursing Assessment

Multiple factors underlie immune problems in the older person. Therefore, a health history and physical examination are essential. The key assessment areas include the following factors:

- Age
- Nutrition

- Recent infections
- Immunization status
- Allergies
- Disorders and diseases
  - Autoimmune disease
  - Neoplastic disease
  - Chronic illness
  - Surgery
- Pain
- Medications
- Blood transfusions
- Lifestyle, stress, and other factors

Nursing Interventions to Improve Immune Status

Nursing interventions that can improve immune status in the older person include the following:

- Consider older people who are under substantial stress at high risk for conditions associated with a decreased immune status.
- Encourage laboratory testing for hormone levels associated with stress to identify older people at high risk.
- Assist people in identifying active, positive coping strategies, especially following stressful events.
- Educate the person, family, and friends about the effects of stress.
- Administer pneumococcal vaccine at or prior to the age of 65 with revaccination as recommended by the primary care provider.
- Stress the importance of obtaining yearly influenza immunizations.
- Encourage daily vitamin and mineral supplements.

- Encourage all older persons to develop an exercise plan appropriate for their physical status.
- Encourage community senior centers to offer education about HIV infection.
- Screen for HIV infection in older people.
- Encourage older adults to seek advice from health-care professionals when symptoms occur.

PATIENT-FAMILY TEACHING GUIDELINES

Prevention of Influenza

1. Can the flu be prevented?

   A flu shot greatly reduces your chances of getting the flu. No vaccine is completely effective, but studies show that older people who get the flu shot are 70% less likely to be hospitalized and 85% less likely to die as a result of getting the flu.

   The flu is highly contagious and spreads easily from person to person. It is caused by viruses that infect the nose, throat, and lungs. When you are out in crowded places like church or the mall, try to avoid contact with people who are coughing and sneezing. Wash your hands often and do not put things found in public places in or near your mouth. The flu can be life threatening in an older person or a person with other chronic illness like diabetes or diseases of the kidneys, liver, heart, or lungs.

2. Who should get a flu shot?

   The Centers for Disease Control (a part of the federal government) recommends the following people receive flu shots each year because these persons are categorized as high risk for serious illness and complications from the flu:

- People over the age of 65
- Residents of nursing homes and other long-term care facilities where older persons live in close contact
- Adults with chronic heart or lung disease
- Adults with diabetes or with kidney, liver, heart, or lung disease
- Healthcare workers in contact with people in high-risk groups
- Caregivers or people who live with someone in a high-risk group

3. Will my insurance cover the cost of the shot?

The cost of the flu shot is covered by Medicare. Many private health insurance plans also pay for the flu shot. You can get a flu shot at your doctor's office or you may receive it from your local health department or at flu shot clinics sponsored by some drug or department stores.

4. When is the best time to get the flu shot?

In the United States, the flu season usually starts in December and ends in April. The best time to get the flu shot is between mid-September and mid-November. It takes about 1 to 2 weeks to develop immunity after you receive the flu shot.

5. What about side effects of the flu shot?

The vaccine is made from killed flu viruses, so you cannot possibly get the flu. The vaccine is grown in eggs, so people who are severely allergic to eggs should not get the flu shot. Some people (fewer than one third who get the flu shot) report soreness, redness, or swelling in the arm where the flu shot was given. These side effects can last

(continued)

up to 2 days and usually are controlled with acet-aminophen.

6. What are the symptoms of the flu?

Flu causes fever, chills, dry cough, sore throat, runny nose, headache, muscle ache, and fatigue. Usually symptoms are worse than symptoms of a cold or upper respiratory infection. If you get the flu, make sure to rest, drink plenty of fluids, and take acetaminophen to control aches and fever. Call your doctor or primary healthcare provider if:

- Your fever (usually over 100°F) lasts for more than a few days.
- You are diagnosed with heart, lung, liver, or kidney problems.
- You are taking drugs to fight off cancer or other drugs that weaken your body's immune response.
- You feel sick and do not seem to be getting better.
- You have a cough with phlegm.
- You or someone caring for you is worried about your condition.

7. How is the flu treated?

Because the flu is caused by a virus, antibiotics (only effective against bacterial infections) are not an effective treatment. The four drugs approved to treat the flu include:

- Amantadine (Symmetrel)
- Rimantadine (Flumadine)
- Zanamivir (Relenza)
- Oseltamivir (Tamiflu)

These drugs must be taken within 48 hours of the onset of symptoms, so it is important to call your doctor or primary healthcare provider if you think you have the flu. These drugs shorten the duration of the illness and prevent complications like pneumonia. They are only available by prescription and are not right for everyone. Other drugs may be given to make you feel better, including cough medication and antibiotics should you develop a bacterial pneumonia as a complication of the flu.

CHAPTER 22

MULTISYSTEM PROBLEMS: CARING FOR FRAIL ELDERS WITH COMORBIDITIES

Medical comorbidities complicate the nursing assessment and treatment of medical conditions and place the frail older person at risk for poor outcomes because of the atypical presentation of disease, delays in the initiation of treatment, need for multiple pharmacological interventions, and diminished organ reserve capacity that inhibits the physiological and psychological responses to stressors. Often, the term **frail** is used to describe an older person with diagnosed chronic illness, loss of organ function, diagnosis of recurrent acute illness, and social risk factors such as poverty, social isolation, and functional or cognitive decline. A frail older person exhibits dependence in one or more activities of daily living and is diagnosed with three or more comorbid conditions and one or more geriatric syndromes (including dementia, delirium, depression, incontinence, falls, osteoporosis, gait disturbance, or pressure ulcers) (Lichtman, 2003). Frailty has also been defined as the presence of three or more of the following criteria:

- Unplanned weight loss (10 lb in the last year)
- Weakness
- Poor endurance and energy

- Slowness
- Low activity

(Young, 2003)

Frailty is an important concept for gerontological nurses and other healthcare providers caring for older people because:

- The frail older adult is the largest consumer of healthcare, community services, and long-term care.
- The number of older persons over the age of 85 is increasing rapidly in the United States, and the prevalence of frailty increases dramatically with age.
- Nurses and other healthcare professionals are interested in identifying frail older persons to initiate specialized geriatric services to meet their needs, including geriatric assessment, multidisciplinary care, and specialized geriatric services (Fried et al., 2001).

RISKS OF FRAILTY

A frail older person is at high risk for dependency, institutionalization, falls, injuries, hospitalization, slow recovery from illness, and mortality. The frail older adult is most in need of and most likely to benefit from specialized geriatric services (Fried, 1994; Fried et al., 2001). The very old (85+), those with physical frailty and cognitive impairment, and those dependent on formal and informal supports to maintain health, function, and autonomy are most at risk for decline. Often the frail older person will suffer a rapid decline and decompensation as a result of acute illness or worsening of a chronic condition. This phenomenon of decline has been termed the **geriatric cascade** and results from the interaction of the frail older person, acute illness, and the stress of institutional care (Fretwell, 1998).

THE PATHS TO FRAILTY

It has been hypothesized (Albert, Im, & Raveis, 2002) that older persons can become frail by one or more of three pathways:

- Changes of aging and loss of organ reserve and function in the very old
- Diagnosis with several chronic illnesses, each of which alone and in combination with others can cause harmful effects on overall physiological function
- Existence in harmful social and psychological environments

Because of the variability in aging and uniqueness of each person's compensatory ability, chronological age should never serve as a sole marker for making treatment decisions. Given the varying rates of aging between individuals and the heterogeneity of the aging process, a particular older patient may have many, some, or no age-related problems or comorbidities (National Institute on Aging & National Cancer Institute, 2004).

COMMON DIAGNOSES ASSOCIATED WITH FRAILTY IN THE OLDER ADULT

Chronic conditions and diseases such as diabetes, cardiovascular diseases, osteoporosis, and arthritis are major causes of frailty and disability in late life. Risks for disease and frailty increase with age and can be exacerbated by poor lifestyle choices and poverty (National Institute on Aging, 2005).

Cumulative Effect of Comorbidities

Often a frail older person will be diagnosed with several underlying chronic conditions and develop an acute condition that disrupts the stability of the chronic conditions. For instance, a person with a mild cognitive impairment might develop a urinary tract infection and might become more confused as a result of the infection. Often, treatment is delayed because nurses and other healthcare providers do not recognize the importance of subtle changes in the frail older person's function. This delay in treatment can make the acute illness more difficult to treat.

Older persons with cognitive impairment cannot adequately report symptoms of acute or chronic illness. Careful assessment of changes from baseline function, vital signs, and information from reliable caregivers is crucial.

The frail older person is more at risk for poor treatment outcomes and even death because of the interaction between normal changes of aging and common illnesses associated with age (Rosenthal, Kaboli, Barnett, & Sirio, 2002). Comorbidity and functional status are important factors in determining medical therapy and nursing interventions. Careful monitoring of the patient's status and effectiveness of the overall plan of care is indicated because frail older persons with poor function are at increased risk of toxicity from multiple medications, **iatrogenesis** or adverse outcomes of therapeutic interventions, and poor treatment outcomes when receiving nursing and medical treatment for acute illness. To meet the special needs of older patients during hospitalization, every effort should be made to correctly diagnose all vague symptoms and problems, treat all relevant diseases, assess the effect of current changes in the older person's health status, including the effect of the acute illness on other diagnosed chronic illnesses, and prevent complications of hospitalization (nosocomial infections, falls, delirium, polypharmacy, nutritional deficiencies) (Saltvedt, Mo, Fayers, Kaasa, & Sletvold, 2002).

Trajectories of Functional Decline

1. *Sudden Death*—Physical function is optimal and a massive unpredictable event such as accident or trauma, heart attack, or stroke occurs suddenly, resulting in immediate death.
2. *Diagnosis with a Terminal Illness*—Physical function is optimal and a terminal illness such as cancer is diagnosed with gradual, progressive, linear decline over a short and predictable period of time.
3. *Organ Failure*—Physical function gradually declines with entry and re-entry into the healthcare system with periods of return home between hospital stays, resulting in a downhill trajectory with periods of plateau.
4. *Frailty*—Lingering, expected deaths occur with a long, gradual downhill progression of already diminished physical function. Twenty percent experienced death with a frailty trajectory.

(Glaser & Strauss, 1968; Lunney et al., 2003)

Frailty and Emotional Health

Chronic conditions and frailty also negatively affect emotional health. New-onset depression is frequent in older patients with significant chronic illnesses. The negative impact of these illnesses on function is increased by the presence of depression (Robertson & Montagnini, 2004).

Cancer

Increasing age is directly associated with increasing rates of cancer, corresponding to an 11-fold increased incidence in persons over the age of 65. Despite these statistics, very few older persons enter into chemotherapy clinical trials. Limited information is available regarding the efficacy of various treatments such as surgery, chemotherapy, and radiation in this age group. The course of cancer treatment has shifted from relatively high mortality risks to patterns of chronic remission and recurrence in many of the most common malignancies, particularly solid tumors, with the advent of therapies that use multiple treatment modalities and collaborative care (Kagan, 2004). Signs and symptoms of frailty in a person with cancer include cachexia or wasting syndrome, functional and cognitive decline, serum albumin less than 2.5 g/100 dl, recurrent diagnoses with secondary infections (pneumonia, skin infections, urinary tract infection), and unremitting pain.

Cardiovascular Disease

Cardiovascular disease is the most common cause of hospitalization and death in the older population. The underlying cause is most often coronary atherosclerosis, which occurs not only as a result of aging processes but also from the cumulative effect of poor personal health habits such as smoking, obesity, sedentary lifestyle, and poorly controlled hypertension (McCance & Huether, 2001). Separating the effects of aging from the effects of pathology is difficult and requires more ongoing study. Better understanding of preventive measures and increasing sophistication in diagnosis and treatment have resulted in decreasing rates of heart disease in both men and women.

Alzheimer's Disease

When cognitive capacity is impaired due to the diagnosis of Alzheimer's disease or another irreversible neurodegenerative dementia, care and treatment decisions become even more difficult. Virtually all patients with dementia have unremitting disease courses inevitably leading to death (Marson, Dymek, & Geyer, 2001). The treatment preferences of persons with dementia are often made by family members on behalf of the patient or upon predetermined wishes such as living wills. In reality, however, treatment choices may not be so simple. There are many factors to consider such as burden of treatment, chance of success of the intervention, relief of symptoms, reduction of a family's burden of care, level of understanding and commitment on the part of families, and level of acuity of the setting in which the care is provided.

Musculoskeletal Problems

Changes in bone and muscle are associated with functional disability in later life. Osteoporosis, osteoarthritis, and age-related loss of muscle mass force many older people to become functionally dependent, suffering weakness, falls, fractures, and other problems related to immobility. Older patients diagnosed with musculoskeletal problems are at risk for frailty because weakness and immobility will compound recovery from surgery, acute illness, or chronic illness. Loss of bone and muscle mass may make position change more difficult, complicate early ambulation attempts after surgery, necessitate the use of bedpans and catheters, and delay trips to the bathroom, thus facilitating urinary and fecal incontinence. The older person is also at risk for falls and significant injury resulting from these falls. Signs of frailty in an older person with musculoskeletal problems may include decreased stamina and physical deconditioning, shortness of breath on exertion, history of falls, dizziness, weakness, poor vision or hearing, cognitive or mood impairment inhibiting judgment and preparation for movement, and diagnoses with comorbidities such as cardiovascular or neurologic disease.

Diabetes

Older persons with diabetes are at risk for frailty because of the complicated nature of managing and treating diabetes and its association with other diseases and problems such as cardiovascular disease and declines in neural, renal, immune, and sensory function. When acute illness is diagnosed in an older person with diabetes, often eating patterns are disrupted, new medications are added, and activity levels are changed. All of these factors can greatly affect the patient's blood glucose levels and medication regimen. Because of declines in the immune system's ability to protect against infection, older adults with diabetes are more at risk for urinary tract infection, otitis media, development of peripheral ulcers, cholecystitis, and respiratory infection. When antibiotics are used in older persons with diabetes, they are usually prescribed at higher doses for longer periods of time to ensure complete eradication of the offending organism. These higher doses place the person at risk for medication side effects and drug interactions, including development of antibiotic-associated diarrhea, fungal infections, decreases in renal excretion of all prescribed medications, and development of hypo- or hyperglycemia. Older persons with diabetes may be considered frail if they exhibit any of the following characteristics: frequent need for treatment of severe hypo- or hyperglycemia indicating poor regulation and control, frequent diagnosed secondary infections, fluctuating vital signs and weight, presence of cognitive or functional impairment, financial and social problems inhibiting access to appropriate medications or treatment, and diagnosis with comorbidities complicating the assessment and treatment of the diabetes.

Long-Term Care

Factors in the long-term care environment may exacerbate behavioral problems. Maintaining the emotional and relational well-being of those with dementia depends on caregivers who see dignity even in those severely affected by their condition. Overly restrictive institutional care facilities designed to protect vulnerable persons with dementia are capable of myriad abuses of power (Post, 1995; Post et al., 2001). With the best intentions, an efficient nursing staff may actually reinforce the resident's dependence (National Institutes of Health, 2000). Many long-term care facilities are understaffed. Nurses and nursing assistants may save time by "doing for" residents rather than encouraging residents to do more for themselves. Nurses should address problem behaviors using social and environmental modifications and creative activities, thereby preserving independence and self-esteem. Drugs for behavioral control should be used cautiously and only for specific purposes such as depression, psychosis, anxiety, and sleep disturbances (Martin & Whitehouse, 1990). Polypharmacy and overmedication are serious problems inherent in the care of patients with dementia.

Palliative care can be provided to seriously ill patients at any time during the disease process. Palliative care emphasizes development of a therapeutic relationship by the provision of stable healthcare providers, alleviation of pain and management of troublesome symptoms, respite for families, reduction in use of acute care hospitals for death and unnecessary hospitalization, and increases in patient and family satisfaction with healthcare delivery (City of Hope & American Association of Colleges of Nursing, 2003).

Cognitively impaired and physically frail patients become even more confused with social isolation, exposure to narcotic pain medications and drugs used for anesthesia, and changes in their usual care routine. They are less able to participate in rehabilitation after surgery. Dementia patients and others with aphasia are much less likely to verbalize pain and request pain medications.

Acute Illness and Hospitalization

Common causes of hospitalization include pneumonia, influenza, heart failure, ischemic heart disease, urinary tract infection, hip fracture, digestive disorders, and dehydration (Malone & Danto-Nocton, 2004). Additional facts about hospitalization include:

- Older persons account for 36% of all hospitalizations and 50% of hospital revenues.
- About 66% of Americans die in hospitals, and over 80% of the deaths occur in persons 65 years of age or older.
- About one fourth of patients who died in hospitals were perceived by their families to have moderate or severe pain at the end of life.
- In the year before death, nearly all older Americans are hospitalized, accounting for 20% of all Medicare expenditures.

(Landefeld, 2004; SUPPORT, 1995)

Adverse drug events can be minimized by implementing preventive strategies. Use of computerized entry systems, monitoring of prescriptions by a clinical pharmacist, and identification of the correct patient and drug using bar-code technology are methods that have been shown to decrease the frequency of medication errors. Adverse drug events can result from the following errors:

- Missed dose (7%)
- Wrong technique (6%)
- Illegible order (5%)
- Duplicate therapy (5%)
- Drug-drug interaction (5%)
- Equipment failure (1%)
- Inadequate monitoring (1%)
- Preparation error (1%)

(Agency for Healthcare Research and Quality, 2001)

Medications that can cause delirium through intoxication or withdrawal include anesthetics, analgesics, antiasthmatics, anticonvulsants, antihypertensives, antimicrobials, antiparkinsonian medications, corticosteroids, gastrointestinal H_2 blockers, muscle relaxants, hypnotics, and psychotropic medications.

Some evidence suggests that sensory deprivation experienced by patients placed in windowless hospital rooms is associated with higher rates of delirium (McCusker et al., 2001). Additional factors include not wearing hearing aids or eyeglasses, separation from personal objects, and lack of clocks and calendars. Falls can occur when older people are moving about in unsafe environments and trying to ambulate with intravenous poles on slippery or wet floors without appropriate footwear. Very old patients may arrive at the hospital in later and more severe stages of illness, may have other diagnosed chronic illness, may have sensory or cognitive impairment, and may be less able to adapt to their new environment. Thus, they are more at risk from adverse events and poor outcomes during hospitalization. Entering the hospital from a nursing home is associated with many of the attributes (including cognitive impairment) predicting poor outcomes during hospitalization (Fretwell, 1998). Nursing home residents are more at risk for adverse events, and nurses are required to provide special monitoring of their progress. Delirium and functional decline should be recognized as signs of the failure or side effects of the treatment regimen and of inadequate efforts to maintain function (Landefeld, 2004).

Common problems experienced by nursing home residents before, during, and after hospitalization include incomplete data, vague reports of signs and symptoms of illness, lack of medical records and poor communication regarding the predetermined wishes and code status of the patient. To facilitate better care of hospitalized nursing home residents, the nurse should attempt to communicate with the nursing home staff and gain as much information as possible. Hospital and nursing home nurses can work together to develop a standardized transfer database to include all necessary information and keep open lines of communication to better meet the needs of nursing home residents requiring acute care.

Two general issues should be considered in caring for older persons in the hospital: (1) determining the goals of care and (2) designing and implementing strategies to achieve those goals (Landefeld, 2004). Failure to address these issues leads to frustration on the part of patients, families, and caregivers. Setting realistic goals is an important opportunity for caregivers to engage in open and honest conversations with patients and families. Care can be designated as aggressive, modified, palliative, or hospice. Code status and goals of care should be discussed, clarified, and clearly noted on the chart as early as possible during the hospital admission process. Disagreements between family, patient, and caregivers are red flags that signal trouble during the caring process. The multidisciplinary team can be mobilized to help resolve conflicts.

Aggressive care is usually appropriately delivered to older persons with high functional ability, satisfactory quality of life, high rehabilitation potential, and the ability to endure and cooperate with the demands of therapy. Modified aggressive treatment is usually appropriate for older persons with higher degrees of frailty or multiple comorbidities who still have sufficient reserve capacity to respond to the treatment. Age alone should not dictate the appropriate level of care. The older person's predetermined wishes in conjunction with his or her underlying degree of frailty and the professional opinions of members of the healthcare team are the key factors.

Proposed screening tests for relevant comorbid conditions upon hospital admission include:

- Mental status testing to quantify the older person's baseline mental status and to identify cognitive deficits that may interfere with the ability to provide informed consent or to participate in the treatment and rehabilitation plan.
- Depression testing to quantify the older person's baseline level of depression, to identify patients needing referral for counseling or treatment with antidepressants, and to identify patients who may lack motivation, incentive, and drive to participate in the plan of care.
- Activities of daily living to identify previous level of function and baseline status. This is helpful information to be considered in discharge planning.

- Social support to identify family, friends, and religious and spiritual advisors who can assist and support the older person during illness and recovery.
- Presence of comorbidities, including heart disease, lung disease, chronic renal insufficiency, hypertension, diabetes, malignancy, collagen disorders, arthritis, visual impairment, and autoimmune disorders. If the patient is capable, he or she should be asked for permission to obtain and review old medical records from other hospitalizations or healthcare clinics.
- Nutrition measures, including weight, height, bone mass index, serum albumin, and cholesterol to provide valuable information and predict responses to drug therapy and aggressive treatment.
- Polypharmacy information regarding the medications taken by the older person to prevent duplication of prescriptions during hospitalization, to avoid interactions, and to predict compliance with the discharge plan.
- End-of-life preferences. Has the older person established a living will or named a healthcare proxy? Is the older person still able to state the kind of treatment he or she would like during this hospitalization and illness?

(Adapted from Lichtman, 2003)

Many hospitals have established acute care of the elderly (ACE) units to provide specialized care to older persons and decrease the risks of adverse events during hospitalization. An ACE unit is based on four key concepts:

1. A safe environment with uncluttered halls to promote mobility, carpeted floors to decrease glare, raised toilet seats to improve continence, and a common lounge area to promote socialization and decrease isolation

2. Patient-centered interdisciplinary care guided by nurse-driven protocols to address key nursing issues such as mobility, skin care, nutrition, and continence
3. Discharge planning with the goal of returning the older patient to his or her former living status
4. Careful medical and nursing interventions to prevent adverse outcomes and avoid iatrogenic problems

ACE units have been shown to prevent functional decline, decrease length of stay, and decrease nursing home placement. Additionally, ACE units have demonstrated improvement in the process of care, including increased implementation of nursing care plans to promote independent function, increased physical therapy consults, and greater satisfaction among patients, caregivers, physicians, and nurses (Counsell et al., 2000; Landefeld, 2004).

Assessing Treatment Burden

The most significant quality-of-life concern arises from the burdens that life-extending treatment can impose on people with frailty or dementia. The caregiver must examine the potential of an intervention from the very ill or disoriented person's point of view. Will the treatment be interpreted as assault or torture? Will it prolong a life with significant behavioral or physical problems? Are there indications that the dementia patient is refusing treatment by continued attempts to remove dialysis and feeding tubes (Post, 1995). Therapeutic interventions that impose considerable burdens on the person with dementia should not be tolerated in a humane and just healthcare system.

The cascade of illness or functional decline is the hypothesized pathway of development of complications during illness (Fretwell, 1998). If the cascade of illness is able to progress unabated, an older person who is admitted to the hospital with mild confusion and stable chronic illness could progress to serious illness functional decline, nursing home placement, or even death as a result of the hospitalization.

Ethical standards that guide healthcare decision making at the end of life support the self-determination of the patient (assuming the patient has made these known before becoming cognitively impaired) or best interests of the patient (in the case of the patient who did not execute advance directives before becoming impaired) (Veatch, 1989). An ethical dilemma that may arise is whether a patient should be treated for a secondary problem, such as infection, if death is pending.

Common reasons for withholding or withdrawing aggressive treatment include patient choice, excessively burdensome care, potential for further reduction in quality of life, prolongation of the dying process, and acknowledgment that the disease progression will inevitably result in death, and treatment is likely to be ineffective (Lesage & Latimer, 1998). Healthcare professionals may find it difficult to stop life-sustaining treatment because they have been educated to "do everything possible" to support life. Although life-sustaining treatments may be appropriate for some patients with frailty and dementia, such treatments may only prolong suffering of other patients. Palliative treatments such as surgery, radiation, or chemotherapy may be appropriate in that they relieve pain and suffering, but the benefit of these treatments should outweigh the burdens to ensure they are morally and ethically justified.

Healthcare treatments for coexisting diseases should be modified early in the course of care for the person with dementia. Because dementia shortens the life span, some interventions designed to reduce long-term risk factors can be avoided. High-risk interventions that are commonly carried out and are associated with limited chance of therapeutic success include cardiopulmonary resuscitation, tube feeding, intravenous therapy, fluid restriction, and invasive laboratory testing (Mitchel, Kiely, & Hamel, 2003; Volicer, Volicer, & Hurley, 1993). Invasive medical treatments often upset the patient's emotional-behavioral adjustment, either because such treatments cannot be understood by the recipient or because the extension of life will add to mental and physical suffering (Post, 1995).

When ethical dilemmas cannot be resolved through the usual care planning and communication process, the ethics committee should be consulted. All healthcare institutions should have access to an ethics committee to provide a forum for reflection and discussion of values, to build a moral community, and to attempt to meet the needs of the patient and family through group process and consensus. Ethics committees often validate or provide options regarding ethical dilemmas and support the care team in relation to already planned options (City of Hope & American Association of Colleges of Nursing, 2003).

Nurses in all settings should practice according to the following guidelines:

- Be aware of drug interactions. Polypharmacy and drug toxicity are key problems for older persons.
- Remember that the presentation of illness is less dramatic and more vague than in other age groups. Key signs and symptoms of heart disease, infection, gastrointestinal problems, depression, and cancer may not be accompanied by the classic signs and

symptoms seen in younger adults. Aggressively investigate falls, weight loss, confusion, fatigue, decline in functional ability, and incontinence.

- Conduct holistic nursing assessments when caring for frail older adults and those with comorbidities. Use valid and reliable assessment tools on admission and periodically thereafter to monitor the effect of treatments and interventions.
- Seek to access and provide the most intensive services to those considered the most frail and those diagnosed with multiple comorbidities. The comprehensive services provided by a multidisciplinary team can benefit the older adult with acute and chronic needs and deliver a full range of services across settings.
- Practice ethically according to professional standards. Try to establish advance directives and identify end-of-life preferences. Educate and empower older patients and families so that they can make more informed treatment decisions, avoid futile care, and refuse interventions that are excessively burdensome, painful, and invasive.
- Promote healthy aging in all clinical settings. Establishing a healthy lifestyle at any age will prevent or delay the onset of disability, make the pharmacological treatment of chronic illness more effective, and improve or maintain functional ability.
- Recognize and treat pain in older persons, including those with dementia or other disabilities that preclude them from adequately expressing their pain.
- Become expert at providing end-of-life care to the seriously ill and dying patient. The nurse can help provide a comfortable death that is free from pain and troubling symptoms in a supportive, caring environment.

- Seek continuing education programs and pursue advanced degrees. Keep current by reading journals. Collaborate with experts in nursing and other health professions, and advocate to improve care and services for older persons with health needs.

(Amella, 2004; Mezey & Fulmer, 1998; Young, 2003; Nurses Improving the Care of the Hospitalized Elderly (NICHE) project. See the Hartford Institute for Geriatric Nursing Website—www.hartfordign.org)

PATIENT-FAMILY TEACHING GUIDELINES

The nurse will often teach older persons and their families about planning for a hospital stay for surgery or treatment of an illness. The following guidelines may help an older person at risk for adverse outcomes to have a safer and more effective hospitalization experience.

1. What should I consider when planning to enter the hospital next week for treatment of my illness?

   Bring complete medical records with you to the hospital. Ask your doctor for a copy of your most recent laboratory values, your last physical examination, and an accounting of your past medical history including all hospitalizations, surgical interventions, invasive testing, and so on. Also bring a list of your current medications and dosing schedule, all of your contact information, contact information for your healthcare proxy, insurance information, and living will (if you have one).

2. What should I tell the nurses at the hospital when I am admitted?

   Tell them why you are there and what goals you would like to accomplish. Also tell them if you have allergies to food or medication, problems walking, bowel or bladder problems, sleep problems, chronic pain, or other important issues relating to your care. If you wear a hearing aid or glasses, please let the nurses know. Answer all of their questions as openly and honestly as you can. Your family or significant other can help, if you wish.

3. What personal items should I bring with me?

   Bring good walking slippers, a bathrobe, medical records, a book if you are a reader, a CD player for music, a small amount of money for incidental purchases, and pictures of your family. Avoid bringing valuable jewelry and large or bulky items. Ask your friends to send flowers when you go home instead of to the hospital because they can be difficult to carry out and can clutter up a small hospital room.

4. Besides my family, who should I notify regarding my hospitalization?

   You may want to let some close friends know and notify them of your visiting preferences. Some hospitalized patients like to have visitors and others prefer phone calls or cards. If you are religious, you should notify your priest, minister, or rabbi.

5. How can I prepare myself to come back to my home after my hospitalization?

   Your nurse and social worker will work with you and your family from the moment you are

(continued)

admitted so that you will be able to return to your previous level of function and living arrangement. Some older people find that after treatment for an illness or an operation they are too weak to go directly home, and a short stay at a rehabilitation facility may be indicated. You should discuss these options with your nurse, physician, and social worker when you reach the hospital.

6. I am worried that they will hitch me up to a machine and if something goes wrong, I will be a burden to my family.

Discuss the goals of your hospitalization and your fears with your healthcare providers and your family. Your predetermined wishes are critical to your care and will be clearly noted on your chart. If you do not have a current healthcare proxy, you will be asked to name one when you reach the hospital in the unlikely event that you will be unable to make decisions for yourself.

References

Agency for Health Care Policy and Research (AHCPR). U.S. Department of Health and Human Services. Panel for the Prediction of Pressure Ulcers in Adults. (1992). *Pressure ulcers in adults: Prediction and prevention. Clinical Practice Guideline No. 3* (AHCPR Bulletin No. 920047). Rockville, MD: Author.

Agency for Health Care Policy and Research. (1995). *Acute pain management: Operative or medical procedures and trauma* (AHCPR Publication No. 92-0032). Rockville, MD: U.S. Department of Health and Human Services.

Agency for Healthcare Research and Quality. (2001). *Reducing and preventing adverse drug events to decrease hospital costs* (AHRQ Publication No. 01-0020). Retrieved September 19, 2004, from www.ahrq.gov/qual/aderia/aderia.htm.

Ala, T. A., Mattson, M. D., & Frey, W. H. (2003). The clinical diagnosis of Alzheimer's disease without the use of head imaging studies. A cliniconeuropathological study. *Journal of Alzheimer's Disease, 5(6),* 463–465.

Albert, S., Im, A., & Raveis, V. (2002). Public health and the second 50 years of life. *American Journal of Public Health, 92(8)* 1–3.

Ali, A., & Lacy, B. (2004). Abdominal complaints and gastrointestinal disorders. C. Landefeld, R. Palmer, M. Johnson, C. Johnston, & W. Lyons, (Eds), In *Current geriatric diagnosis and treatment.* New York: Lange Medical Books/McGraw-Hill.

Amella, E. (2004). Presentation of illness in older adults. *American Journal of Nursing, 104(10),* 40–51.

American Academy of Ophthalmology. (2003). *Take care of your family's eyes at every stage of life.* Retrieved July 10, 2003, from www.aao.org/aao/news/release/091702.cfm.

American Association of Clinical Endocrinologists. (2002). AACE clinical practice guidelines for the evaluation and treatment of hyperthyroidism and hypothyroidism. *Thyroid Guidelines Task Force,* 1–23.

American Diabetes Association. (2001). Clinical practice recommendations. *Diabetes Care, 24* (S1–S1320).

American Geriatrics Society (AGS) Panel on Chronic Pain in

Older Persons. (2002). The management of persistent pain in older persons. *Journal of the American Geriatrics Society, 50,* S205–S224.

American Medical Association. (1992). *Diagnostic and treatment guidelines on elder abuse and neglect.* Chicago: Author.

American Medical Directors Association. (2001). *Altered nutritional status: Clinical practice guideline.* Washington, DC: Author.

American Nurses Association. (1994). *Position Statement: Assisted Suicide.* Retrieved April 14, 2002, from http://nursingworld.org.

American Nurses Association. (ANA) (2004). *Nursing: Scope and standards of practice.* Washington, DC: American Nurses Publishing.

American Pain Society. (1999). *Principles of analgesic use in the treatment of acute pain and cancer pain.* Glenview, IL: American Pain Society.

American Pain Society Quality of Care Committee. (1995). Quality improvement guidelines for the treatment of acute pain and cancer pain. *Journal of the American Medical Association, 274,* 1874–1880.

American Psychiatric Association, Committee on Nomenclature and Statistics. (2000). *Diagnostic and statistical manual of mental disorders* (4th ed., text revision) (*DSM-IV-TR*). Washington, DC: Author.

American Psychological Association. (1998). What practitioners should know about working with older adults. *Professional Psychology: Research and Practice, 29*(5), 413–427.

American Psychological Association. (2003). What practitioners should know about working with older adults. *Professional Psychology: Research and Practice, 29*(5), 413–427.

American Thoracic Society. (2002). *Diagnosis and care of patients with COPD.* Retrieved September 17, 2002, from www.thoracic.org.

American Thoracic Society. (2004). *Statement on cardiopulmonary exercise testing.* Retrieved November 9, 2004, from www.thoracic.org.

Ang-Lee, M. K., Moss, J., & Yuan, C. (2001). Herbal medicines and perioperative care. *Journal of the American Medical Association, 286,* 208–216.

Annon, J. (1974). *The behavioral treatment of sexual problems: Volume I, Brief therapy.* Honolulu, HI: Enabling Systems.

Applebaum, G. E., King, J. E., & Finucane, T. E. (1990). The outcome of cardiopulmonary resuscitation initiated in nursing homes. *Journal of the American Geriatrics Society, 38,* 197–200.

Aravanis, S. C., Adelman, R. D., Breckman, R., Fulmer, T., Holder, E., Lachs, M. S., et al. (1993). Diagnostic and treatment guidelines on elder abuse and neglect. *Archives of Family Medicine, 2*(4), 371–388.

Assad, L. A. D. (2000). Urinary incontinence in older men. *Topics in Geriatric Rehabilitation, 16*(1), 33–53.

Atchison, K. (1997). The general oral health assessment index (the geriatric oral health assessment index). In G. D. Slade (Ed.), *Measuring oral health and quality of life.* Chapel Hill: University of North Carolina, Dental Ecology.

Awoke, S., Mouton, C., & Parrott, M. (1992). Outcomes of skilled cardiopulmonary resuscitation in a long-term care facility: Futile therapy? *Journal of the American Geriatrics Society, 40,* 593–595.

Baatile, J., Langbein, W. E., Weaver, F., Maloney, C., & Jost, M. B. (2000). Effect of exercise on perceived quality of life of individuals with Parkinson's disease. *Journal of Rehabilitation Research & Development, 37,* 529–534.

Baddor, L. (2000). Cellulitis syndromes: An update. *International Journal of Antimicrobial Agents, 14*(2), 113–116.

Bailey, J. L., & Sands, J. M. (2003). Renal disease. In W. R. Hazzard, J. P. Blass, J. B. Halter, J. G. Ouslander, & M. E. Tinetti (Eds.), *Principles of geriatric medicine and gerontology* (5th ed., pp. 551–568). New York: McGraw-Hill.

Balducci, L., Pow-Sang, J., Friedland, J., & Diaz, J. I. (1997). Prostate cancer. *Clinics in Geriatric Medicine, 13*(2), 283–306.

Baranoski, S. (2001). Skin tears: Guard against the enemy of frail skin. *Nursing Management, 32*(8), 25–31.

Barzilai, N. (2003). Disorders of carbohydrate metabolism. In M. Beers & R. Berkow (Eds.), *Merck manual of geriatrics.* Internet Edition Merck & Co. Retrieved February 14, 2003, from http://www.merck.com/pubs/mm.

Beck, L. H. (1999). Aging changes in renal function. In W. R. Hazzard, J. P. Blass, W. H. Ettinger, J. B. Halter, & J. G. Ouslander (Eds.), *Principles of geriatric medicine and gerontology* (4th ed., pp. 767–776). New York: McGraw-Hill.

Beck-Little, R., & Weinrich, S. (1998). Assessment and management of sleep disorders in the elderly. *Journal of Gerontological Nursing, 24*(4), 21–29.

Becker, R. (2004). Hypercoagulability and anticoagulation. In M. Beers & R. Berkow (Eds.), *Merck manual of geriatrics.* Retrieved September 14, 2004, from www.merck.com.

Beers, M H., & Berkow, R. (2000). *The Merck manual of geriatrics* (3rd ed.). Whitehouse Station, NJ: Merck Research Laboratories.

Behrman, A. L., Light, K. E., Flynn, S. M., & Thigpen, M. T. (2002). Is the functional reach test useful for identifying falls risk among individuals with Parkinson's disease? *Archives of Physical Medicine & Rehabilitation, 83,* 538–542.

Beitz, J. M., & Zuzelo, P. R. (2003). The lived experience of having a neobladder. *Western Journal of Nursing Research, 25,* 294–316.

Berenbeim, D., Parrott, M., Purnell, J., & Pennachio, D.

(2001). How to manage diabetes in the older patient. *Patient Care*/January 30. Retrieved August 9, 2002, from www.patientcareonline.com.

Berne, R., & Levy, M. (2000). Blood and hemostasis. In *Principles of physiology* (3rd ed.). Boston: Mosby.

Bille-Brahe, U., & Andersen, K. (2001). Suicide among the Danish elderly. In D. De Leo (Ed.), *Suicide and euthanasia in older adults: A transcultural journey* (pp. 47–56). Seattle, WA: Hogrefe & Huber.

Blackwell, S., & Hendrix, P. (2001). Common anemias. *Clinical Reviews, 11* (3), 53–64.

Blair, E. (1999). Diabetes in the older adult. *Advance for Nurse Practitioners, 7*(7), 33–36.

Blehar, M., & Oren, D. (1997). Gender differences in depression. *Medscape Women's Health Journal, 2*(1). Retrieved on June 14, 2000, from www.medscape.com/urewartich/408844.

Block, S. D. (2001). Perspectives on care at the close of life. Psychological considerations, growth and transcendence at the end of life: The art of the possible. *Journal of the American Medical Association, 285,* 2898–2906.

Bogardus, S.T., Yueh, B., & Shekelle, P. (2003). Screening and management of adult hearing loss in primary care. *Journal of the American Medical Association, 289*(15), 1986–1990.

Bootzin, R. R., Epstein, D., & Wood, J. M. (1991). Stimulus control instructions. In P. J. Hauri (Ed.), *Case studies in insomnia* (pp. 19–28). New York: Plenum.

Borum, M. (2004). Esophageal disorders. In M. Beers & R. Berkow (Eds.), *Merck manual of geriatrics.* Retrieved January 18, 2004, from www.merck.com.

Bottomley, J. M. (2000). Complementary nutrition in treating urinary incontinence. *Topics in Geriatric Rehabilitation, 16,* 61–77.

Boustani, M., Peterson, B., Hanson, L., Harris, R., Lohr, K. N., & U.S. Preventive Services Task Force. (2003). Screening for dementia in primary care: A summary of the evidence for the U.S. Preventive Services Task Force. *Annals of Internal Medicine, 138,* 927–937.

Boynton, P. R., Jaworski, D., & Paustian, C. (1999). Meeting the challenges of healing chronic wounds in older adults. *Nursing Clinics of North America, 34*(4), 921–932.

Braden, B., & Bergstrom, N. (1994). Predictive validity of the Braden scale for pressure sore risk in a nursing home population. *Research in Nursing and Health, 17,* 459–479.

Bravo, C. V. (2000). Aging of the urogenital system. *Reviews in Clinical Gerontology, 10,* 315–324.

Bromley, S. (2000). Smell and taste disorders: A primary care approach. *American Family Physician, 61,* 427–436.

Brown, A. D. G., & Cooper, T. K. (1998). Gynecologic orders in the elderly—sexuality and aging. In

R. Tallis, H. Fillit, & J. C. Brocklehurst (Eds.), *Brocklehurst's textbook of geriatric medicine and gerontology* (5th ed, pp. 987–997). Edinburgh Scotland: Churchill Livingstone.

Brown, D. B. (1999). Managing sleep disorders. *Clinician Reviews, 9*(10), 51–71.

Brown, J., Vittinghoff, E., Wyman, J., Stone, K., Nevitt, M., Ensrud, K., et al. (2000). Urinary incontinence: Does it increase risk for falls and fractures. *Journal of the American Geriatrics Society, 48*(7), 721–725.

Brownell, P. (1999). Mental health and criminal justice issues among perpetrators of elder abuse. *Journal of Elder Abuse and Neglect, 11*(4), 81–94.

Burger, S. G., Kayser-Jones, J., & Bell, J. P. (2001). Food for thought. Preventing/treating malnutrition and dehydration. *Contemporary Long Term Care, 24,* 24–28.

Burke, T. (2002). *A grey area: Colour specification in dementia-specific accommodation.* Retrieved December 10, 2002, from www.dementia.com.au/papers/TimBurkeFINALVERSION.htm.

Burman, K. (2000). *Clinical management of hypothyroidism.* Retrieved September 14, 2001, from www.medscape.com.

Burman, K. (2001). Graves' disease in women. *Women's Health in Primary Care, 4*(4), 306–317.

Butler, R. N., & Lewis, M. I. (2003). Sexuality and aging. In

W. R. Hazzard, J. P. Blass, J. B. Halter, J. G. Ouslander, & M. E. Tinetti (Eds.), *Principles of geriatric medicine and gerontology* (5th ed., pp. 1277–1282). New York: McGraw-Hill.

Caboral, M., & Mitchell, J. (2003). New guidelines for heart failure focus on prevention. *Nurse Practitioner, 28*(1), 13, 16, 22–23.

California Advocates for Nursing Home Reform. (2002). *Elder abuse: What can you do to prevent elder abuse.* Retrieved November 10, 2004, from www.canhr.org/abuse/abuse_prevent.htm.

California Healthcare Foundation/American Geriatrics Society Panel on Improving Care for Elders with Diabetes. (2003). *Journal of the American Geriatrics Society, 51*(5), S5265–5280.

Calle, E. E., Thun, M. J., Petrelli, J. M., Rodriguez, C., & Heath, C. W. (1999). Body-mass index and mortality in a prospective cohort of U.S. adults. *New England Journal of Medicine, 341,* 1097–1105.

Camilleri, M., Lee, J., Viramontes, B., Bharucha, A., & Tangalos, E. (2000). Insights into the pathophysiology and mechanisms of constipation, irritable bowel syndrome and diverticulosis in older people. *Journal of the American Geriatrics Society, 48,* 1142–1150.

Capezuti, E. (2002). Side rail use and bed-related fall outcomes among nursing home residents. *Journal of the*

American Geriatrics Society, 50(1), 90–96.

Capezuti, E., Brush, B. L., & Lawson, W. T. (1997). Reporting elder mistreatment. *Journal of Gerontological Nursing, 23*(7), 24–32.

Carbone, D. J., & Seftel, A. D. (2002). Erectile dysfunction: Diagnosis and treatment in older men. *Geriatrics, 57*(9), 18–24.

Cassell, C., & Foley, K. (1999). *Principles of care of patients at the end of life: An emerging consensus among the specialties of medicine.* New York: Millbank Memorial Fund.

Castells, A. (2004). Gastrointestinal tumors. In M. Beers & R. Berkow (Eds.), *Merck manual of geriatrics.* Retrieved January 22, 2004, from www.merck.com.

Centers for Disease Control. (1999). *Special focus: Healthy aging.* Retrieved August 19, 2000, from www.cdc.gov/nccdphp.

Centers for Disease Control. (2001). *Oral health for older Americans.* Retrieved November 12, 2004, from www.cdc.gov.

Centers for Disease Control. (2003). *Questions and answers about TB.* www.cdc.gov.

Centers for Medicare and Medicaid Services. (2002). *Minimum Data Set manual, version 2.0.* Retrieved June 16, 2003, from http://www.cms.hhs.gov/medicaid/mds20/mds0900b.pdf.

Chalmers, J. (2000). Behavior management and communication strategies for dental professionals when caring for patients with dementia. *Special Care Dentistry, 20,* 147–154.

Chen, H. X., Ryan, P. A., & Ferguson, R. P. (1998). Characteristics of acquired immunodeficiency syndrome in older adults. *Journal of the American Geriatrics Society, 46*(2), 153–156.

Cheng, C., Umland, E., & Muirhead, G. (2000, June 15). New and old drugs to treat insomnia. *Patient Care,* 34–43. Retrieved March 12, 2001, from http://www.patientcareonline.com.

Chesson, A. (2000). Practice parameters for the evaluation of insomnia. *Sleep, 23*(4), 237–241.

Chia-Hui, C., Schilling, L. S., & Lyder, C. H. (2001). A concept analysis of malnutrition in the elderly. *Journal of Advanced Nursing, 36*(1), 131–142.

Chow, R. D. (2001). Benign prostatic hyperplasia: Patient evaluation and relief of obstructive symptoms. *Geriatrics, 56*(3), 33–38.

City of Hope & American Association of Colleges of Nursing. (2003). *ELNEC graduate curriculum.* End of Life Nursing Care at the End of Life. Education Consortium, Nat'l Cancer Institute, Bethesda, MD.

Cobin, R., Weisen, M., & Trotto, N. (1999). Hypothyroidism, hyperthyroidism, hyperparathyroidism. *Patient Care, 9,* 185–206.

Cockcroft, D. W., & Gault, M. H. (1976). Prediction of creatinine clearance from serum creatinine. *Nephron, 16,* 31.

Coleman, P. (2002). Improving oral health care for the frail elderly: A review of widespread problems and best practices. *Geriatric Nursing, 23*(4), 189–198.

Connell, B., McConnell, E., & Francis, T. (2002). Tailoring the environment of oral health care to the needs and abilities of nursing home residents with dementia. *Alzheimer's Care Quarterly, 3*(1), 19–25.

Copstead, L. C., & Banasik, J. L. (2000). *Pathophysiology, biological and behavioral perspectives* (2nd ed., pp. 184–218). Philadelphia: Saunders.

Council for Nutrition Clinical Strategies in Long-Term Care. (2001). Anorexia in the elderly: An update. *Annals of Long-Term; Care,* Supplement; 2–14.

Counsell, S., Holder, C., Liebenauer, L., Palmer, R., Fortunsky, R., Kresevic, D., Quinn, L. et al. (2000). Effects of a multicomponent intervention on functional outcomes and process of care in hospitalized older patients: A randomized controlled trial of acute care for elders (ACE) in a community hospital. *Journal of the American Geriatrics Society, 48*(12), 1572–1581.

Covinsky, K. E. (2002). Malnutrition and bad outcomes. *Journal of General Internal Medicine, 17,* 956–957.

Covinsky, K. E., Covinsky, M. H., Palmer, R. M., & Sehgal, A. R. (2002). Serum albumin concentration and clinical assessments of nutritional status in hospitalized older people: Different sides of different coins? *Journal of the American Geriatrics Society, 50,* 631–637.

Coyle, C. (2003). Current management of diabetes mellitus in adults. *Advance for Nurse Practitioners, 11*(5), 33–38.

Craven, R. F. (2000). Physiologic adaptation with aging. In S. L. Woods, E. S. S. Froelicher, & S. A. Motzer (Eds.), *Cardiac nursing* (4th ed., pp. 180–185). Philadelphia: Lippincott.

Cunningham, S. (2000a). High blood pressure. In S. L. Woods, E. S. S. Froelicher, & S. A. Motzer (Eds.), *Cardiac nursing* (4th ed., pp. 777–817). Philadelphia: Lippincott.

Dahlin, C. (2004). Oral complications at the end of life. *American Journal of Nursing, 104*(7), 40–47.

Danner, C. J., & Harris, J. P. (2003). Hearing loss and the aging ear. *Geriatrics and Aging, 6*(5), 40–43.

Del Bene, S., & Vaughan, A. (2000). Diagnosis and management of myocardial infarction. In S. L. Woods, E.S.S. Froelicher, & S. A. Motzer (Eds.), *Cardiac nursing* (4th ed., pp. 513–540). Philadelphia: Lippincott.

Dembner, A. (2004, September 14). Hospices widen care services. *Boston Globe,* B24.

Demers, K. (2001). *Hearing screening. Try this: Best practices in nursing to care for older adults,* Hartford Institute for Geriatric Nursing, 12.

Demling, R., & DeSanti, L. (2001). Protein-energy malnutrition, and the non-healing cutaneous wound. *CME.* Retrieved 2003, from www.medscape.com/ viewprogram/714?

Department of Health and Human Services Office of Inspector General. (2001). *Psychotropic Drug Use in Nursing Homes.* Retrieved February 12, 2005, from www.oig.hhs.gov/oei/reports/ oei-02-00-00490.pdf.

Diabetes Guidelines Work Group. (1999). *Massachusetts guidelines for adult diabetes care.* Boston: Massachusetts Department of Public Health, Massachusetts Health Promotion Clearinghouse.

Digiovanna, A. G. (2000). *Human aging, Biological perspectives* (2nd ed., pp. 46–47, 312–326). New York: McGraw-Hill.

Drickamer, M. A., & Lachs, M. S. (1992). Should patients with Alzheimer's disease be told their diagnosis. *New England Journal of Medicine, 326,* 947–951.

Duda, J. E. (2004). Pathology and neurotransmitter abnormalities of dementia with Lewy bodies. *Dementia & Geriatric Cognitive Disorders, 17,* 3–14.

Duffy, L. M. (1998). Lovers, loners, and lifers: Sexuality and the older adult. *Geriatrics, 53* (Suppl. 1), S66–S69.

Dunlop, B., Rothman, M. B., Condon, K. M., Hebert, K. S., & Martinez, I. L. (2000). Elder abuse: Risk factors and use of case data to improve policy and practice. *Journal of Elder Abuse and Neglect, 12*(3/4), 95–122.

Duthie, E., Mark, D., Tresch, D., Kartes, S., Neahring, J., & Aufderheide, T. (1993). Utilization of cardiopulmonary resuscitation in nursing homes in one community: Rates and nursing home characteristics. *Journal of the American Geriatrics Society, 41,* 384–388.

Eastley, R., Wilcock, G. K., & Bucks, R. S. (2000). Vitamin B-12 deficiency in dementia and cognitive impairment: The effects of treatment on neuropsychological function. *International Journal of Geriatric Psychiatry, 15,* 226–233.

End-of-Life Nursing Education Consortium (ELNEC). (2003). Care Curriculum. American Association of College of Revising and City of Hope National Medical Center, Los Angeles, City.

Epocrates.com. (2003). *Prescription medication information program.* Retrieved March 14, 2003, from www.Epocrates.com.

Epocrates.com. (2004). *Adverse drug events—hemolytic anemia.* Retrieved September 14, 2004, from www.epocrates.com.

Epocrates.com. (2004). Drug and formulary reference.

Retrieved October 14, 2004, from www.epocrates.com.

Epocrates.com. (2004). Epocrates essentials, drug information program. Retrieved November 13, 2004, from www.epocrates.com.

Ettinger, W. (2003a). Local joint, tendon, and bursa disorders. In M. Beers & R. Berkow (Eds.), *The Merck manual of geriatrics* (3rd ed., pp. 489–493). Whitehouse Station, NJ: Merck Research Laboratories.

Evans, W. (1997). Functional and metabolic consequences of sarcopenia. *Journal of Nutrition, 127,* 998S–1003S.

Expert Consensus Panel. (2004). Treatment of agitation in older persons with dementia. Expert Knowledge Systems. Alexopoulos, G., Silver, J., Kahn, D., Frances, A., & Carpenter, D. (Eds). Retrieved December 13, 2004, from www.psychguides.com.

Fahey, V. A. (1999). *Vascular nursing* (3rd ed.). Philadelphia: W. B. Saunders.

Fahey, V. A., & McCarthy, W. J. (1999). Arterial reconstruction of the lower extremity. In V. A. Fahey, *Vascular nursing* (3rd ed., pp. 233–269). Philadelphia: W. B. Saunders.

Fair, J. M., & Berra, K. A. (2000). Lipid management and coronary heart disease. In S. L. Woods, E. S. S. Froelicher, & S. A. Motzer (Eds.), *Cardiac nursing* (4th ed., pp. 819–834). Philadelphia: Lippincott.

Fairfield, K. M. & Fletcher, R. H. (2002). Vitamins for chronic disease prevention in adults:

Scientific review. *Journal of the American Medical Association, 287,* 3116–3126.

Farlow, M. R. (2003). Update on rivastigmine. *Neurologist, 9(5),* 230–234.

Feldman, H., Gauthier, S., Hecker, J., Vellas, B., Subbiah, P., Whalen, E., et al. (2001). A 24-week, randomized, double-blind study of donepezil in moderate to severe Alzheimer's disease. *Neurology, 57,* 613–620.

Fielo, S. (2001). Focus on feet. *Nursing Spectrum, 5*(12NE), 12–15.

Fine, S. L., Berger, J.W., Maguire, M. G., & Ho, A. C. (2000). Age-related macular degeneration. *New England Journal of Medicine, 342*(7), 483–492.

Finucane, T. E., Christmas, C., & Travis, K. (1999). Tube feeding in patients with advanced dementia: A review of the evidence. *Journal of the American Medical Association, 282,* 1365–1370.

Floyd, J. (1999). Sleep promotion in adults. *Annual Review of Nursing Research, 17*(6)27–56.

Fretwell, M. (1998). Acute hospital care for frail older patients. In W. Hazzard, E. Bierman, J. Blass, W. Ettinger, & J. Halter (Eds.), *Principles of geriatric medicine and gerontology.* New York: McGraw-Hill.

Fried, L. (1994). Frailty. In W. Hazzard, E. Bierman, J. Blass, W. Ettinger, & J. Halter (Eds.), *Principles of geriatric medicine and gerontology.* New York: McGraw-Hill.

Fried, L., Tangen, C., Walston, J., Newman, A., Hirsch, C., Gottdiener, J., et al. (2001). Frailty of older adults: Evidence for a phenotype. *Journals of Gerontology: Biological Sciences and Medical Sciences, 56A*(3), M146–156.

Friedman, M. (2004). Aging and the blood; Anemias; Hematologic malignancies; Lymphomas. In M. Beers & R. Berkow (Eds.), *Merck manual of geriatrics.* Retrieved September 14, 2004, from www.merck.com.

Frisoni, G. B., Franzoni, S., Bellelli, G., Morris, J., & Warden, V. (1998). Overcoming eating difficulties in the severely demented. In L.Volicer & A. Hurley (Eds.), *Hospice care for patients with advanced progressive dementia* (pp. 48–67). New York: Springer.

Fulmer, T., & O'Malley, T. (1987). *Inadequate care of the elderly: A health care perspective on abuse and neglect.* New York: Springer.

Fulmer, T., Feldman, P. H., Kim, T. S., Carty, B., Beers, M., Molina, M., & Putnam, M. (1999). An intervention study to enhance medication compliance. *Journal of Gerontological Nursing, 25*(8), 6–14.

Fune, L., Shua-Haim, J. R., Ross, J. S., & Frank, E. (1998). Infectious diseases in the elderly. *Clinical Geriatrics, 6*(3), 31–50.

Gambert, S. R. (2001). Prostate cancer: When to offer screening in the primary care setting. *Geriatrics, 56,* 22–31.

Garfinkle, D., Zisapel, N., Wainstein, J., & Laudon, M. (1999). Facilitation of benzodiazepine discontinuation by melatonin. *Archives of Internal Medicine, 159*(20), 1–11.

Georgetown University. (2004). *Cultural competence in health care: Is it important for people with chronic conditions?* Institute for Health Care Research and Policy, Issue Brief 5. Georgetown University Center for Research and Policy, Washington, DC.

Geronurse Online. (2004). *Mealtime difficulties.* Retrieved September 9, 2004, from www.geronurseonline.org.

Gilchrist, B., & Chiu, N. (2000). Pressure sores. In M. Beers & R. Berkow (Eds.), *The Merck manual of geriatrics* (chap. 14, pp. 155–169): Merck & Co. Whitehouse Station.

Glaser, B., & Strauss, A. (1968). *A time for dying.* Chicago: Aldine.

Gordon, M. (1994). *Nursing diagnosis: Process and application.* St. Louis, MO: Mosby.

Gray, P., & Hildebrand, K. (2000). Fall risk factors in Parkinson's disease. *Journal of Neuroscience Nursing, 32,* 222–228.

Halpin-Landry, J., & Goldsmith, S. (1999). Feet first. Diabetes care. *American Journal of Nursing, 99*(2), 26–34.

Hamers, J. P. H., Gulpers, M. J. M., & Strik, W.

(2004). Use of physical restraints with cognitively impaired nursing home residents. *Journal of Advanced Nursing, 45,* 246–251.

Hartford Institute for Geriatric Nursing. (1999). *Best nursing practices in care for older adults.* Retrieved October 17, 2003, from www.hartfordign.org.

Hartford Institute for Geriatric Nursing. (1999). *Best nursing practices in care of older adults.* New York: New York University.

Hartford Institute for Geriatric Nursing. (2001). *Incorporating essential gerontologic content into baccalaureate nursing education and staff development* (3rd ed.). New York: Author.

Hazzard, W. R., Blass, J. P., Ettinger, W. H., Halter, J. B., & Ouslander, J.G. (1999). *Principles of geriatric medicine and gerontology.* New York: McGraw-Hill.

Health Resources and Services Administration. (1996). *A national agenda for geriatric education: White papers* (Vol. 1). Washington, DC: U.S. Department of Health and Human Services.

Hegge, M., & Fischer, C. (2000). Grief responses of senior and elderly widows: Practice implications. *Journal of Gerontological Nursing, 26*(2) February, 35–43.

Horowitz, M. (2004). Aging and the gastrointestinal tract. In M. Beers & R. Berkow (Eds.), *Merck manual of geriatrics.* Retrieved August 4, 2004, from www.merck.com.

Howard, L., West, D., & Ossip-Klein, D. (2000). Chronic constipation management for institutionalized older adults. *Geriatric Nursing, 21*(2), 78–82.

Hu, P., Seeman, T., Harris, T.B., & Reuben, D. B. (2003). Does inflammation or undernutrition explain the low cholesterol-mortality association in high-functioning older persons? MacArthur studies of successful aging. *Journal of the American Geriatrics Society, 51,* 80–84.

Huebscher, R. (1999). Natural, alternative, and complementary therapies for sleep. *Nurse Practitioner Forum, 10*(3), 117–119.

Huffman, G. B. (2002). Evaluating and treating unintentional weight loss in the elderly. *American Family Physician, 65,* 640–650.

Hunt, S. A., Baker, D. W., Chin, M. W., Cinquegrani, M. P., Feldman, A. M., Francis, G.S., et al. (2001). ACC/AHA guidelines for the evaluation and management of chronic heart failure in the adult: Executive summary. *Journal of the American College of Cardiology, 38,* 2101–2113.

Hutton, B., Feine, J., & Morais, J. (2002). Is there an association between edentulism and nutritional state? *Journal of the Canadian Dental Association, 68*(3), 182–187.

Institute of Medicine. (2002). *Confronting chronic neglect: The education and training of health professionals on family violence.* Washington, DC: National Academy Press.

Institute of Medicine, Food and Nutrition Board. (1997). *Dietary reference intakes for calcium, phosphorus, magnesium, vitamin D and fluoride.* Washington, DC: National Academy Press.

Institute of Medicine, Food and Nutrition Board. (1998). *Dietary reference intakes for thiamine, riboflavin, niacin, vitamin B-6, folate, vitamin B-12, pantothenic acid, biotin and choline.* Washington, DC: National Academy Press.

Institute of Medicine, Food and Nutrition Board (2000). *Dietary reference intakes for Vitamin C, Vitamin E, Selenium and Carotenoids.* Washington, DC: National Academy Press.

Institute of Medicine, Food and Nutrition Board. (2004). *Dietary reference intakes for water, potassium, sodium, chloride, and sulfate.* Washington, DC: National Academy Press.

Jackler, R. K. (2003). A 73-year-old man with hearing loss. *Journal of the American Medical Association, 289*(12), 1557–1565.

Jao, D., & Alessi, C. (2004). Sleep disorders. In C. Landefeld, R. Palmer, M. Johnson, C. Johnston, & W. Lyons (Eds.), *Current geriatric diagnosis and treatment.* New York: Lange Medical Books/McGraw-Hill.

Jarvis, C. (2004). *Physical examination and health assessment* (4th ed.). Philadelphia: Saunders.

Jassal, V., Fillit, H., & Oreopoulos, D. G. (1998). Diseases of the aging kidney. In R. Tallis, H. Fillit, & J. C. Brocklehurst (Eds.), *Brocklehurst's textbook of geriatric medicine and gerontology* (5th ed., pp. 949–971). Edinburgh: Churchill Livingstone.

Jenike, M. (1999). *Depression in the elderly. Geriatric medicine.* Boston: Harvard Medical School, Division on Aging.

Johns, A. F., & Sabatino, C. P. (2002). Wingspan—The second national guardianship conference recommendations. *Stetson Law Review, 31*(3), 595–609.

Joint Commission on Accreditation of Healthcare Organizations. (2003). *Improving the Quality of Pain Management through Measurement and Action.* Oakbrook Terraa, IL: Department of Publications, Joint Commission Resources.

Joint National Committee on Prevention, Detection, Evaluation, and Treatment of High Blood Pressure & National High Blood Pressure Education Program Coordinating Committee. (2003). *The seventh report of the Joint National Committee on Prevention, Detection, Evaluation, and Treatment of High Blood Pressure.* Retrieved November 9, 2004, from www.nhlbi.nih.gov/guidelines/hypertension.

Journal of the American Medical Association. (2000). *JAMA Patient Page: Psychiatric illness in older adults, 283*(21), 2886.

Kado, D., Karlamangla, A., Huang, M., Troen, A., Rowe, J.,

Selhub, J., & Seeman, T. (2004). *Homocysteine versus the vitamins folate, B_6 and B_{12} as predictors of cognitive function and decline in older high functioning adults: Macarthur studies of successful aging.* Retrieved December 6, 2004, from ars.usda.gov.

Kagan, S. (2004). *The advanced practice nurse in an aging society. The 2004 sourcebook for advanced practice nurses.* Lippincott Williams & Wilkins. Philadelphia, PA. Retrieved 9/21/2004. www.tnpj.com.

Kane, R., Ouslander, J., & Abrass, I. (1999). *Essentials of clinical geriatrics* (3rd ed.). New York: McGraw-Hill.

Kane, R. L., Ouslander, J. G., & Abrass, I. B. (2004). *Essentials of clinical geriatrics* (5th ed.). New York: McGraw-Hill.

Kase, E., & Ostrov, B. (2001). Intricacies in the diagnosis and treatment of gout. *Patient Care, 33*–47. Retrieved November, 2002, from www.patientcare. com.

Kayser-Jones, J., & Pengilly, K. (1999). Dysphagia among nursing home residents. *Geriatric Nursing, 20*(2), 77–84.

Kayser-Jones, J., & Schell, E. (1997). The mealtime experience of a cognitively impaired elder: Ineffective and effective strategies. *Journal of Gerontological Nursing, 23*(7), 33–39.

Kennedy-Malone, L., Fletcher, K. R., & Plank, L. M. (2000). *Management guidelines for gerontological nurse practitioners.* Philadelphia: F. A. Davis.

Kerr, L. D. (2003). Inflammatory arthritis in the elderly. *Mount Sinai Journal of Medicine, 70*(1), 23–26.

Kimmick, G., & Muss, H. B. (1997). Breast cancer in older women. *Clinics in Geriatric Medicine, 13*(2), 265–282.

Krasner, D., & Sibbald, G. (1999). Nursing management of chronic wounds. *Nursing Clinics of North America, 34*(4), 933–948.

Krogh, R. H., & Bruskewitz, R. C. (1998). Disorders of the lower genitourinary tract. *Clinical Geriatrics, 6*(13), 19–25.

Kuritzky, L. (2001). Hypothyroidism. *American Journal for Nurse Practitioners,* May, 26–41.

Kyba, F. (1999). Improving care at the end of life: Barriers, challenges and resources. *Texas Nursing,* September, 6–13.

Lachs, M. S., & Pillemer, K. A. (1995). Abuse and neglect of elderly persons. *New England Journal of Medicine, 332*(7), 437–443.

Lachs, M. S., Williams, C., O'Brien, S., Hurst, L., & Horwitz, R. I. (1997). Risk factors for reported elder abuse and neglect: A nine-year observational cohort study. *Gerontologist, 37*(4), 469–474.

Landefeld, C. (2004). Hospital care. In C. Landefeld, R. Palmer, M. Johnson, C. Johnston, & W. Lyons (Eds.), *Current geriatric diagnosis and treatment*. New York: Lange Medical Books.

Laurent-Bopp, D. (2000). Heart failure. In S. L. Woods, E. S. S. Froelicher, & S. A. Motzer (Eds.), *Cardiac nursing* (4th ed., pp. 560–579). Philadelphia: Lippincott.

Leber, K., Perron, V., & Sinni-McKeehan, B. (1999). Common skin cancers in the United States: A practical guide for diagnosis and treatment. *Nurse Practitioner Forum, 10*(2), 106–112.

Lee, A. G., & Beaver, H. A. (2003). Visual loss in the elderly — Part 1: Chronic visual loss: What to recognize and when to refer. *Clinical Geriatrics, 11*(6), 46–53.

Lekan-Rutledge, D., & Colling, J. (2003). Urinary incontinence in the frail elderly. *American Journal of Nursing, 103*(Suppl. 3), 36–46.

LeMone, P., & Burke, K. (2004). *Medical-surgical nursing: Critical thinking in client care* (3rd ed.). Upper Saddle River, NJ: Prentice Hall Health.

Lesage, P., & Latimer, E. (1998). An approach to ethical issues. In N. MacDonald (Ed.), *Palliative medicine: A case-based approach*. New York: Oxford University Press.

Letran, J. L., & Brawer, M. K. (1999). Disorders of the prostate. In W. R. Hazzard, J. P. Blass, W. H. Ettinger, J. B. Halter, & J. G. Ouslander (Eds.), *Principles of geriatric medicine and gerontology* (4th ed., pp. 809–821). New York: McGraw-Hill.

Li, I., & Smith, R. V. (2003). Driving and the elderly. *Clinical Geriatrics, 11*(5), 40–46.

Lichtenberg, P. A. (1997). Clinical perspectives on sexual issues in nursing homes. *Topics in Geriatric Rehabilitation, 12*(4), 1–10.

Lichtman, S. (2003). Guidelines for the treatment of elderly cancer patients. *Cancer Control, 10*(6), 445–453.

Lockwood, A. H., Salvi, R. J., & Burkard, R. F. (2002). Tinnitus. *New England Journal of Medicine, 347*(12), 904–910.

Logsdon, R. G., Teri, L., McCurry, S. M., Gibbons, L. E., Kukull, W. A., & Larson, E. B. (1998). Wandering: A significant problem among community-residing individuals with Alzheimer's disease. *The Journal of Gerontology, 53*, P294–P299.

Lopez, O. L., Becker, J. T., Wisniewski, S., Saxton, J., Kaufer, D. I., & DeKosky, S. T. (2002). Cholinesterase inhibitor treatment alters the natural history of Alzheimer's disease. *Journal of Neurology, Neurosurgery & Psychiatry, 72*, 310–314.

Lozada, C., & Altman, R. (2001). Osteoarthritis. In L. Robbins, C. Burckhardt, & R. Dehoratius (Eds.), *Clinical care in the rheumatic diseases* (pp. 113–119). Atlanta, GA: Association of Rheumatology Health Professionals.

Lunney, J., Lynn, J., Foley, D., Lipson, S., & Guralnik, J. (2003). Patterns of functional decline at the end of life. *Journal of the American*

Medical Association, 289(18), 2387–2392.

Mahoney, E. K., Hurley, A. C., Volicer, L., Bell, M., Gianotis, P., Harsthorn, M., et al. (1999). Development and testing of the resistiveness to care scale. *Research in Nursing and Health, 22,* 27–38.

Malone, M., & Danto-Nocton, E. (2004). Improving the hospital care of nursing facility residents. *Annals of Long-Term Care, 12*(5), 42–49.

Manolagas, S. (2003). Aging and the musculoskeletal system. In M. Beers & R. Berkow (Eds.), *The Merck manual of geriatrics.* Whitehouse Station, NJ: Merck Research Laboratories.

Manthorpe, J., & Watson, R. (2003). Poorly served? Eating and dementia. *Journal of Advanced Nursing, 41,* 162–169.

Marcincuk, M. C., & Roland, P. S. (2002). Geriatric hearing loss: Understanding the causes and providing appropriate treatment. *Geriatrics, 57*(4), 44.

Marcus, M. B. (2002). Aging of AIDS. *U.S. News and World Report, 133*(6), 40.

Marson, D., Dymek, M., & Geyer, J. (2001). Informed consent and competency. *Neurologist, 7,* 317–326.

Martin, R., & Whitehouse, P. (1990). Evaluation of dementia. *Neurology, 40,* 439–443.

Marui, W., Iseki, E., Kato, M., Akatsu, H., & Kosaka, K. (2004). Pathological entity of dementia with Lewy bodies and its differentiation from Alzheimer's disease. *Acta*

Neuropathologica, 108, 121–128.

Matear, D. (2000). How should we deliver and assess oral health education in seniors' institutions? *Journal of the Gerontological Nursing Association, Perspectives, 24*(2), 15–21.

McCaffery, M., & Pasero, C. (1999). *Pain: Clinical Manual* (2nd ed.). St. Louis, Mo: Mosby.

McCague, P. A. (1999). Taste and smell losses in normal aging and disease. *Journal of Dental Hygiene, 73*(2), 105.

McCance, K., & Huether, S. (2001). *Pathophysiology: The biologic basis for disease in adults and children.* St. Louis, MO: Mosby.

McCance, K., & Mourad, L. (2000). Alterations in musculoskeletal function. In S. Huether & K. McCance (Eds.), *Understanding pathophysiology* (pp. 1031–1074). St. Louis, MO: Mosby.

McCrea, L. (2003). *Anatomy and physiology of constipation. New approaches to the management of constipation.* Symposium highlights, Medical Association Communications, Wrightstown, PA.

McCue, J. D. (1999). Treatment of urinary tract infections in long-term care facilities: Advice, guidelines, and algorithms. *Clinical Geriatrics, 7*(8), 11–17.

McCusker, J., Cole, M., Abrahamowicz, M., Han, L., Podoba, J., & Ramman-Haddad, L. (2001). Environmental risk factors for delirium in hospitalized older people. *Journal of the American Geriatrics Society, 49,* 1327–1334.

Medline Plus. (2004). *Medical encyclopedia: Sickle cell anemia.* U.S. National Library of Medicine and the National Institutes of Health. Retrieved September 14, 2004, from www.nlm.nih.gov.

Meiner, S. (2001). Gouty arthritis: Not just a big toe problem. *Geriatric Nursing, 22,* 132–134.

Merck manual of geriatrics. (2001). Rahway, NJ: Merck Sharp & Dohme Research Laboratories.

Merritt, S. (2000). Putting sleep disorders to rest. *RN, 63*(7), 26–30. Retrieved March 12, 2001, from www.rnweb.com.

Messinger-Rapport, B. J., & Thacker, H. L. (2001). Prevention for the older woman: A practical guide to hormone replacement therapy and urogynecologic health. *Geriatrics, 56*(9), 32–42.

Metter, E., Lynch, N., Conwit, R., Lindle, R., Tobin, J., & Hurley, B. (1999). Muscle quality and age: Cross-sectional and longitudinal comparisons. *Journals of Gerontology Series A: Biological Sciences and Medical Sciences Online, 54*(5), B207–218.

Mezey, M., & Fulmer, T. (1998). Quality care for the frail elderly. *Nursing Outlook, 46*(6), 291–292.

Miller, D. (2001). Pharmacologic interventions in

the 21st century. In L. Robbins, C. Burckhardt, & R. Dehoratius (Eds.), *Clinical care in the rheumatic diseases* (pp. 169–177). Atlanta, GA: Association of Rheumatology Health Professionals.

Miller, M. (2000). Nocturnal polyuria in older people: Pathophysiology and clinical implications. *Journal of the American Geriatrics Society, 48,* 1321–1329.

Mini Nutrition Assessment. (2003). *Tool and information on usage.* Retrieved June 16, 2003, from http://www.mna-elderly. com.

Mitchell, S., Kiely, D., & Hamel, M. (2003). Dying with advanced dementia in the nursing home. *Archives of Internal Medicine, 164,* 321–326.

Mitchell, S. L., Teno, J. M., Roy, J., Kabumoto, G., & Mor, V. (2003). Clinical and organizational factors associated with feeding tube use among nursing home residents with advanced cognitive impairment. *Journal of the American Medical Association, 290,* 73–80.

Monga, T. N., Monga, U., Tan, G., & Grabois, M. (1999). Coital positions and sexual functioning in patients with chronic pain. *Sexuality and Disability, 17,* 287–297.

Mooradian, A., McLaughlin, S., Boyer, C., & Winter, J. (1999). Diabetes care for older adults. *Diabetes Spectrum, 12*(2), 70–77.

Morbidity and Mortality Weekly Report. (2003).

Influenza and pneumococcal vaccination coverage among persons > 65 years and persons 18–64 years with diabetes and asthma. (Vol. 53: No. 43). Retrieved December 15, 2004, from Center for Disease Control www.cdc.gov/mmwr/pdf/wk/mm5343.pdf.

Mortimer, J., & McElhaney, J. (2004). Cancers in the geriatric population. In C. Landefeld, R. Palmer, M. Johnson, In C. Johnston, & W. Lyons, (Eds.). *Current geriatric diagnosis and treatment.* New York: Lange Medical Books/McGraw-Hill.

Mouton, C., & Espino, D. (2000). Ethnic diversity of the aged. In J. Gallo, J. Busby-Whitehead, P. Rabins, R. Silliman, & J. Murphy (Eds.), *Reichel's care of the elderly: Clinical aspects of aging* (5th ed., pp. 595–608). Baltimore: Lippincott Williams & Wilkins.

Munster, P. N., & Hudis, C. A. (1999). Systemic therapy for breast cancer in the elderly *Clinical Geriatrics, 7*(7), 70–80.

Murphy, C., Schubert, C. R., Cruickshanks, K. J., Klein, B. E., Klein, R., & Nondahl, D. M. (2002). Prevalence of olfactory impairment in older adults. *Journal of the American Medical Association, 288,* 2307–2312.

Nadeau, C., & Varrone, J. (2003). Treat DVT with low molecular weight heparin. *Nurse Practitioner, 28*(10), 22–29.

National Cancer Institute. (2002). *What you need to know about oral cancer.* Retrieved November 12, 2004, from www.cancer.gov.

National Cancer Institute. (2003). *Physician data query.* Bethesda, MD: Author. Retrieved 11/14/2003 www.cancer.gov/cancerinfo/pdq.

National Center on Elder Abuse at the American Public Human Services Association (formerly the American Public Welfare Association) in collaboration with Westat. (1998). *The National Elder Abuse Incidence Study; final report: September 1998.* Washington, DC: National Aging Information Center.

National Consensus Project (NCP) for Quality Palliative Care. (2004). *Clinical practice guidelines for quality palliative care.* Retrieved September 14, 2004, from www.national consensusproject.org.

National Diabetes Education Program. (2003). *Four steps to control your diabetes for life.* Retrieved August 16, 2004, from www.ndep.nih.gov/diabetes/control/4steps.htm.

National Guideline Clearinghouse. (2001). *Cataract in the adult eye.* Retrieved August 14, 2003, from www.guideline.gov.

National Heart, Lung, and Blood Institute (NHLBI). (2002). *The lungs in health and disease.* National Institutes of Health, U.S. Department of Health and Human Services, No. 97-3279.

National Heart, Lung, and Blood Institute (NHLBI). (2002b). *Considerations for diagnosing and managing asthma in the elderly.* National Asthma Education and Prevention

Program, National Institutes of Health, No. 96-3662.

National Heart, Lung, and Blood Institute. (2004). *Your guide to lowering blood pressure: The DASH diet.* Retrieved November 9, 2004, from www.nhlbi.nih.gov.

National Hospice and Palliative Care Organization. (2000). *Hospice fact sheet.* Alexandria, VA: Author. Retrieved September 14, 2002, from www.nhpco.org.

National Institute of Allergy and Infectious Diseases. (2002). *Tuberculosis.* National Institutes of Health, U.S. Department of Health and Human Services. Retrieved November 12, 2003, from www.niaid.nih.gov.

National Institute of Diabetes and Digestive and Kidney Diseases (NIDDK). National Diabetes Information Clearinghouse. (2004). *Diabetes overview.* Retrieved August 16, 2004, from www.diabetes. NIDDK.NIH.gov.

National Institute on Aging. (2004). *Age page. Aging and your eyes.* Retrieved April 23, 2003, from www.nia.nih.gov.

National Institute on Aging. (2005). *Portfolio for progress: Reducing disease and disability.* Retrieved January 9, 2005, from www.nia publications.org/pubs/ portfolio/html/reducing.htm.

National Institute on Aging & National Cancer Institute. (2004). *Working group 3: Effects of comorbidity on cancer.* Retrieved August 16, 2004, from www.nia.nih.gov/ health.

National Institutes of Health. (2000). *National Center on Sleep Disorders Research, Test your sleep IQ* (Publication No. 00-3797). Washington, DC: U.S. Government Printing Office.

National Osteoporosis Foundation. (2002). *Physician guide to osteoporosis prevention and treatment.* Washington, DC: Author.

Nelson, H. D., Humphrey, L. L., Nygren, P., Teutsch, S. M., & Allan, J. D. (2002). Postmenopausal hormone replacement therapy: Scientific review. *Journal of the American Medical Association, 288,* 872–881.

Nicolle, L. E. (2003). Urinary tract infections in the elderly. In W. R. Hazzard, J. P. Blass, J. B. Halter, J. G. Ouslander, & M. E. Tinetti (Eds.), *Principles of geriatric medicine and gerontology* (5th ed., 1107–1116). New York: McGraw-Hill.

Nir, Z., Zolotogorsky, Z., & Sugarman, H. (2004). Structured nursing intervention versus routine rehabilitation after stroke. *American Journal of Physical Medicine & Rehabilitation, 83,* 522–529.

Norred, C.L., & Brinker, F. (2001). Potential coagulation effects of preoperative complementary and alternative medicines. *Alternative Therapy Health Medicine, 7,* 58–67.

North American Nursing Diagnosis Association (NANDA). (2001). *Nursing diagnoses: Definitions & classification 2001-2002.* Philadelphia: Author.

Nurses Asthma Education Partnership Project. (2003). Nurses: Partners in Asthma Care. National Heart, Lung, and Blood Institute, National Institutes of Health. Retrieved November 12, 2003, from www.nhlbi.nih.gov.

O'Dell, M. (1998). Skin and wound infections: An overview. *American Family Physician, 57*(10), 2424–2432.

Oh, R., & Brown, D. (2003). Vitamin B_{12} deficiency. *American Family Physician, March 1, 67*(5). Retrieved December 6, 2004, from www.aafp.org.

Omnibus Budget Reconciliation Act. (1987). *Public Law 100-203. Subtitle C: Nursing home reform.* Washington, DC: U.S. Department of Health and Human Services: 52 Fed. Reg. 38582, 38584.

Ouslander, J. G. (2000). Urinary incontinence. In D. Osterweil, K. Brummel-Smith, & J. C. Beck (Eds.), *Comprehensive geriatric assessment* (pp. 555–572). New York: McGraw-Hill.

Ovington, L. (2001). Wound management: Cleansing agents and dressings. In M. J. Morison (Ed.), *The prevention and treatment of pressure ulcers* (pp. 135–154). Edinburgh: Mosby.

Pace, B., Lynn, C., & Glass, R. (2001). Breathing problems during sleep. *Journal of the American Medical Association, 285*(22), 2936.

Palmer, M. H. (2000). Interdisciplinary approaches to the treatment of urinary incontinence in older adults. *Topics in Geriatric Rehabilitation, 16,* 1–9.

Palumbo, M. V. (2000). Increasing awareness of the hearing impaired. Hearing Access 2000. *Journal of Gerontological Nursing, 16* (9), 26–30.

Parkinson Study Group. (2000). A randomized controlled trial comparing pramipexole with levodopa in early Parkinson's disease: Design and methods of the CALM-PD Study. *Clinical Neuropharmacology, 23,* 34–44.

Payette, H., Gray-Donald, K., Cyr, R., & Boutier, V. (1995). Predictors of dietary intakes in a functionally dependent elderly population in the communities. *American Journal of Public Health, 85,* 677–683.

Pearson, L., & Hutton, J. (2002). A controlled trial to compare the ability of foam swabs and toothbrushes to remove dental plaque. *Journal of Advanced Nursing, 39*(5), 480–489.

Persson, M. D., Brismar, K. E., Katzarski, K. S., Nordenstrom, J., & Cederholm, T. E. (2002). Nutritional status using mini nutritional assessment and subjective global assessment predict mortality in geriatric patients. *Journal of the American Geriatrics Society, 50,* 1996–2002.

Pillemer, K. A., & Finkelhor, D. (1988). The prevalence of elder abuse: A random sample survey. *Gerontologist, 28*(1), 51–57.

Pillemer, K. A., & Moore, D. W. (1989). Abuse of patients in nursing homes: Findings from a survey of staff. *Gerontologist, 29*(3), 314–320.

Position of the American Dietetic Association: Ethical and legal issues in nutrition, hydration and feeding. (2002). *Journal of the American Dietetic Association, 102,* 716–726.

Post, L., Mitty, E., Bottrell, M., Dubler, N., Hill, T., Mezey, M., & Ramsey, G. (2001). Guidelines for end-of-life care in nursing facilities: Principles and recommendations. *NAELA Quarterly,* vol. no. 14(2) Spring, 24–30.

Post, S. (1995). *The moral challenge of Alzheimer disease.* Baltimore: Johns Hopkins University Press.

Potts, H. W., Richie, M. F., & Kaas, M. J. (1996). Resistance to care. *Journal of Gerontological Nursing, 22,* 11–16.

Prather, C. (2004). Constipation, diarrhea and fecal incontinence. In M. Beers & R. Berkow (Eds.), *Merck manual of geriatrics.* Retrieved August 16, 2004, from www.merck.com.

Raia, P. (1999). Habilitation therapy: A new starscape. In L.Volicer & L. Bloom-Charette (Eds.), *Enhancing the quality of life in advanced dementia* (pp. 38–55). Philadelphia: Taylor & Francis.

Rasul, I., & Kandel, G. (2001). An approach to iron deficiency anemia. *Canadian Journal of Gastroenterology, 15*(11), 739–747.

Ray, S., Secrest, J., Ch'ien, A., & Corey, R. (2002). Managing gastroesophageal reflux disease. *Nurse Practitioner, 27*(5), 36–50.

Reichmuth, K., & Meyer, K. (2003). Management of community-acquired pneumonia in the elderly. *Annals of Long-Term Care, 11*(7), 27–31.

Reisberg, B., Doody, R., Stoffler, A., Schmitt, F., Ferris, S., Mobius, H. J., et al. (2003). Memantine in moderate-to-severe Alzheimer's disease. *New England Journal of Medicine, 348,* 1333–1341.

Rempusheski, V. F., & Hurley, A. C. (2000). Advance directives and dementia. *Journal of Gerontological Nursing, 26*(10), 27–33.

Resnick, N., & Yalla, S. (1985). Current concepts: Management of urinary incontinence in the elderly. *New England Journal of Medicine, 313,* 800–805.

Reuben, D., Herr, K., Pacala, J., Potter, J., Pollock, B., & Semla, T. (2002). *Gastrointestinal diseases: Geriatrics at your fingertips.* Malden, MA: Blackwell.

Reuben, D., Herr, K., Pacala, J., Pollick, B., Potter, J., & Semla, T. (2003). *Geriatrics at your fingertips.* Malden, MA: American Geriatrics Society, Blackwell.

Reuben, D., Herr, K., Pacala, J., Potter, J., Pollock, B., & Semla, T. (2002). *Geriatrics at your fingertips.* Malden, MA: Blackwell. American Geriatrics Society.

Riccio, P., Knight, B., & Cody, M. S. (1999). Medication use with implications for sleep in elderly dementia caregivers. *Home Health Care Managed Practice, 12*(1), 42–49.

Ries, L. A. G., Eisner, M. P., Kosary, C. L., Hankey, B. F., Miller, B. A., Clegg, L., & Edwards, B. K. (Eds.). (2002). *SEER cancer statistics review, 1973–1999*. Bethesda, MD: National Cancer Institute. Retrieved September 19, 2003, from http://seer.cancer.gov/csr/1973_1999/.

Robertson, R., & Montagnini, M. (2004). Geriatric failure to thrive. *American Family Physician, 70*(2), 343–350.

Rojas, A. I., & Phillips, T. J. (1999). Patients with chronic leg ulcers show diminished levels of vitamins A and E, carotenes and zinc. *Dermatologic Surgery, 25,* 601–604.

Rosenthal, G., Kaboli, P., Barnett, M., & Sirio, C. (2002). Age and risk of in-hospital death: Insights from a multihospital study of intensive care patients. *Journal of the American Geriatrics Society, 50,* 1205–1212.

Russell, R. M., Rasmussen, H., & Lichtenstein, A. H. (1999). Modified food guide pyramid for people over 70 years of age. *Journal of Nutrition, 129,* 751–753.

Saltvedt, I., Mo, E., Fayers, P., Kaasa, S., & Sletvold, O. (2002). Reduced mortality in treating acutely sick, frail older patients in a geriatric evaluation and management unit. A prospective randomized trial. *Journal of the American Geriatrics Society, 50,* 792–798.

Saxon, S. V., & Etten, M. J. (2002). *Physical changes and aging: A guide for the helping professions* (4th ed.). New York: Tiresias Press.

Schiffman, S. S. (1997). Taste and smell losses in normal aging and disease. *Journal of the American Medical Association, 278*(16), 1357–1362.

Schlegel, D. J., Tanne, D., Demchuk, A. M., Levine, S. R., Kasner, S. E., & Multicenter rt-PA Stroke Survey Group. (2004). Prediction of hospital disposition after thrombolysis for acute ischemic stroke using the National Institutes of Health Stroke Scale. *Archives of Neurology, 61,* 1061–1064.

Schmader, K., Hanlon, J. T., Weinberger, M., Landsman, P. B., Samsa, G. P., Lewis, I., et al. (1994). Appropriateness of medication prescribing in ambulatory elderly patients. *Journal of the American Geriatrics Society, 42,* 1241–1247.

Schnelle, J., Alessi, C., Al-Samarrai, N., Fricker, R., & Ouslander, J. (1999). The nursing home at night: Effects of an intervention on noise, light and sleep. *Journal of the American Geriatrics Society, 47,* 430–438.

Schober-Flores, C. (2001). The sun's damaging effects. *Dermatology Nursing, 13*(4), 279–286.

Schultz, S. K., Ellingrod, V. L., Turvey, C., Moser, D. J., & Arndt, S. (2003). The influence of cognitive impairment and behavioral dysregulation on daily functioning in the nursing home setting. *American Journal of Psychiatry, 160,* 582–584.

Schulz, J. (2004). Anorectal disorders. In M. Beers & R. Berkow (Eds.), *Merck manual of geriatrics.* Retrieved January 15, 2004, from www.merck.com.

Schwartz, J. B. (1999). Clinical pharmacology. In W. R. Hazzard, J. P. Blass, W. H. Ettinger, J. B. Halter, & J. G. Ouslander (Eds.), *Principles of geriatric medicine and gerontology* (4th ed., pp. 303–331). New York: McGraw-Hill.

Scott, C., & Popovich, D. (2001, January). Undiagnosed alcoholism & prescription drug misuse among the elderly. *Caring Magazine, 20*(1), 20–25.

Ship, J. A. (2002). Diagnosing, managing and preventing salivary gland disorders. *Oral Diseases, 8,* 77–89.

Ship, J.A., Pillemer, S. R., & Baum, B. J. (2002). Xerostomia and the geriatric patient. *Journal of the American Geriatrics Society, 50*(3), 535–543.

Shumaker, S., Legault, C., Rapp, S., Thal, L., Wallace, R., Ockene, J., Hendrix, S., et al. (2003). Estrogen plus progestin and the incidence of dementia and mild cognitive impairment in postmenopausal women. *Journal of the American Medical Association, 289,* 2651–2662.

Silverstein, N. L., & Flaherty, G. (1996). Deadly mix: Dementia and wandering. *Gerontologist, 36,* 156–157.

Smith, D., & Newman, D. (1989). The bran solution. *Contemporary Long Term Care, 12,* 66.

Smith, D. A., & Ouslander, J. G. (2000). Pharmacologic management of urinary incontinence in older adults. *Topics in Geriatrics Rehabilitation, 16,* 54–60.

Smith, D. R. (2003). Update on Alzheimer drugs. *Neurologist, 9,* 225–229.

Smith, S. J. (1998). Providing palliative care for the terminal Alzheimer patient. In L.Volicer & A. Hurley (Eds.), *Hospice care for patients with advanced progressive dementia* (pp. 247–256). New York: Springer.

Solomon, D. (2003). Metabolic and thyroid disorders. In M. Beers & R. Berkow (Eds.), *Merck manual of geriatrics.* Rahway, NJ: Merck.

Solomon, R., & Donnenfeld, E. D. (2003). Recent advances and future frontiers in treating age-related cataracts. *Journal of the American Medical Association, 290*(2), 248–251.

Stanford University Geriatric Education Resource Center. (2000). *Tools for geriatric care.* Board of Trustees of the Leland Stanford Junior University. Retrieved October 3, 2004, from www.geri-resources@lists. stanford.edu.

Steers, W. D. (1999). Meeting the urologic needs of the aging population. *Clinical Geriatrics, 7*(5), 62–64, 73.

Stern, M. F. (1997). Erectile dysfunction in older men. *Topics in Geriatric Rehabilitation, 12*(4), 40–52.

Stevens, J., Cai, J., Pamuk, E. R., Williamson, D. F., Thun, M. J., & Wood, J. L. (1998). The effect of age on the association between body-mass index and mortality. *New England Journal of Medicine, 338,* 1–7.

Stone, J. T., & Wyman, J. F. (1999). Falls. In J. T. Stone, J. F. Wyman, & S. A. Salisbury (Eds.), *Clinical gerontological nursing: A guide to advanced practice* (2nd ed., pp. 341–366). Philadelphia: W. B. Saunders.

Strandberg, T. E., Ylikorkala, O., & Tikkanen, M. J. (2003). Differing effects of oral and transdermal hormone replacement therapy on cardiovascular risk factors in healthy postmenopausal women. *American Journal of Cardiology, 92*(2), 212–214.

Sullivan, D. H., Bopp, M. M., & Roberson, P. K. (2002). Protein-energy undernutrition and life-threatening complications among the hospitalized elderly. *Journal of General Internal Medicine, 17,* 923–932.

Sullivan, D. H., Sun, S., & Walls, R. C. (1999). Protein-energy undernutrition among elderly hospitalized patients. *Journal of the American Medical Association, 281,* 2013–2019.

SUPPORT. (1995). A controlled trial to improve care for seriously ill hospitalized patients. The study to understand prognoses and preferences for outcomes and risks of treatment. *Journal of the American Medical Association, 274*(20), 1591–1598.

Swagerty, D. L. (1999). Elder mistreatment. *American Family Physician, 59*(10), 2804–2808.

Szirony, T. A. (1999). Infection with HIV in the elderly population. *Journal of Gerontological Nursing, 25*(10), 25–31.

Tabloski, P., & Church, O. M. (1999). Insomnia, alcohol and drug use in community-residing elderly persons. *Journal of Substance Use, 3*(4), 147–154.

Tabloski, P., Cooke, K., & Thoman, E. (1998). A procedure for withdrawal of sleep medication in elderly women who have been long-term users. *Journal of Gerontological Nursing, 24*(9), 20–28.

Tanne, D., Kasner, S. E., Demchuk, A. M., Koren-Morag, N., Hanson, S., Grond, M., et al. (2002). Markers of increased risk of intracerebral hemorrhage after intravenous recombinant tissue plasminogen activator therapy for acute ischemic stroke in clinical practice: The Multicenter rt-PA Stroke Survey. *Circulation, 105,* 1679–1685.

Tefferi, A. (2004). Chronic myeloid disorders. In M. Beers & R. Berkow (Eds.), *Merck manual of geriatrics.* Retrieved December 6, 2004, from www.merck.com.

Thomas, D. R. (2001). Improving outcome of pressure ulcers with nutritional interventions: A review of the evidence. *Nutrition, 17,* 121–125.

Thomas, D., Flaherty, J., & Morley, J. (2001). The management of chronic pain in long-term care settings. *Supplement to the Annals of Long-Term Care,* November. Newtown Square, PA: MultiMedia HealthCare/Freedom.

Thomas, D., Goode, P. S., & LaMaster, K. (2003). Clinical consensus: The constipation crisis in long-term care. *Supplement to the Annals of Long-Term Care, (S),* October, 2–12.

Thompson, J. (2000). A practical guide to wound care. *RN, 63*(1), 48–57.

Tinetti, M. (2003). Chronic dizziness and postural instability. In M. Beers & R. Berkow (Eds.), *The Merck manual of geriatrics* (Chap. 19). Whitehouse Station, NJ: Merck Research Laboratories.

Titler, M., & Mentes, J. (1999). Research utilization in gerontological nursing practice. *Journal of Gerontological Nursing, 25*(6), pp. 6–9.

Tompkins, R. (2004). Acute abdomen and surgical gastroenterology. In M. Beers & R. Berkow (Eds.), *Merck manual of geriatrics.* Retrieved January 22, 2004, from www.merck.com.

Toy, P. (2004). Anemia. In C. Landefeld, R. Palmer, M. Johnson, C. Johnston, & W. Lyons, (Eds.). *Current geriatric diagnosis and treatment.* New York: Lange Medical Books/McGraw-Hill.

Trudeau, S. A. (1999). Prevention of physical limitations in advanced Alzheimer's disease. In L.Volicer & L. Bloom-Charette (Eds.), *Enhancing quality of life for persons with advanced Alzheimer's disease* (pp. 80–90). Philadelphia: Taylor & Francis.

U.S. Preventive Services Task Force. (2003). *Guide to clinical preventive services, 3rd edition: Periodic updates.* Rockville, MD: Agency for Health Care Research and Quality. Retrieved November 14, 2003, from www. ahcpr.gov/clinic/uspstf/uspsprca.htm.

U.S. Surgeon General. (2003). *Executive summary. Mental health: Culture, race and ethnicity.* U.S. Department of Health and Human Services, U.S. Public Health Service. Retrieved September 27, 2003, from www.surgeongeneral.gov.

Uphold, C. R., & Graham, M. V. (2003). *Clinical guidelines in adult health* (3rd ed.). Gainesville, FL: Barmarre Books.

Veatch, R. M. (1989). *The patient as partner: A theory of human-experimentation ethics.* Bloomington and Indianapolis: Indiana University Press.

Vellas, B., Guigoz, Y., Garry, P. J., Nourhashemi, F., Bennahum, D., Lauque, S., & Albarede, J. L. (1999). The Mini Nutritional Assessment and its use in grading the nutritional state of elderly patients. *Nutrition, 15,* 116–122.

Volicer, L., & Hurley, A. C. (1998). *Hospice care for patients with advanced progressive dementia.* New York: Springer.

Volicer, L., Brandeis, G. H., & Hurley, A. C. (1998). Infections in advanced dementia. In L.Volicer & A. Hurley (Eds.), *Hospice care for patients with advanced progressive dementia* (pp. 29–47). New York: Springer.

Volicer, L., Mahoney, E., & Brown, E. J. (1998). Nonpharmacological approaches to the management of the behavioral consequences of advanced dementia. In M. Kaplan & S. B. Hoffman (Eds.), *Behaviors in dementia: Best practices for successful management* (pp. 155–176). Baltimore: Health Professions Press.

Volicer, L., Seltzer, B., Rheaume, Y., Karner, J., Glennon, M., Riley, M. E., et al. (1989). Eating difficulties in patients with probable dementia of the Alzheimer type. *Journal of Geriatric Psychiatry and Neurology, 2*(4), 169–176.

Volicer, L., Volicer, B., & Hurley, A. (1993). Is hospice care appropriate for Alzheimer patients? *Caring, 11,* 50–55.

Volpato, S., Leveille, S. G., Corti, M., Harris, T. B., & Guralnik, J. M. (2001). The value of serum albumin and high-density lipoprotein cholesterol in defining mortality risk in older persons with low serum cholesterol. *Journal of the American Geriatrics Society, 49,* 1142–1147.

Wagner, L., Greenberg, S., & Capezuti, E. (2002). Elder abuse and neglect. In V. T. Cotter & N. E. Strumpf (Eds.), *Advanced practice nursing with older adults clinical guidelines.* New York: McGraw-Hill.

Wald, A. (2004). Lower gastrointestinal tract disorders. In M. Beers & R. Berkow (Eds.), *Merck manual of geriatrics.* Retrieved January 22, 2004, from www.merck.com.

Walton, J., Miller, J., & Tordecilla, L. (2001). Elder oral assessment and care. *MEDSURG Nursing, 10*(1), 37–44.

Walton, J., Miller, J., & Tordecilla, L. (2002). Elder oral assessment and care. *ORL— Head and Neck Nursing, 20*(2), 12–19.

Watson, R. (2000). Assessing neurological functioning in older people. *Elderly Care, 12*(4), 25–27.

Waye, J. (2004). Endoscopic gastrointestinal procedures. In M. Beers & R. Berkow (Eds.), *Merck manual of geriatrics.* Retrieved January 20, 2004, from www.merck.com.

Wellons, M. F., Sanders, L., Edwards, I. J., Bartlett, J. A., Heald, A. E., & Schmader, K. E. (2002). HIV infection: Treatment outcomes in older and younger adults. *Journal of the American Geriatrics Society, 50*(4), 603–607.

Wells-Federman, C. (1999). Care of the patient with chronic pain: Part I. *Clinical Excellence in Nursing Practice, 3*(4), 192–204.

Weston, B. C., Aliabadi, Z., & White, G. L. (2000). Glaucoma — Review for the vigilant clinician. *Clinician Reviews, 10*(8), 58–74.

Whitaker, R., Whitaker, V. B., & Dill, C. (1998). Glaucoma:

What the nurse practitioner should know. *Nurse Practitioner Forum, 9*(1), 7–12.

White, R., & Ashworth, A. (2000). How drug therapy can affect, threaten and compromise nutritional status. *Journal of Human Nutrition and Dietetics, 13,* 119–129.

Wilson, B. A., Shannon, M. T., & Stang, C. L. (2002). *AgingEye Times.* Retrieved October 15, 2003, from www.agingeye.net/visionbasics/eye&meds.php.

Wilson, B., Shannon, M., & Stang, C. (2003). *Nurse's drug guide 2003.* Upper Saddle River, NJ: Prentice Hall Health.

Woods-Smith, D., Arnstein, P., Rosa, K., & Wells-Federman, C. (2002). Effects of integrating therapeutic touch into a cognitive behavioral pain treatment program: *Report of a pilot clinical trial. Journal of Holistic Nursing, 20,* 367–387.

Workman, M. L. (2000). Immune mechanisms in rheumatic disease. *Nursing Clinics of North America, 35*(1), 175–188.

Wyman, J. F. (2003). Treatment of urinary incontinence in men and older women. *American Journal of Nursing, 103* (Suppl. 3), 26–35.

Yesavage, J. A., & Brink, T. L. (1983). Development and validation of a geriatric depression screening scale: A preliminary report. *Journal of Psychiatric Research, 17,* 37–49.

Yoneyama, T., Yshoda, M., Ohrui, T., Mukaiyama, H., Okamoto, H., Hoshiba, K., et al. (2002). Oral care reduces pneumonia in older patients in nursing homes. *Journal of the American Geriatrics Society, 50,* 430–433.

Young, H. (2003). Challenges and solutions for care of frail older adults. *Online Journal of Issues in Nursing, 8*(2), Manuscript 4. Retrieved December 12, 2004, from www.nursingworld.org/ojin/topic21/tpc21_4.htm.

INDEX